CUMMINGS

REVIEW OF
OTOLARYNGOLOGY

CUMMINGS

REVIEW OF
OTOLARYNGOLOGY

HARRISON W. LIN, MD
Assistant Professor
Department of Otolaryngology—Head and Neck Surgery
University of California, Irvine
Irvine, California

DANIEL S. ROBERTS, MD, PhD
Division of Otolaryngology—Head and Neck Surgery
University of Connecticut
Farmington, Connecticut

JEFFREY P. HARRIS, MD, PhD
Distinguished Professor
Division Chief
Division of Otolaryngology—Head and Neck Surgery
University of California, San Diego
San Diego, California

Foreword by
CHARLES W. CUMMINGS, MD
Distinguished Service Professor
Department of Otolaryngology—Head and Neck Surgery
Professor, Department of Oncology
Johns Hopkins Medical Institutions
Baltimore, Maryland

ELSEVIER

ELSEVIER

1600 John F. Kennedy Blvd.
Ste 1800
Philadelphia, PA 19103-2899

CUMMINGS REVIEW OF OTOLARYNGOLOGY   ISBN: 978-0-323-40194-4

Library of Congress Cataloging-in-Publication Data

Names: Lin, Harrison W., author. | Roberts, Daniel S. (Daniel Stewart), 1974- author. | Harris, Jeffrey P. (Jeffrey Paul), 1949- author.
Title: Cummings review of otolaryngology / Harrison W. Lin, Daniel S. Roberts, Jeffrey P. Harris ; foreword by Charles W. Cummings.
Other titles: Review of otolaryngology
Description: Philadelphia, PA : Elsevier, [2017] | Includes index.
Identifiers: LCCN 2016027590 (print) | LCCN 2016028336 (ebook) | ISBN 9780323401944 (pbk. : alk. paper) | ISBN 9780323427999 ()
Subjects: | MESH: Otorhinolaryngologic Diseases | Otorhinolaryngologic Surgical Procedures | Outlines
Classification: LCC RF46 (print) | LCC RF46 (ebook) | NLM WV 18.2 | DDC 616.2/1–dc23
LC record available at https://lccn.loc.gov/2016027590

Content Strategist: Belinda Kuhn
Content Development Specialist: Kathryn M. DeFrancesco and Cara-Beth Lillback
Publishing Services Manager: Hemamalini Rajendrababu
Project Manager: Dr. Atiyaah Muskaan
Design Direction: Renee Duenow
Marketing Manager: Melissa Fogarty

Printed in China

Last digit is the print number: 9   8   7   6   5   4   3   2   1

Contributors

Amir Afrogheh, BChD, MChD
Clinical Research Fellow
Head and Neck Pathology
Massachusetts General Hospital
Harvard Medical School
Boston, Massachusetts
Consultant Pathologist, NHLS
Senior Lecturer/Specialist
University of the Western Cape
Cape Town, South Africa
Chapter 11 Head and Neck Pathology

Brian S. Chen, MD
Staff Surgeon, Otology and Neurotology
Department of Otolaryngology—Head and Neck Surgery
William Beaumont Army Medical Center
El Paso, Texas
Chapter 2 Otology and Neurotology

Jennifer Derebery, MD
Associate, House Ear Clinic
Clinical Professor of Otolaryngology
University of Southern California
Los Angeles, California
Chapter 8 Otolaryngic Allergy

Jayme Rose Dowdall, MD
Instructor
Department of Otology and Laryngology
Harvard Medical School
Boston, Massachusetts
Chapter 7 Laryngology

William C. Faquin, MD, PhD
Director, Head and Neck Pathology
Massachusetts General Hospital
Massachusetts Eye and Ear Infirmary
Associate Professor of Pathology
Harvard Medical School
Boston, Massachusetts
Chapter 11 Head and Neck Pathology

Daniel Fink, MD
Assistant Professor, Laryngology and Voice Disorders
Department of Otolaryngology—Head and
    Neck Surgery
Louisiana State University Health Sciences Center
Baton Rouge, Louisiana
Chapter 7 Laryngology

M. Boyd Gillespie, MD, MSc
Professor
Department of Otolaryngology—Head and
    Neck Surgery
Medical University of South Carolina
Charleston, South Carolina
Chapter 9 Sleep Medicine

John L. Go, MD
Associate Professor
Director of Head and Neck Imaging
Department of Radiology
Division of Neuroradiology
University of Southern California
Los Angeles, California
Chapter 12 Head and Neck Radiology

Sachin Gupta, MD
Attending, Otology and Neurotology
Department of Otolaryngology—Head and Neck Surgery
Walter Reed National Military Medical Center
Washington, DC
Chapter 2 Otology and Neurotology

Allen S. Ho, MD
Assistant Professor of Surgery
Department of Surgery
Cedars-Sinai Medical Center
Los Angeles, California
Chapter 5 Head and Neck Surgery

Marc H. Hohman, MD
Facial Plastic and Reconstructive Surgeon
Associate Director, Otolaryngology Residency Program
Madigan Army Medical Center
Tacoma, Washington
Assistant Professor
Department of Surgery
Uniformed Services University of the Health Sciences
Bethesda, Maryland
Chapter 3 Facial Plastic and Reconstructive Surgery

Kiran Kakarala, MD
Assistant Professor
Department of Otolaryngology—Head and Neck Surgery
University of Kansas School of Medicine
Kansas City, Kansas
Chapter 5 Head and Neck Surgery

Elliot Kozin, MD
Department of Otolaryngology
Harvard Medical School
Boston, Massachusetts
Chapter 8 Otolaryngic Allergy
Chapter 9 Sleep Medicine

Shelby Leuin, MD
Assistant Clinical Professor
Pediatric Otolaryngology
Rady Children's Hospital
University of California, San Diego
San Diego, California
Chapter 6 Pediatric Otolaryngology

Aaron Lin, MD, MA
Pediatric Otolaryngologist
Department of Head and Neck Surgery
Southern California Permanente Medical Group
Downey, California
Chapter 6 Pediatric Otolaryngology

James Lin, MD
Associate Professor
Department of Otolaryngology
Kansas University Medical Center
Kansas City, Kansas
Chapter 2 Otology and Neurotology

Theodore McRackan, MD
Assistant Professor
Director, Lateral Skull Base Surgery
Department of Otolaryngology
Medical University of South Carolina
Charleston, South Carolina
Chapter 2 Otology and Neurotology

Anandh G. Rajamohan, MD
Assistant Professor
Department of Radiology
Division of Neuroradiology
University of Southern California
Los Angeles, California
Chapter 12 Head and Neck Radiology

Douglas D. Reh, MD
Associate Professor
Otolaryngology—Head and Neck Surgery
Johns Hopkins Medicine
Baltimore, Maryland
Chapter 4 Rhinology and Endoscopic Sinus Surgery

Brian Kip Reilly, MD
Assistant Professor of Otolaryngology
Children's National Medical Center
Washington, DC
Chapter 6 Pediatric Otolaryngology

Peter M. Sadow, MD, PhD
Associate Director, Head and Neck Pathology
Pathology Service
Massachusetts General Hospital
Associate Professor
Department of Pathology
Harvard Medical School
Associate Director, Head and Neck Pathology
Department of Otolaryngology
Massachusetts Eye and Ear Infirmary
Boston, Massachusetts
Chapter 11 Head and Neck Pathology

Ryan J. Smart, MD, DMD
Oral and Maxillofacial Surgeon
Clinical Instructor of Surgery-University of North Dakota
    School of Medicine, Staff Surgeon
Essentia Health
West Fargo, North Dakota
Chapter 10 Oral Surgery

Srinivas M. Susarla, MD, DMD
Department of Plastic Surgery
Johns Hopkins Hospital
Baltimore, Maryland
Chapter 3 Facial Plastic and Reconstructive Surgery
Chapter 10 Oral Surgery

Jonathan Ting, MD, MS
Department of Otolaryngology—Head and Neck Surgery
Indiana University School of Medicine
Zionsville, Indiana
Chapter 4 Rhinology and Endoscopic Sinus Surgery

Aaron Wieland, MD
Assistant Professor of Surgery
Department of Surgery
Division of Otolaryngology—Head and Neck Surgery
University of Wisconsin
Madison, Wisconsin
Chapter 5 Head and Neck Surgery

Foreword

The mission of the comprehensive text Cummings Otolaryngology/Head and Neck Surgery is to present, in accessible fashion, information that allows the readership exposure to the most current core content of the specialty. This review mirrors that mission. Congratulations to Drs. Lin, Roberts, and Harris for their excellent work. Medical contributions are expanding at a rate that makes currency of knowledge almost unattainable. Clinical- and compliance-related demands leach away discretionary time previously used to "keep up." This review book consolidates and highlights the content of its parent to allow rapid review and acquisition of new knowledge. It also presents a vehicle for specialty board examination preparation. Kudos to the editors for this most helpful initiative.

Charles W. Cummings
2016

Preface

Cummings Review of Otolaryngology is a review book designed for physicians taking the otolaryngology written and oral board, recertification, and in-service examinations; the otolaryngology intern, resident, and fellow trainees looking to augment their knowledge base; and medical students preparing for subinternships and residency training. If you are reading this book, you likely have performed at a high level on written examinations for most of your life. Although *Cummings Review of Otolaryngology* and other texts will prepare you for written examinations in the field of otolaryngology in a systematic and logical way, excelling on clinical rounds and on oral board examinations is a skill that improves with familiarity of oral testing formats and compartmentalizing your fund of knowledge in an organized, easily accessible manner.

We believe that this book is the primary and go-to resource that a medical student or resident will read before clinical rounds with the attending surgeon, a complex surgical case, a mock oral board examination, or the *American Board of Otolaryngology* examinations. The learning and information conveyed through the book will allow readers to have the most important clinical information—such as a differential diagnosis, clinical algorithm, treatment options, or a list of how-to's—instantly accessible in their memory to respond quickly to questions in a clinical or testing situation, to facilitate teaching of other residents and medical students, and to assist in patient management. This organized and structured way of thinking is central to success in the oral board format, as well as in clinical rotations and patient care.

Harrison W. Lin
Daniel S. Roberts
Jeffrey P. Harris

Acknowledgments

We would like to acknowledge all of our teachers and mentors, who have dedicated their lives to both the highest level of patient care and passing on their craft to subsequent generations of surgeons. They serve as continued inspiration toward our academic pursuits. In addition, we wish to thank the students and trainees whose probing questions constantly push us to stay current and to serve as a stimulus for our own creativity.

Harrison W. Lin
Daniel S. Roberts
Jeffrey P. Harris

Contents

Preparing for Clinical Rounds and Board Examinations

INTRODUCTION

Most residents who completed a general surgical internship will remember the "five W's" that can cause post-operative fever, including *wind* (pneumonia or atelectasis), *water* (urinary tract infection), *walking* (deep venous thrombosis), *wound* (wound infection), and *wonder drug* (drug reaction). Those that are undergoing or completed otolaryngology training will furthermore recall being asked to recount the auditory pathway and peaks of the auditory brainstem response, to describe the innervation and actions of the laryngeal muscles, or to discuss the reconstructive ladder, among many other questions in the clinic, on rounds, or in the operating room. Undoubtedly, these well-described and time-tested clinical pearls are critically important in the context of both examinations and everyday patient care, particularly to the resident trainee rotating through busy clinical services while trying to simultaneously read, learn how to operate, and provide the highest quality clinical care. Time is a luxury students and residents unfortunately do not have, and consequently they are best served by learning quickly, efficiently, and effectively.

We wrote the *Cummings Review of Otolaryngology* in an effort to provide a highly-efficient learning instrument to its readers. Clinical pearls such as the "five W's", "E.C.O.L.I.", and the reconstructive ladder *organize* and *compartmentalize* information into packets that most anyone at this level of education and training can swiftly consume, digest and incorporate into their long-term memory. This book provides this compartmentalization of otolaryngology and all of its depth, breadth, and complexity, and offers readers the foundation upon which they can build and expand their fund of knowledge with articles, textbooks, and discussions with senior residents and attendings. Although this text will importantly augment the knowledge base of the reader in a systematic and organized manner, success on clinical rounds and on in-service and board examinations will be further optimized with better understanding of how to prepare for attending rounds and improved familiarity of the testing formats. This chapter provides a systematic approach to these tasks.

ORAL EXAMINATIONS

Familiarity with the format of oral exams will provide the infrastructure upon which the examinee can prepare for success. For most residents and medical students, written exams have been the mainstay of testing, with far less training in the oral exam format. To begin, the American Board of Otolaryngology oral examination takes place over a weekend in a hotel in the city of Chicago, Illinois, near O'Hare International Airport. You have the option of staying in the hotel, in a neighboring hotel walking or shuttle distance away, or in your own accommodations. Based on the first letter of your last name, you will have your exam on Saturday morning, Saturday afternoon, Sunday morning, or Sunday afternoon. At the exam, you receive a number and a list of five examiners who will likely be among the most prominent and published names in our field. Over 40 minutes, you will be tested on three cases in each of five rooms with different sub-specialty topics, which include head and neck surgical oncology, otology and neurotology, facial plastic and reconstructive surgery, and two general otolaryngology rooms. General cases encompass rhinology, sleep, allergy, pediatric otolaryngology, laryngology, and other general otolaryngology topics. One room will focus on allergy, rhinology, and sleep, and the other will focus on laryngology and pediatric otolaryngology. The examiners will be accessing your ability to discuss eloquently the diagnostic workups, treatment options, complications, and, at times, management of emergencies for each of the presented cases.

Success on the oral board exam depends on an ability to communicate an organized and structured thought process. Oral board formats are similar to the workup of a patient in a clinic. Points are attained by starting with the chief complaint and obtaining a thorough history of the present illness, past medical history, past surgical history, family history, social history, list of medications and allergies, and review of systems. After completing the full history, the examinee should ask to perform a physical exam, first asking for the patient's vital signs. If there is an emergency, you will be expected to discuss basic life support and assess the patient's *airway*, *breathing*, and *circulation*. A brief summary statement with pertinent information from the history and physical, along with a comprehensive differential diagnosis, should be provided at some point after the initial assessment is completed. Asking for additional information such as laboratory tests, imaging, and audiograms will also be necessary in many cases. Pathology is typically incorporated into several cases during the testing day. Imaging, pathologic slides, and test results will give you an opportunity to refine your differential diagnosis as needed.

As you discuss the case with your examiner, he or she may focus, narrow, expedite, or redirect your questioning if necessary. When medical treatment or surgery is indicated, you should be able to recite the various options in management, the risks and benefits of each, and the postoperative care protocols. You may need to recognize and manage complications in the postoperative setting.

PEARLS FOR SUCCESS ON ORAL EXAMS

- Stay organized. You are provided a pencil and paper and are welcome to take notes as needed.
- Do not go directly to the diagnosis, even if it may seem obvious to you. Rather, the goal during a case is to obtain points (check marks) by logically moving through the workup of a patient and verbally stating all history questions you should ask, studies you should obtain, diagnoses you should consider, and treatment options you may offer. Demonstrate an organized and linear thought process.

- This review book provides you with the lists to be memorized so that you have easy access to what you want and need to say for many questions that may arise in your oral exam. If you are presented with a patient with hoarseness, simply recite the list of key history questions for a patient with hoarseness. If you are presented with a patient with ear drainage, ask the key questions to ask of all patients presenting to an otology clinic. If your patient has pediatric hearing loss, describe the list of tests you could offer and recommend to the parents. If you are performing parotid surgery and are asked how you would go about finding the facial nerve, simply recount the list of five ways to find the trunk of the facial nerve. If you believe that a rhinoplasty patient could benefit from an increase in tip projection, mention the three ways you could accomplish that. Memorizing the lists in this book will arm you with an organized and comprehensive depth and breadth of knowledge that will help you to remain cool, calm, and collected and succeed in your exam.
- When providing a differential diagnosis use a mnemonic to stay organized. Although this may seem to you artificial, it is an effective way to recite calmly and easily a thorough list of possible diagnoses. Pick one of the examples and stick with it, write it down on your provided piece of paper, and refer to it when needed to guide you.
  - "KITTENS" (K—congenital; I—infectious, iatrogenic; TT—toxins, trauma; E—endocrine; N—neoplastic; S—systemic)
  - "VITAMIN-C" (V—vascular; I—infectious, inflammatory; T—toxins, trauma; A—autoimmune; M—metabolic; I—iatrogenic; N—neoplastic; C—congenital)
  - "VINDICATE" (V—vascular; I—infectious, inflammatory; N—neoplastic; D—drugs; I—iatrogenic; C—congenital; A—autoimmune; T—trauma, toxins; E—endocrine)
- For pathology questions, describe the finding you see on the image, even if you are unable to provide the correct diagnosis. After all, you are not a pathologist and neither is your examiner. The correct diagnosis is obviously preferred, but some credit may possibly be obtained for an accurate description of the pathological specimen.
- Ask for one test or imaging study at a time. If you are correct in asking for the study, you will be presented the results and will need to interpret them accurately in an organized fashion that demonstrates to your examiner your knowledge and abilities.
- Review computed tomography (CT) and magnetic resonance (MR) images by stating (1) the type of imaging, (2) the view, (3) the type of sequences if applicable, and (4) roughly where the slice is within the series. For example, you could state, "this is an axial CT of the neck, soft-tissue windows, with contrast, at the level of the larynx," or "this is an MR of the temporal bone, coronal cuts, T1 imaging with contrast, at the level of the internal auditory canal." You may be provided with and asked to interpret a stack of images from the same scan, and not just one isolated image. Be systematic and help yourself by stating the normal anatomy, which both demonstrates to your examiner your familiarity with the anatomy and helps build a mental image in your brain of where you are. As you should have learned by now, recognition and familiarity with *normal* help you identify *abnormal*. Partial credit can be given for an accurate radiologic description of the abnormal findings whether or not the correct diagnosis is obtained.
- Take advantage of any opportunity to take mock examinations. Do not miss formal mock exams that may be provided by your residency programs during your chief year, and if doing a fellowship, consider getting together with your co-fellows in other subspecialties to practice together. If you are not in a fellowship, consider going on Google Talk or Skype to practice with your co-residents or other residents preparing for the exam. If you take the time to prepare mock exam case files (on Microsoft PowerPoint, for instance) with radiology and pathology images from your own files, publications, or Google searches, and practice going through the formal routine of taking an oral board exam, the actual exam will seem much more familiar and easier.
- Bringing other viewpoints, standards of care, and opinions is another benefit of talking to and studying with co-fellows or residents of other programs. This is especially true for graduates of smaller residency programs who may have only been exposed to a limited number of subspecialty-trained attending physicians. Discussing the "board answers," that is, what you should say in the board exam, rather than your local surgeon's independent viewpoint, would serve you well. For instance, your otology-attending physician may have gone forward with a stapedectomy in the setting of a persistent stapedial artery or overhanging facial nerve, but the "board answer" may be to abort. It would be appropriate to bring up the fact that you may have witnessed a successful completion of this case by a more experienced surgeon, but you would abort the case and refer it to a more seasoned otologist.
- Examiners are on your side. If you feel yourself starting to panic or tighten up, ask for a second and relax. You are likely doing better than you think.
- You need to pass the written exam to take the oral exam. If you passed the written exam, chances are heavily in your favor that you will pass the oral exam.

DIFFERENTIAL DIAGNOSIS AND CLINICAL ROUNDS

Cummings Review of Otolaryngology is a powerful tool for rapid learning and review for medical students, interns, and junior residents rounding in the hospital and preparing for "pimp" questions, as well as for residents studying for oral and written in-service and board exams. Even though other review books provide summaries of information of what could be said during an oral examination or in response to a "pimp" question, our book provides a logical, systematic approach that can be applied to any oral exam format; to frequently asked questions by chief residents, fellows, and attending physicians; and to address any clinical situation: *what questions should you ask in the history, what findings are you looking for on physical exam, what is the differential diagnosis, what are the critical findings on radiology and pathology studies, what are the treatment options, what is your best option, what are ways to perform this, and what is your postoperative management?* Once these lists are reviewed and memorized, the reader will have an armamentarium of knowledge that can be instinctively accessed and effectively used in any clinical or examination scenario.

For further detail, you will often need to go to the reference books and other texts to explain in more detail many of the key "buzzwords" that are in this review book. Obviously, the more senior in training you are, the better these terms will make sense to you and stay with you. However, these lists, if memorized early in training, can serve the trainee exceedingly well on rounds, in the clinic, in the operating room, and on exams. For instance, a medical student or intern may have difficulty explaining exactly where the *soft-tissue triangles* are located, but a sub-intern will routinely be asked to recite the subunits of the nose by facial-plastics attending physicians. Similarly, a student may not know exactly where the *greater superficial petrosal nerve* travels, but may be asked to name all branches of the facial nerve or surgical landmarks of the middle cranial fossa. Being able to learn such packets of information from this review book and accurately recite them when put on the spot could easily and favorably affect the enthusiasm of the attending and resident physicians for the sub-intern and dramatically elevate the student's position on the program's rank list.

PEARLS FOR SUCCESS ON WRITTEN EXAMS AND CLINICAL ROUNDS

- Preparation and repetition are the keys to success. Use the list format to "pimp" question your fellow residents and medical students early and often. Cross off lists that are already memorized, and work to memorize as much of the book as possible. In doing so, the number of humiliatingly awkward silences that follow being asked a "pimp" question will be minimized.
- The American Board of Otolaryngology written examination is a long test, comprising eight 50-minute sections, and is completed on a computer at a local testing center. After signing in, providing all required forms of identification, and putting all of your belongings in a locker, you will be taken to the testing room, where you are provided a whiteboard, marker, and eraser for any notes you may want to take. The clock starts once you log in and click to start a section, and the "break clock" starts once you complete each section. You are given a total of 60 minutes of break time to spend as you wish, and you will need to allot sufficient time to eat lunch, which you will need to bring and store in the locker.
- Undoubtedly, to become a medical student and otolaryngology resident, you will have had to perform at the highest levels on written exams at nearly all points of your education. Most of you will unlikely need to follow the test-taking suggestions in this book, or already have your own effective test-preparation routines. That said, however, it is anecdotally reported that 10-15% of examinees fail the otolaryngology written board exam every year. Accordingly, do not underestimate the difficulty of and level of performance needed to pass the exam. It has been shown that performance on in-service examinations correlates closely with performance on the board examination, and, consequently, you and your program director should be able to determine the intensity at which you should prepare for the written exam.
- Given the length of the exam, prepare your mental endurance as the test date approaches by taking full weekend days during which you study for 3 to 4 consecutive hours without breaks in the morning and again in the afternoon after a brief lunch break. Determine how much caffeine you will need to optimize your attentiveness and minimize mental fatigue as you enter the seventh and eighth hours of study and test taking. Remember that those final questions are worth just as much as the first set of questions.

- Do not perseverate on one or a handful of questions and jeopardize your ability to read and intelligently answer all questions fully. As with most computer tests you have previously taken, you can always go back within a section to questions about which you are unsure. If you have absolutely no idea what the answer may be, just guess, and minimize time wasted. If you have narrowed it down to two or three choices, take a short amount of time to decide what the best guess would be.
- Oftentimes the question will ask for the "best" answer or "next" course of action. Try to avoid overthinking the question; for example, you may be tempted to establish the diagnosis of an unvaccinated child acutely presenting with drooling and stridor, and want to visualize the supraglottis, but the "next" and "best" course of action may be to establish the airway and intubate the child.
- "Pimping" on clinical rounds is often formulated toward one answer, or a short list (eg, what would you need to see on pathology for a follicular thyroid carcinoma diagnosis, or what are the subsites of the hypopharynx?), and because of the limited time of early morning rounds, you will be expected to answer quickly. Unfortunately, the questions can often be in a frustrating "what am I thinking?" format (eg, what exam finding in particular would you expect in a patient with necrotizing otitis externa, or what is special about adenoid cystic carcinoma, or what else could it be?); being able to list off a differential diagnosis or key findings for a particular pathology quickly would maximize your chance of naming the desired answer.
- Remember to include a differential diagnosis in your presentations because this will help you in your learning.
- Remember your patients. Success on written exams and with frequently encountered "pimp" questioning is facilitated by correlating your clinical experiences with your medical knowledge. Use a key figure or a list of pathologic features presented in this book to associate with a clinical experience. You will never forget facts that are associated with patient care.
- The radiology and pathology images in *Cummings Review of Otolaryngology* are arranged in a high-yield format for exams in otolaryngology. Review these images before your in-service, written, and oral board exams. These images represent some of the most frequently encountered pathologies in our field, and you may find many on your exams.

We wish you success on your written and oral examinations and congratulate you in your choice of a career in otolaryngology, head and neck surgery.

2 Otology and Neurotology

TEMPORAL BONE ANATOMY

Temporal bone portions
  a. Squamous
  b. Petrous
  c. Tympanic
  d. Mastoid

LATERAL VIEW OF THE LEFT TEMPORAL BONE (Fig. 2.1)

Key Points

- The *temporal line* approximates the floor level of the middle fossa ±5 mm.
- The sigmoid and lateral sinuses are typically anterior and superior to the emissary vein, respectively.
- The *Macewen triangle*, which is located posterior and superior to the spine of Henle, approximates the lateral landmark of the mastoid antrum.

SUPERIOR VIEW OF THE LEFT TEMPORAL BONE (Fig. 2.2)

Key Points

- The *arcuate eminence* typically corresponds to the superior semicircular canal, but not always.
- The *greater superficial petrosal nerve* (GSPN) exits from the geniculate ganglion of the facial nerve; the geniculate ganglion is dehiscent without bony covering in about 10-20% of temporal bones.

MEDIAL VIEW OF LEFT TEMPORAL BONE (Fig. 2.3)

Key Points

- The lateral portion of the internal auditory canal (IAC) is called the *fundus*, and the medial portion is called the *porus*.
- Bill's bar is named after William House. It separates the facial nerve from the superior vestibular nerve at the fundus of

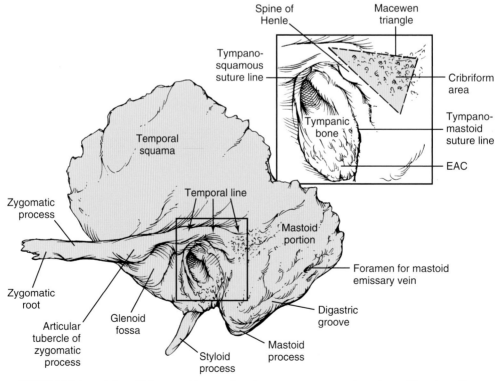

FIGURE 2.1 Lateral view of left temporal bone surface shows squamous, tympanic, and mastoid portions. (From Francis HW, Niparko JK. *Temporal Bone Dissection Guide*. New York, NY: Thieme; 2011 and Flint PW, Haughey BH, Lund VJ, et al. *Cummings Otolaryngology—Head and Neck Surgery*. 6th ed. Philadelphia, PA: Saunders; 2015, fig. 127-1.)

the IAC. Identification of Bill's bar allows early identification of the facial nerve, likely uninvolved with pathology (ie, a vestibular schwannoma arising from a vestibular nerve).

INFERIOR VIEW OF THE LEFT TEMPORAL BONE (Fig. 2.4)

Key Points
- The styloid process is anteromedial to the stylomastoid foramen.
- Medial and superior to the mastoid tip is the digastric groove, which is the origin of the posterior belly of the digastric muscle. The anterior border of the digastric groove is the stylomastoid foramen.
- The cochlear aqueduct is inferior and parallel to the IAC.

THE AURICLE

BLOOD SUPPLY
- External carotid artery
  - Superficial temporal artery (anterior)
  - Posterior auricular (posterior)

EAR CANAL
- Lateral one-third is cartilaginous (has cerumen glands and hair follicles)
- Medial two-thirds are bony (no cerumen glands or hair follicles)
- Bony-cartilaginous junction is a route of disease spread
- Fissures of Santorini: natural fissures in anterior cartilaginous ear canal that allows the spread of disease to the superficial parotid
- Foramen of Huschke: anteroinferior bony defect that typically obliterates during development; patency allows the spread of disease to the deep parotid lobe/temporomandibular joint (TMJ)

EARDRUM (Fig. 2.5)
1. Manubrium (handle of malleus)
2. Anterior malleolar fold
3. Posterior malleolar fold
4. Pars flaccida (has no fibrous layer between the keratinizing squamous epithelium and middle ear mucosa); space medial to pars flaccida and lateral to malleus neck: *Prussack's space*

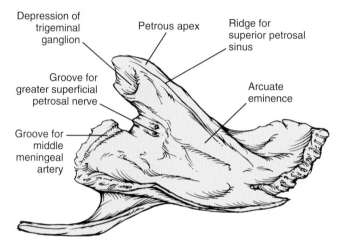

FIGURE 2.2 Superior view of left temporal bone shows petrous and squamous portions forming the floor of the middle fossa and anterior limit of the posterior fossa. (From Francis HW, Niparko JK. *Temporal Bone Dissection Guide*. New York, NY: Thieme; 2011 and Flint PW, Haughey BH, Lund VJ, et al. *Cummings Otolaryngology—Head and Neck Surgery*. 6th ed. Philadelphia, PA: Saunders; 2015, fig. 127-2.)

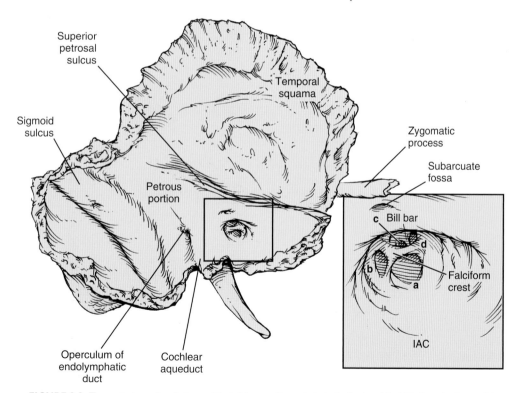

FIGURE 2.3 The posterior surface features of the left temporal bone include the fundus of the IAC. Foramina for cranial nerve VIII: cochlear (*a*), inferior vestibular (*b*), and superior vestibular (*c*) divisions and cranial nerve VII (*d*) are shown. (From Francis HW, Niparko JK. *Temporal Bone Dissection Guide*. New York, NY: Thieme; 2011 and Flint PW, Haughey BH, Lund VJ, et al. *Cummings Otolaryngology—Head and Neck Surgery*. 6th ed. Philadelphia, PA: Saunders; 2015, fig. 127-3.)

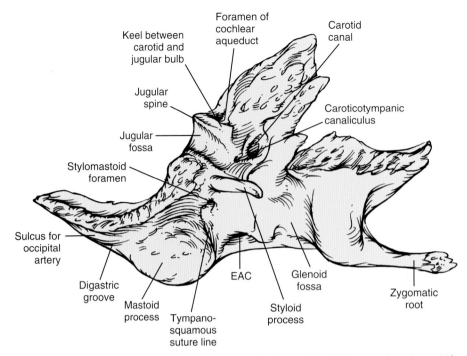

FIGURE 2.4 Inferior View of the Left Temporal Bone. Note the linear relationship between the stylomastoid foramen, digastric groove, and styloid process. (From Francis HW, Niparko JK. *Temporal Bone Dissection Guide*. New York, NY: Thieme; 2011 and Flint PW, Haughey BH, Lund VJ, et al. *Cummings Otolaryngology—Head and Neck Surgery*. 6th ed. Philadelphia, PA: Saunders; 2015, fig. 127-5.)

5. Long process of the incus
6. Promontory behind the eardrum
7. Fibrous tympanic annulus (not present along the pars flaccida)
8. Umbo
9. Lateral or short process of the malleus
10. Opening of the Eustachian tube

MIDDLE EAR

1. Epitympanum (superior to the annulus)
   a. Prussack's space
   b. Anterior epitympanum (Supratubal recess) - compartment anterior to the malleus head
   c. Posterior epitympanum compartment posterior to the cog (communicates with the mastoid via the aditus ad antrum into the antrum)
2. Mesotympanum (at the level of the annulus, superiorly/inferiorly)
3. Hypotympanum (below the level of the annulus)
4. Eustachian tube (protympanum): connects and ventilates the anterior mesotympanic space to the nasopharynx
5. Above the Eustachian tube is the *supratubal recess* (STR)
   a. The posterior boundary *cochleariform process* (inferiorly) and the *cog* (superiorly); the former is where the tensor tympani tendon takes a 90-degree turn from the medial wall of the middle ear and inserts onto the malleus
   b. The medial wall will house the geniculate ganglion; it may be dehiscent by the cholesteatoma
6. Sinus tympani in the posterior mesotympanic space, medial to the descending facial nerve, posterior to the oval window (separated by the *ponticulus*) and round window niche (separated by the *subiculum*) and of variable posterior extension; cholesteatoma may hide here
7. Facial recess is lateral to the vertical facial nerve but medial to the chorda tympani nerve, which, in turn, is medial to the annulus

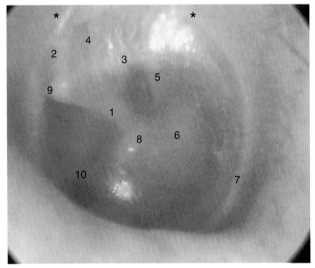

FIGURE 2.5 Surface features of the left TM include the manubrium of the malleus (mallear stria, *1*); anterior mallear fold (*2*); posterior mallear fold (*3*); pars flaccida, or Shrapnell membrane (*4*); long process of incus (*5*); pars tensa, through which the promontory and round window are visible (*6*); tympanic annulus (*7*); umbo (*8*); lateral process (*9*); Eustachian tube opening (*10*); and anterior and posterior tympanic spines (*asterisks*). The anterior and posterior tympanic spines are the borders of the bony gateway to the epitympanum (*notch of Rivinus*). (From Flint PW, Haughey BH, Lund VJ, et al. *Cummings Otolaryngology—Head and Neck Surgery*. 6th ed. Philadelphia, PA: Saunders; 2015, fig. 127-8.)

8. The suspensory ligaments and mesenteries of the ossicles separate the aeration of the epitympanum and mesotympanum, and connect
   a. Anterior to the stapes (*isthmus tympani anticus*)
   b. Posterior to the stapes (*isthmus tympani oticus*)
9. The long process of the incus has a single blood supply without collaterals predisposing it to erosion
10. The stapedius tendon is innervated by the facial nerve, and it comes out of the *pyramidal eminence* and inserts onto the neck of the stapes.

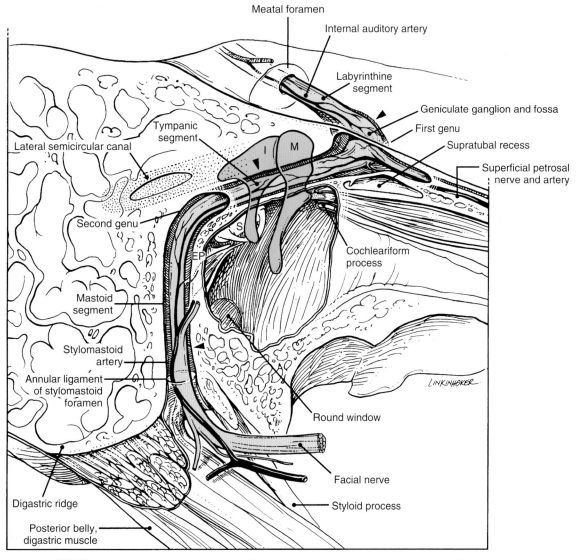

FIGURE 2.6 Anatomy of the Infratemporal Portion of the Facial Nerve and Associated Middle Ear Structures. Shown are sites of vulnerability to injury (*arrowheads*). *Perigeniculate region:* Susceptibility of the genicular fossa to fracture also increases the risk of nerve injury via nerve compression and ischemia in the narrow meatal foramen and labyrinthine segment. The first genu of the facial nerve is tethered by the GSPN, which increases susceptibility to shearing injuries; vascular watershed area between branches of the external carotid artery and posterior circulation, the geniculate ganglion is susceptible to injury during surgical dissection in the STR of the anterior epitympanum. *Tympanic segment:* The nerve is most frequently dehiscent above the oval window and distal tympanic segment; the second genu is susceptible to injury in cholesteatoma surgery because of pathologic dehiscence or distorted anatomy and failure to identify important surgical landmarks. *Mastoid segment:* In the lower portion of its vertical course and just distal to the stylomastoid foramen, the nerve is positioned lateral to the tympanic annulus and is therefore susceptible to injury during surgery of the EAC. *EP,* Eminence pyramidale; *I,* incus; *M,* malleus; *S,* stapes. (From Francis HW. Facial nerve emergencies. In Eisele D, McQuone S, eds. *Emergencies of the Head and Neck.* St. Louis, MO: Mosby; 2000 and Flint PW, Haughey BH, Lund VJ, et al. *Cummings Otolaryngology—Head and Neck Surgery.* 6th ed. Philadelphia, PA: Saunders; 2015, fig. 127-9.)

11. Tensor tympani innervation by V3 and inserts into the neck of the malleus

COURSE OF THE FACIAL NERVE, RIGHT-EAR PARASAGITTAL VIEW (Fig. 2.6)

KEY POINTS

1. Exits the brainstem (cisternal or the cerebellopontine angle [CPA] portion) 14-17 mm
2. Enters the porus of the IAC and courses to the fundus (meatal portion, 8-10 mm)
3. Intratemporal facial nerve's bony housing = fallopian canal
4. Labyrinthine segment, 3-5 mm, the narrowest portion, and completely enclosed in bone, leaving it most susceptible to compression from edema (Bell's) and trauma (temporal bone fracture)
5. Geniculate ganglion at the first genu of the facial nerve
6. Facial nerve in the inner ear enters just posterior and superior to the cochleariform process
7. Courses over the superior border of the oval window (*tympanic segment,* 10-12 mm)
   a. Dehiscent here up to 25-55% of the temporal bones, leaving it susceptible to injury/inflammatory mediators
8. Second or mastoid genu
9. *Mastoid or descending facial nerve,* 12-15 mm
10. Exits at the stylomastoid foramen
    a. Exit is surrounded by the posterior belly of the digastric and skull-base periosteum

11. Facial nerve functions
    a. Special visceral efferent (facial nucleus to the stapedius, posterior belly digastric, stylohyoid muscle, and muscles of facial expression)
    b. General visceral efferents (superior salivatory nucleus in the nervus intermedius to the geniculate ganglion to the lacrimal gland, nasal mucosa, and submandibular and sublingual glands)

c. Special sensory fibers (anterior two-thirds tongue taste to the solitary nucleus)
d. Somatic sensory fibers (posterior external auditory canal [EAC] and conchal skin of the auricle to the spinal trigeminal nucleus)
e. Visceral afferent fibers (nasal mucosa to solitary nucleus)

MASTOID AND PETROUS APEX

REGIONS OF TEMPORAL BONE PNEUMATIZATION

1. Mastoid
2. Petrous apex
3. Perilabyrinthine
4. Accessory (zygomatic, squamous, occipital, and styloid)

AIR CELL TRACTS

1. Posterosuperior (sinodural)
2. Posteromedial (retrofacial and retrolabyrinthine)
3. Subarcuate
4. Perilabyrinthine
5. Peritubal

AUDITORY ANATOMY AND PHYSIOLOGY

EXTERNAL EAR

1. Auricle resonance frequency 5300 Hz
2. Ear canal resonance frequency 3000 Hz
3. Allows localization via
    a. Interaural time difference
    b. Interaural intensity difference

EARDRUM/OSSICULAR CHAIN (Fig. 2.7)

1. Eardrum: footplate ratio 20:1 (26 dB advantage)
2. Ossicular chain lever ratio 1.3:1 (2.3 dB advantage)
3. *Theoretical* gain of eardrum/ossicular chain: 28 dB
4. *Actual* gain or eardrum/ossicular chain: 20 dB

COCHLEA (Fig. 2.8)

1. Vibratory wave: oval window → scala vestibuli (perilymph filled) → helicotrema → scala tympani (perilymph filled) → round window

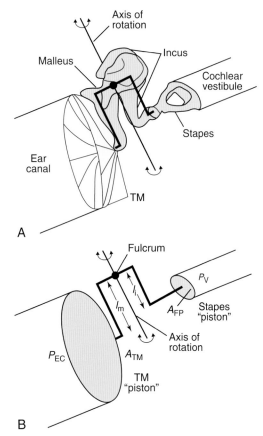

FIGURE 2.7 Schematic of the Middle Ear System. (**A**) Motion of the ossicular chain along its axis of rotation is illustrated. (**B**) Area of the TM (A_{TM}) divided by area of the footplate (A_{FP}) represents the *area ratio* (A_{TM}/A_{FP}). The length of the manubrium (l_m) divided by the length of the incus long process (l_i) is the *lever ratio* (l_m/l_i). P_{EC}, External canal sound pressure; P_V, sound pressure of the vestibule. (From Merchant SN, Rosowski JJ. Auditory physiology. In Glasscock ME, Gulya AJ, eds. *Glasscock-Shambaugh Surgery of the Ear*. 5th ed. Hamilton, ON: Decker; 2003:64, fig. 129-2.)

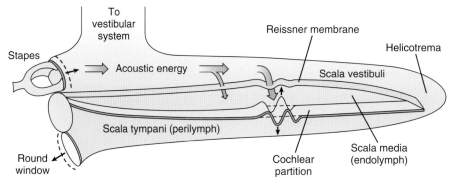

FIGURE 2.8 Schematic Showing Sound Propagation in the Cochlea. As sound energy travels through the external and middle ears, it causes the stapes footplate to vibrate. The vibration of this footplate results in a compressional wave on the inner ear fluid. Because the pressure in the scala vestibuli is higher than that in the scala tympani, this sets up a pressure gradient that causes the cochlear partition to vibrate as a traveling wave. Because the basilar membrane varies in its stiffness and mass along its length, it is able to act as a series of filters that respond to specific sound frequencies at specific locations along its length. (From Geisler CD. *From Sound to Synapse: Physiology of the Mammalian Ear*. New York, NY: Oxford University Press; 1998:51 and Flint PW, Haughey BH, Lund VJ, et al. *Cummings Otolaryngology—Head and Neck Surgery*. 6th ed. Philadelphia, PA: Saunders; 2015, fig. 129-6.)

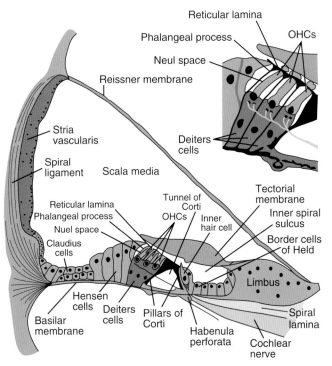

2. Basilar membrane (Fig. 2.9) is
   a. Tonotopic: high frequencies at basal region (stiffer)
   b. Lower frequencies at apical region (more flexible)
   c. Stiffness difference allows it to be a frequency filter
3. Vibratory wave → deflection of hair cell stereocilia → potassium influx → depolarization (resting potential in endolymph +60-100 mV relative to perilymph) → action potential at first level neurons of spiral ganglion (Fig. 2.10)
4. Potassium recirculated back through supporting cells and back into the perilymph via the stria vascularis

CENTRAL AUDITORY PATHWAYS (Fig. 2.11)

1. Auditory nerve
2. Cochlear nuclei
   a. Dorsal cochlear nucleus
   b. Anterior ventral cochlear nucleus
   c. Posterior ventral cochlear nucleus (the majority of auditory fibers cross the midline)
3. Superior olivary complex
4. Lateral lemniscus
5. Inferior colliculus
6. Medial geniculate body
7. Auditory cortex

STAPEDIUS REFLEX

1. Auditory nerve → cochlear nucleus → interneurons → bilateral facial motor nuclei → bilateral stapedius tendons

FIGURE 2.9 Cross section of the organ of Corti showing the major cellular structures. (From Flint PW, Haughey BH, Lund VJ, et al. *Cummings Otolaryngology—Head and Neck Surgery*. 6th ed. Philadelphia, PA: Saunders; 2015, fig. 128-2.)

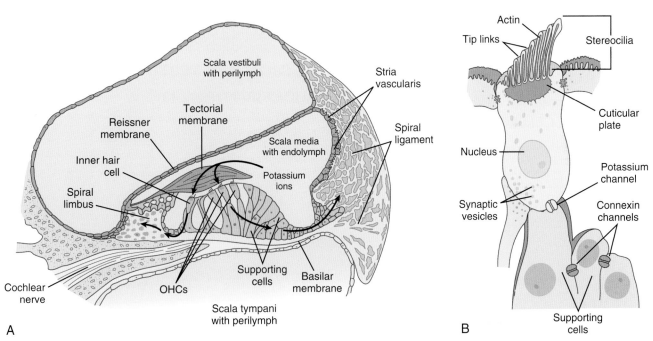

FIGURE 2.10 Mechanoelectrical transduction of the auditory signal depends on the recycling of potassium ions in the organ of Corti. (**A**) Schematic cross-sectional view of the human cochlea. The scala media (cochlear duct) is filled with endolymph, and the scala vestibuli and tympani are filled with perilymph. The endolymph of the scala media bathes the organ of Corti, located between the basilar and tectorial membranes and containing the inner and OHCs. A relatively high concentration of potassium in the endolymph of the scala media relative to the hair cell creates a cation gradient maintained by the activity of the epithelial supporting cells, spiral ligament, and stria vascularis. (**B**) Cells contain stereocilia along the apical surface and are connected by tip links. The potassium gradient is essential to enable depolarization of the hair cell following influx of potassium ions in response to mechanical vibration of the basilar membrane, deflection of stereocilia, displacement of tip links, and opening of gated potassium channels. Depolarization results in calcium influx through channels along the basolateral membrane of the hair cell, which causes degranulation of neurotransmitter vesicles into the synaptic terminal and propagates an action potential along the auditory nerve. Gap junction proteins between the hair cells (potassium channel, *yellow*) and epithelial supporting cells (connexin channels, *red*) allow for the flow of potassium ions back to the stria vascularis, where they are pumped back into the endolymph. (From Willems PJ. Genetic causes of hearing loss. *N Engl J Med*. 2000;342(15):1101-1109 and Flint PW, Haughey BH, Lund VJ, et al. *Cummings Otolaryngology—Head and Neck Surgery*. 6th ed. Philadelphia, PA: Saunders; 2015, fig. 129-4.)

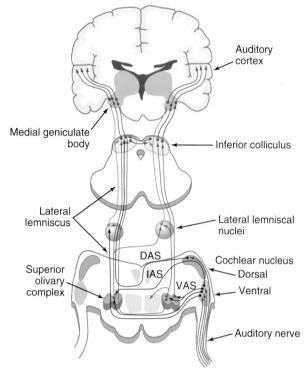

FIGURE 2.11 Illustration of the major central ascending auditory pathways for sound entering via the right cochlea. Commissural pathways and descending feedback projections from higher centers are not depicted. *DAS,* Dorsal acoustic stria; *IAS,* intermediate acoustic stria; *VAS,* ventral acoustic stria. (From Flint PW, Haughey BH, Lund VJ, et al. *Cummings Otolaryngology—Head and Neck Surgery.* 6th ed. Philadelphia, PA: Saunders; 2015, fig. 128-6.)

VESTIBULAR ANATOMY AND PHYSIOLOGY

COPLANAR SEMICIRCULAR CANALS (ANGULAR ACCELEROMETERS) (Fig. 2.12)

1. Horizontal canals
2. Left anterior (superior), right posterior
3. Right anterior (superior), left posterior
   a. Basal firing rate from each ampulla

b. Excitatory with angular acceleration in the direction of the leading canal, and inhibitory in the coplanar, lagging canal; therefore,
   i. Ampullopetal flow of the perilymph in the lateral canals is excitatory
   ii. Ampullofugal flow of the perilymph in the superior and posterior canals is excitatory

OTOLITHIC ORGANS (LINEAR ACCELEROMETERS)

1. Saccule: vertical acceleration
2. Utricle: horizontal acceleration, head tilt

INNERVATION

1. Superior vestibular nerve
   a. Utricle
   b. Superior semicircular canal
   c. Lateral semicircular canal
2. Inferior vestibular nerve
   a. Saccule
   b. Posterior semicircular canal

EUSTACHIAN TUBE

1. Two-thirds cartilaginous; one-third bony
2. Tensor veli palatini is the primary dilator
3. Aging leads to increased slope of the tube, as well as increased length, diameter, and efficiency of the opening
4. *Ostmann fat pad:* metabolically sensitive adipose in the lateral wall of the Eustachian tube distally (rapid weight loss can cause atrophy of the fat pad and results in patulous Eustachian tube syndrome)

AUDIOLOGIC TESTING

AUDIOGRAM (Fig. 2.13)

- O = right-ear air conduction
- X = left-ear air conduction
- Δ = right-ear air masked
- □ = left-ear air masked
- < = right unmasked bone
- > = left unmasked bone

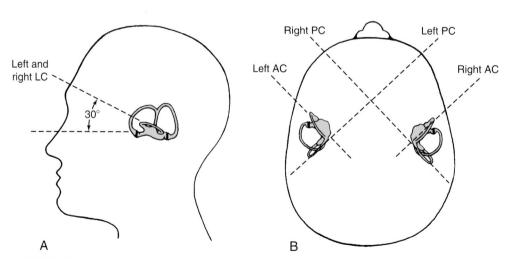

FIGURE 2.12 Orientation of Semicircular Canals. (A) The horizontal canal is tilted 30 degrees upward from a horizontal plane at its anterior end. (**B**) Vertical canals are oriented at roughly 45 degrees from the midsagittal plane. *AC,* Anterior canal; *LC,* lateral canal; *PC,* posterior canal. (Modified from Barber HO, Stockwell CW. *Manual of Electronystagmography.* St. Louis, MO: Mosby-Year Book; 1976 and Flint PW, Haughey BH, Lund VJ, et al. *Cummings Otolaryngology—Head and Neck Surgery.* 6th ed. Philadelphia, PA: Saunders; 2015, fig. 130-2.)

- [= right masked bone
-] = left masked bone

CROSSOVER

1. Bone: 0-10 dB
2. Air (headphones): 35-50 dB
3. Air (insert headphones): 60-65 dB

OBJECTIVE MEASURES UP THE AUDITORY PATHWAY

1. Otoacoustic emissions (OAEs) (spontaneous, transient evoked, distortion product: outer hair cell (OHC) function
2. Ecog: summating potential/action potential (SP/AP) ratio; AP = wave I auditory brainstem response (ABR); >0.35-0.5 abnormal (hydrops or inner ear third window)
3. ABR (five waves):
   a. Distal eighth nerve
   b. Proximal eighth nerve
   c. Cochlear nuclei
   d. Superior olivary complex
   e. Lateral lemniscus
      i. Tumor diagnosis:
         (1) No wave V
         (2) Prolongation I-III (interaural)
         (3) Prolongation I-V (interaural)
         (4) <1 cm tumor only 60% sensitive
      ii. Auditory neuropathy/dyssynchrony
         (1) No ABR
         (2) Present OAEs
4. Vestibular evoked myogenic potential (VEMP): acoustic energy → saccule → inferior vestibular nerve → vestibular nuclei → ipsilateral spinal accessory nucleus → relaxation of sternocleidomastoid (SCM)

IMAGING OF THE SKULL BASE AND TEMPORAL BONE COMPUTED TOMOGRAPHY: THE STUDY OF CHOICE FOR BONY ANATOMY

1. Atresia
2. Canal cholesteatoma

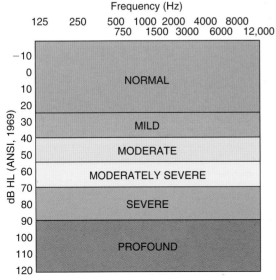

FIGURE 2.13 Audiogram Showing a Range of Hearing Loss. *ANSI,* American National Standards Institute; *dB HL,* decibel hearing level. (From Flint PW, Haughey BH, Lund VJ, et al. *Cummings Otolaryngology—Head and Neck Surgery.* 6th ed. Philadelphia, PA: Saunders; 2015, fig. 133-1.)

3. Exostoses
4. Osteoma
5. Glomus tympanicum
6. Aberrant carotid artery
7. Cholesteatoma, uncomplicated
8. Uncomplicated chronic otitis media (OM)
9. Coalescent mastoiditis
10. Glomus tympanicum versus jugulare if visible lesion is below the annulus (examine the jugular plate)
11. Inner ear malformations
   a. Lateral canal dysplasia
   b. Enlarged vestibular aqueduct
   c. Cochlear dysplasia
12. Labyrinthitis ossificans
13. Superior canal dehiscence/inner ear third windows

MAGNETIC RESONANCE IMAGING IS BETTER FOR SOFT-TISSUE ANATOMY: THE STUDY OF CHOICE FOR INTRACRANIAL PATHOLOGY

1. CPA lesions
   a. Vestibular schwannoma
   b. Meningioma
   c. Epidermoid
   d. Eighth nerve deficiency (highly weighted T2 images: FIESTA or CISS sequences)
   e. Early cochlear fibrosis (ie, early labyrinthitis ossificans before calcification)

WHEN MAGNETIC RESONANCE IMAGING AND COMPUTED TOMOGRAPHY ARE COMPLEMENTARY

1. Complicated OM/cholesteatoma
2. Glomus jugulare tumors
3. Endolymphatic sac tumors
4. Cholesterol granuloma
5. Facial nerve lesions (schwannoma/hemangioma)

IMAGING CHARACTERISTICS OF PETROUS APEX LESIONS (Table 2.1)

The most common petrous apex lesions encountered are: asymmetric pneumatization, retained secretions, cholesterol granuloma, mucoceles and cholesteatomas. Please refer to Table 2.1 for the CT and MRI characteristics of ear entity.

Imaging Characteristics of Cerebellopontine Angle Lesions (Table 2.2)

The most common cerebellopontine angle lesions are acoustic neuromas, meningiomas, arachnoid cysts, epidermoids and lipomas. Please refer to Table 2.2 for the CT and MRI characteristics of each entity.

OTITIS EXTERNA

EXTERNAL AUDITORY CANAL DEFENSE

1. Acidic pH 6.0-6.5
2. Migratory nature of keratin debris (drum is centrifugally out)

NORMAL FLORA

1. *Staphylococcus auricularis*
2. *Staphylococcus epidermidis*
3. *Corynebacterium*
4. *Streptococcus*
5. *Enterococcus*

6. Rarely *Pseudomonas*
7. Rarely fungus

ACUTE OTITIS EXTERNA

1. 90% bacterial
   a. *Pseudomonas*
   b. *S. epidermidis*
   c. *Staphylococcus aureus*
2. 2-10% fungus/other
   a. *Aspergillus*
   b. *Candida*
3. Treatment: always remove debris ("bacterial/fungal potato chips")
   a. Mild otitis externa (OE): acidify ½ white vinegar/distilled water ± rubbing alcohol
   b. Moderate OE (with more edema and purulence): add antibiotic topical drop ± steroid; wick may be necessary if drum is not visible
   c. Severe OE (extension to periauricular and auricular tissues): antibiotic topical drop ± steroid; wick may be necessary; add systemic antibiotic with pseudomonal coverage (quinolone likely)
   d. Fungal OE: antibiotics may precipitate and steroids worsen; debride and antifungal (nystatin cream, ampho B powder/cream, and clotrimazole powder/cream)
4. Complications
   a. Chondritis (*Pseudomonas*)
   b. Perichondritis
   c. Cellulitis
   d. Malignant OE: *Pseudomonas* is the most common at 90%
5. Other acute otitis externa causes
   a. Herpes zoster virus (HZV) (Ramsay Hunt)
   b. Erysipelas (beta hemolytic strep)
   c. Furuncle (*S. aureus*)

d. Bullous myringitis (viral vs. mycoplasma vs. *Streptococcus*)
   i. Can have sensorineural hearing loss (SNHL) component 65%, resolution with infection resolution 60%
6. Malignant OE buzzwords
   a. Diabetic, immunosuppressed
   b. *Pseudomonas* #1; fungal less likely
   c. Granulation at the bony-cartilaginous junction or tympanomastoid suture line
   d. Biopsy needed: r/o malignancy
   e. Imaging
      i. Computed tomography (CT) scan: bony erosion
      ii. Magnetic resonance imaging (MRI): soft-tissue involvement (likely study of choice)
      iii. Technetium scan: can diagnose bony activity and will show long-term change, even after resolution
      iv. Follow with gallium scan or indium scan with tagged white blood cells
   f. Labs
      i. Erythrocyte sedimentation rate: follow disease
      ii. C-reactive protein
   g. Treatment: intravenous antibiotics, surgery only for definitive biopsy; let infectious disease follow

CHRONIC OTITIS MEDIA, MASTOIDITIS, APICITIS, AND COMPLICATIONS OF THE OTITIS MEDIA

ACQUIRED CHOLESTEATOMA DEVELOPMENT THEORIES

1. Invagination (retraction pocket)
2. Basal cell hyperplasia (a defect in the basal membrane allows ingrowth of epithelial cells)

Table 2.1 Imaging Characteristics of Petrous Apex Lesions

Lesion	CT	T1	T2	T1+ Contrast	Notes
Asymmetric pneumatization	Bone marrow filled, no air cells	Hyperintense to intermediate intensity	Hyperintense	No enhancement	T1 signal disappears with fat suppression
Retained secretions	Air cell trabecular preservation, nonexpansile	Hypointense	Hyperintense	No enhancement	
Cholesterol granuloma	Air cell trabecular breakdown, expansile	Hyperintense	Hyperintense	No enhancement	T2 hyperintensity unchanged with fat saturation
Mucocele	Air cell trabecular breakdown, expansile	Hypointense	Hyperintense	Rim enhancement	
Cholesteatoma	Air cell trabecular breakdown, expansile	Hypointense	Hyperintense	May have rim enhancement if granulation tissue is present	DWI restriction (bright signal)

CT, Computed tomography; *DWI*, diffusion-weighted imaging.
From Flint PW, Haughey BH, Lund VJ, et al. *Cummings Otolaryngology—Head and Neck Surgery*. 6th ed. Philadelphia, PA: Saunders; 2015, table 135-1.

Table 2.2 Imaging Characteristics of Cerebellopontine Angle Lesions

Lesion	T1	T2	T1+ Contrast	Notes
Vestibular schwannoma	Isointense to brain	Slightly hyperintense	Enhances	
Meningioma	Isointense to brain	Hypointense/hyperintense	Enhances	T2 signal depends on calcium content
Arachnoid cyst	Hypointense	Hyperintense	No enhancement	Signal characteristics mirror those of CSF
Epidermoid	Hypointense	Hyperintense	No enhancement	T2 signal is slightly more dense than CSF is; DWI shows restriction (bright signal)
Lipoma	Hyperintense	Hyperintense	No enhancement	T1 signal disappears with fat suppression

CSF, Cerebrospinal fluid.
From Flint PW, Haughey BH, Lund VJ, et al. *Cummings Otolaryngology—Head and Neck Surgery*. 6th ed. Philadelphia, PA: Saunders; 2015, table 135-2.

3. Migration theory (through a perforation without contact inhibition into the middle ear)
4. Squamous metaplasia of middle ear mucosa

PETROUS APEX DRAINAGE TRACTS

1. Posterior petrous apex (30% of them pneumatized in temporal bones)
   a. Subarcuate
   b. Sinodural
2. Anterior petrous apex (10% pneumatized in temporal bones)
   a. Peritubal
   b. Retrofacial
   c. Infralabyrinthine
   d. Infracochlear
   e. Glenoid fossa (Ramandier and Lempert)

GRADENIGO SYNDROME (TRIAD)

1. Draining ear
2. Retro-orbital pain
3. Ipsilateral abducens palsy

COMPLICATIONS OF ACUTE AND CHRONIC OTITIS MEDIA

1. Extracranial
   a. Acute mastoiditis
   b. Coalescent mastoiditis (erosion of mastoid air cell septations)
   c. Chronic mastoiditis
   d. Masked mastoiditis (partially treated with antibiotics but still painful)
   e. Subperiosteal abscess
      i. Postauricular (through the cribriform area, with direct extension through bone, and/or thrombophlebitic)
      ii. Bezold (medial wall of mastoid tip medial to SCM muscle into the neck)
      iii. Luc's (zygomatic root)
   f. Petrous apicitis
   g. Labyrinthine fistula
   h. Facial paralysis
   i. Suppurative labyrinthitis
   j. Encephalocele
   k. Cerebrospinal fluid (CSF) leakage
2. Intracranial
   a. Meningitis
   b. Epidural abscess
   c. Subdural empyema
   d. Brain abscess
   e. Lateral/sigmoid sinus thrombosis
   f. Otitic hydrocephalus

TEMPORAL BONE TRAUMA

WHAT YOU SHOULD CARE ABOUT

1. Facial motion present/not present on initial evaluation
2. Otorrhea: that is, CSF
3. Potential carotid canal injury
4. Dizziness

TYPES OF FRACTURES

1. Old system
   a. Longitudinal fracture (80%)
      i. Conductive hearing loss (CHL) > SNHL
      ii. Tympanic membrane (TM) tears/EAC lacerations
      iii. Less facial weakness

   b. Transverse (20%): more force and blow to occiput
      i. SNHL is more likely
      ii. Facial weakness is more likely
   c. Oblique: a mixture of fracture types
2. New system
   a. Otic capsule sparing
      i. CHL/mixed hearing loss (HL) > SNHL
      ii. Less facial weakness (6-14%)
      iii. Less risk CSF leakage
   b. Otic capsule disrupting
      i. SNHL likely
      ii. Facial weakness (30-50%)
      iii. Increased risk CSF leak (8x otic capsule sparing)

FACIAL NERVE TRAUMA (Fig. 2.14)

1. Sunderland classification
   a. First degree: neuropraxia (conduction block)
   b. Second degree: axonotmesis (axons cut, but their endoneurium stays intact; no synkinesis)
   c. Third degree: neurotmesis (endoneurium disrupted; synkinesis possible on regeneration)
   d. Fourth degree: neurotmesis transects entire trunk (endoneurium and perineurium); epineurium intact
   e. Fifth degree: neurotmesis (all three layers cut; endo-, peri-, and epineurium)

CEREBROSPINAL FLUID OTORHINORRHEA (Fig. 2.15)

1. Very rarely will traumatic CSF otorhinorrhea require surgery
2. The use of antibiotics prophylaxis for meningitis is controversial

HEARING LOSS FROM TEMPORAL BONE TRAUMA

- Ossicular injuries
  1. Incudostapedial joint separation (82%)
  2. Dislocation incus (57%)
  3. Fracture stapes crura (30%)
  4. Fixation ossicles in epitympanum (25%)
  5. Malleus fracture (11%)
- Bottom-line evaluation of temporal bone fractures
  1. Any facial function on admission? If not documented, assume there was no facial function
  2. Otorrhea? Observe and put on bed rest and conservative measures to avoid drops; can become confused with "CSF otorrhea"
  3. Dizzy/HL? Take supportive measures and observe CHL for at least 6 months because subluxations can resolve; for SNHL, can try steroids if allowable given other injuries
  4. Get a CT of temporal bones: at the very least, ensure that there are no carotid canal injuries/sphenoid sinus fluid (The latter may be more indicative of carotid injury than carotid canal fracture); if either are noted perform CT angiography (CTA) versus true angiogram.

HEARING LOSS IN ADULTS

HISTORY

1. Tinnitus
2. Vertigo
3. Disequilibrium
4. Otalgia

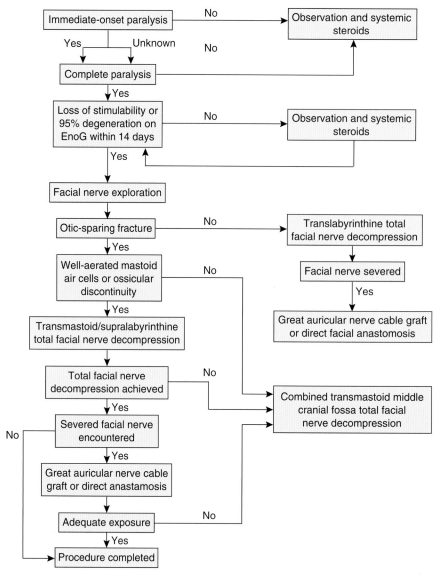

FIGURE 2.14 Management of Traumatic Facial Paralysis. Of note, some otologists may offer decompression surgery for traumatic delayed-onset, complete paralysis with >95% degeneration on ENoG and absent EMG potentials. *EnoG,* Electroneuronography. (From Flint PW, Haughey BH, Lund VJ, et al. *Cummings Otolaryngology—Head and Neck Surgery.* 6th ed. Philadelphia, PA: Saunders; 2015, fig. 145-11.)

5. Otorrhea
6. Headaches
7. Ophthalmologic symptoms
8. Neurologic complaints
9. History of surgery
10. Trauma
11. Noise exposure
12. Family history of HL/syndromes
13. Cardiovascular disorders
14. Rheumatologic disorders
15. Endocrine disorders
16. Neurologic disorders

EXAM

1. Speech
2. Gross hearing
3. Communication type
4. Auricles, ear canals, and eardrums
5. Tuning forks
   a. Weber
   b. Rinne

6. Cranial nerves
7. Remainder head and neck

POTENTIAL CAUSES

1. Genetic
   a. Too numerous to count
2. Infectious
   a. HZV (Ramsay Hunt)
   b. Measles
   c. Mumps
   d. *Cytomegalovirus* (CMV)
   e. Syphilis
   f. Rocky mountain spotted fever
   g. Lyme disease
3. Vascular
4. Neoplastic
5. Traumatic
   a. Physical trauma
   b. Noise
      i. Transient threshold shift (TTS) recovers 24-48 hours
      ii. Permanent threshold shift does not recover

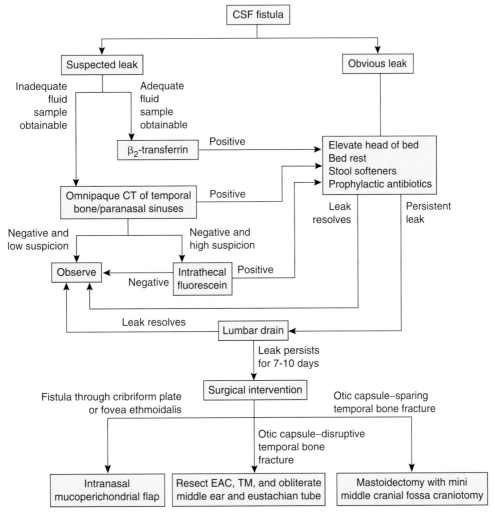

FIGURE 2.15 Management of Traumatic Cerebrospinal Fluid Fistula. *CT*, Computed tomography. (From Flint PW, Haughey BH, Lund VJ, et al. *Cummings Otolaryngology—Head and Neck Surgery.* 6th ed. Philadelphia, PA: Saunders; 2015, fig. 145-13.)

iii. The Occupational Safety and Health Act (OSHA) (noise intensity doubles every 3 dB; OSHA rounded to 5 dB)
1. 90 dB exposure 8-hour limit
2. 95 dB exposure 4-hour limit
3. 100 dB exposure 2-hour limit
4. 105 dB exposure 1-hour limit
5. 110 dB exposure 0.5-hour limit
6. Toxic
   a. Aminoglycosides
      i. Vestibulotoxicity is greater than cochleotoxicity for streptomycin and gentamicin
      ii. Cochleotoxicity is greater than vestibulotoxicity for: kanamycin, tobramycin, amikacin, neomycin, and dihydrostreptomycin
7. Iatrogenic
8. Degenerative
9. Immunologic
   a. Cogan syndrome (eye/ear disorder)
   b. Polyarteritis nodosa
   c. Relapsing polychondritis
   d. Wegener granulomatosis
   e. Scleroderma
   f. Temporal arteritis
   g. Systemic lupus erythematosus
   h. Sarcoidosis
   i. Vogt-Koyanagi-Harada
   j. Primary autoimmune inner ear disease
   k. Antibodies to 68 kDa protein in 50-70%
10. Sudden SNHL
    a. Etiology is mostly idiopathic. Thought to be either a viral or vascular insult.
    b. Must rule out retrocochlear lesion with MRI
    c. Treat with oral prednisone ASAP
    d. If fails, can offer intratympanic dexamethasone injection
    e. No advantage for antivirals in placebo controlled studies

TINNITUS

- Differentiate tinnitus versus bothersome tinnitus
- 40% comorbidity with hyperacusis
- Subjective versus objective tinnitus

Pulse Synchronous

1. Arteriovenous fistula/arteriovenous malformation
2. Paraganglioma
3. Carotid artery stenosis
4. Other atherosclerotic disease
5. Arterial dissection
6. Persistent stapedial artery
7. Intratympanic carotid artery
8. Vascular compression of VIII
9. Hypermetabolic state (pregnancy and thyrotoxicosis)

10. Intraosseous hypervascularity (Paget and otosclerosis)
11. Pseudotumor cerebri
12. Venous hum
13. Dural venous sinus abnormalities, jugular bulb high riding, and diverticulae

Pulse Asynchronous

1. Palatalmyoclonus
2. Middle ear spasm

Nonpulsatile

1. Spontaneous otoacoustic emission
2. Abnormally patulous Eustachian tube

Subjective Tinnitus Types

1. From HL (eg, noise-induced hearing loss and presbycusis)
2. Somatic tinnitus
   a. TMJ
   b. Neck disorder
   c. Gaze evoked
   d. Cutaneous evoked
3. Typewriter tinnitus
4. Fatigue induced
5. Musical/complex
6. Intrusive
7. Associated affective disorder

Treatments for Tinnitus

1. Ambient stimulation
2. Personal listening software
3. Total masking
4. Tinnitus retraining therapy (acoustic stimulation with education and counseling)
5. Acoustic sensitization protocol (neuromonics)
6. Cognitive behavioral therapy
7. Transcranial magnetic stimulation
8. Transcutaneous electrical nerve stimulation (on mastoid)
9. Electrical stimulation
10. Cochlear implantation
11. Pharmacologic (*nothing* is proven)
    a. Studies on gabapentin
    b. Sertraline

NOISE-INDUCED HEARING LOSS

Definition

1. Permanent SNHL with damage to cochlear hair cells, primarily OHCs
2. History of long-term exposure to dangerous noise levels >85 dB/sound-pressure level (SPL) for 8 hours/day on average
3. Gradual loss of hearing over the first 5-10 years of exposure
4. HL initially involves high frequencies (3-8 kHz)
5. Speech-recognition scores consistent with audiometric loss
6. HL stabilizes after noise exposure is terminated

Random Noise-Induced Hearing Loss Facts

- 3 or 4 kHz notch a result of resonant frequency EAC
- TTS: causes buckling of pillar cells (24-48 hours)
- Medial olivocochlear bundle and OHCs may have protective effect by "conditioning" cochlea to noise exposure and changes of basilar membrane stiffness

INFECTIONS OF THE LABYRINTH

CONGENITAL VIRAL

1. CMV: #1 nongenetic cause of HL
2. Rubella: worldwide important cause
3. Herpes simplex virus

CONGENITAL NONVIRAL

1. Syphilis
2. Toxoplasmosis

ACQUIRED LABYRINTHINE INFECTIONS

1. Mumps
2. Measles
3. Syphilis
4. Bacterial meningogenic labyrinthine infections
5. Cryptococcal
6. Varicella zoster
7. No strong correlation with other viral meningitis

OTOTOXIC AND VESTIBULOTOXIC MEDICATIONS

1. Aminoglycosides (likely from reactive oxygen species injuring the outer hair cells)
2. Cisplatin (likely from reactive oxygen species injuring the stria vascularis and the outer hair cells)
3. Carboplatin (less ototoxic compared with cisplatinum)
4. Difluoromethylornithine (antitumor agent and used to treat West African sleeping sickness)
5. Loop diuretics (affects the stria vascularis)
   a. Lasix
   b. Ethacrynic acid
   c. Less so bumetanide
   d. Less so torsemide
6. Macrolides
   a. Erythromycin: possibly reversible
   b. Azithromycin: likely reversible
7. Desferoxamine: possibly reversible SNHL and a chelating agent
8. Hydrocodone: from mostly abuse/recreational use
   a. Rapidly progressive, bilateral
   b. Not responsive to corticosteroids
   c. Cochlear implants work and typically help
9. Methadone: possibly reversible, according to case report(s)
10. Vancomycin: questionable ototoxicity
11. Quinines: possibly permanent, but has a reversible component
12. Acetylsalicylic acid: typically reversible, and it affects the motor protein prestin in OHCs

CENTRAL NEURAL AUDITORY PROSTHESES

AUDITORY BRAINSTEM IMPLANT

- Two manufacturers
  1. Cochlear auditory brainstem implant (ABI) (approved in the United States)
  2. Med-El ABI (not approved in the United States)
- Two indications
  1. Neurofibromatosis II (NF2) (only indication in the United States): does not do as well with ABI as indication #2 does
  2. Cannot perform a cochlear implant (Michel deformity, cochlear nerve agenesis, and ossified cochlea): not yet an indication in the United States
- Two types
  1. Surface paddle electrode on the cochlear nucleus
  2. Penetrating ABI (theoretically should be better, but is not better than surface)
- Two approaches
  1. Translabyrinthine (especially when removing a vestibular schwannoma)
  2. Retrosigmoid

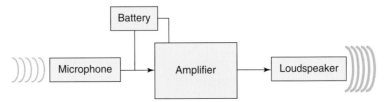

FIGURE 2.16 Schematic Representation of the Components of a Hearing Aid. (From Flint PW, Haughey BH, Lund VJ, et al. *Cummings Otolaryngology—Head and Neck Surgery.* 6th ed. Philadelphia, PA: Saunders; 2015, fig. 162-3.)

AUDITORY MIDBRAIN IMPLANT

1. Stimulates the inferior colliculus

HEARING AID AMPLIFICATION

TYPES

1. BTE: behind the ear
2. ITE: in the ear
3. ITC: in the canal
4. CIC: completely in the canal

COMPONENTS (Fig. 2.16)

The basic components of hearing aids are a microphone, a transducer, an amplifier and a speaker. All hearing aids now are digital.

Transducers (Convert One Form of Energy into Electrical Energy)

1. Microphone (most common, acoustic to electrical)
2. Telecoil (t-coil, electromagnetic energy to electrical)
3. Wireless transducer (eg, frequency modulation or Bluetooth)

TERMINOLOGY

1. Gain: the amount of energy added to the input signal
2. Linear gain (Fig. 2.17)
3. *Compressed*, nonlinear gain (Fig. 2.18)
4. Dynamic range: an individual's threshold of sound perception to discomfort
   a. Compression allows a hearing aid to amplify into a smaller dynamic range (Fig. 2.19)

OTHER IMPORTANT HEARING AID TERMS

1. Feedback: speaker output ⇒ microphone leads to this. Separating them helps.
   a. BTE: better physical separation
   b. Venting ITE, ITC, and CIC increases likelihood but decreases occlusion
   c. Better software limits feedback
   d. Receiver in the canal or *RIC*: the receiver, or speaker, is placed in the ear canal for BTE hearing aids and provides sharper sounds and separation from the microphone to reduce feedback
2. Occlusion (helped by venting)
   a. Reduction of natural acoustic energy by the aid plugging the ear
   b. Resonance of lower frequencies is worsened

APPLIED VESTIBULAR PHYSIOLOGY

1. The vestibular system has basal firing rates from the end organs on both sides
   a. Irritative lesion increases firing rates (Meniere in 30%, early labyrinthitis)

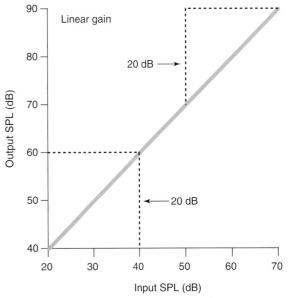

FIGURE 2.17 The relationship of sound input to output in a linear hearing aid circuit. Gain remains at a constant 20 dB regardless of input level. (From Flint PW, Haughey BH, Lund VJ, et al. *Cummings Otolaryngology—Head and Neck Surgery.* 6th ed. Philadelphia, PA: Saunders; 2015, fig. 162-4.)

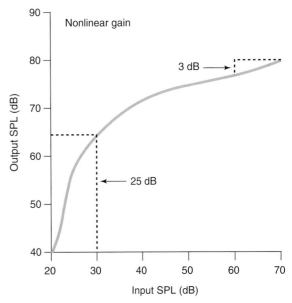

FIGURE 2.18 The relationship of sound input to output in a nonlinear hearing aid circuit. The amount of gain changes as a function of input level. (From Flint PW, Haughey BH, Lund VJ, et al. *Cummings Otolaryngology—Head and Neck Surgery.* 6th ed. Philadelphia, PA: Saunders; 2015, fig. 162-5.)

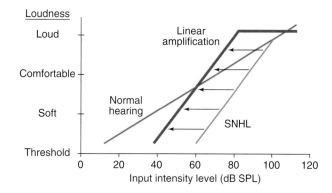

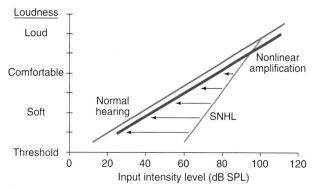

FIGURE 2.19 Representation of the difference between linear and nonlinear amplification in an ear with SNHL and nonlinear loudness growth. (From Stach B. *Clinical Audiology: An Introduction.* San Diego, CA: Singular Publishing; 1998:486 and Flint PW, Haughey BH, Lund VJ, et al. *Cummings Otolaryngology—Head and Neck Surgery.* 6th ed. Philadelphia, PA: Saunders; 2015, fig. 162-6.)

    b. Destructive lesion decreases firing rates
    c. Unequal firing rates due to a peripheral lesion causes the sensation of movement toward the side with relatively higher firing rate

EWALD'S LAWS

1. A stimulation of the semicircular canal causes a movement of the eyes in the plane of the stimulated canal (*relative to the head, not the orbit!*)
    a. A semicircular canal is excited by head rotation about the axis of that canal that brings the forehead toward the ipsilateral side
2. In the horizontal semicircular canals, an ampullopetal endolymph movement causes a greater stimulation than an ampullofugal one does (ampullofugal actually suppresses from the baseline firing rate); acceleration to excitation of the ipsilateral canal is stronger than inhibition is
3. In the vertical (superior and posterior canals) semicircular canals, the reverse is true; the difference between rule 2 and 3 is due to the orientation of the ampullae themselves; turning your head to the right leads to ampullopetal flow, and turning your head down to the right (stimulating the right superior canal) leads to ampullofugal flow

OTHER KEY POINTS

1. Central vestibular nuclei store velocity info (nystagmus from rotation will continue after the endolymph and cupula reach the same speed and the cupula is no longer deflected)
    a. Damage to peripheral vestibular input weakens the storage system

2. Alexander's law: nystagmus from a *peripheral* vestibular lesion is worsened with gaze in the direction of the fast phase.
3. Compensation
    a. Brain increases firing rate on lesioned side acutely
    b. Fine tuning of firing rate under stress (head movement) occurs over time and with activity

EVALUATION OF THE PATIENT WITH DIZZINESS (Fig. 2.20)

HISTORY

1. Onset of dizziness?
2. Vertigo (spinning or nautical), lightheadedness, or "foggy sensation"?
3. Episodic or continuous
    a. Length of episodes
    b. Remitting and exacerbating factors
4. Lifestyle (stress, sleep, and diet)
5. Environment (pressure changes, lights, and noise-induced)
6. Headache?
7. Head trauma?
8. HL?
9. Accompanying symptoms (with episodic dizziness)?

EXAM

1. Otoscopy with insufflation (check for fistula)
2. Cranial nerves, especially extraocular muscle
3. Remaining head and neck
4. Tuning forks (CHL or pseudoconductive in third windows): check tuning fork on medial malleolus for sickle cell disease
5. Cerebellar function (finger to nose, rapid alternating movements, heal/shin tests
6. Head thrust (check vestibulo-ocular reflex [VOR])
7. Romberg, tandem
8. Fukuda step test
9. Hallpike

ANCILLARY TESTING

1. Audiogram asymmetric HL, pseudoconductive loss, and reflexes?
2. Video goggles (videonystagmography)
    a. Spontaneous nystagmus
    b. Gaze nystagmus
    c. Saccades
    d. Smooth pursuit
    e. Optokinetic nystagmus
    f. Positional
        i. Hallpike
        ii. Lateral head, center
        iii. Lateral body
    g. Caloric (lateral canal/superior vestibular nerve test only)
    h. Fistula test with pressure
3. Video head impulse testing
    a. Ability to test gain of each individual canal
4. Rotary chair
    a. VOR: phase, gain, and symmetry
    b. Visual fixation test: ability to suppress VOR
    c. Visually enhanced vestibular-ocular reflex: enhanced VOR by including optokinetic nystagmus
5. cVEMP: acoustic sound → saccule → inferior vestibular nerve → spinal accessory, ipsilateral → relaxation of ipsilateral SCM
6. oVEMP: acoustic sound or bone oscillation → utricular stimulation → superior vestibular nerve → contralateral oculomotor nucleus → contralateral inferior oblique stimulation

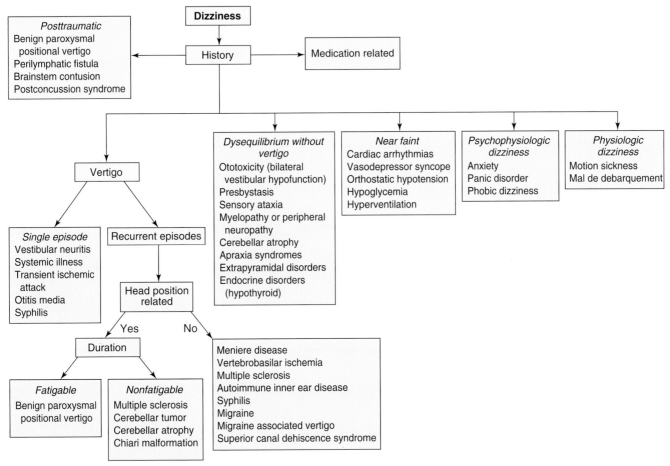

FIGURE 2.20 Algorithm for the differential diagnosis of dizziness based on information from the patient's history. (Modified from Baloh RW, Fife TD, Furman JM, Zee DS. The approach to the patient with dizziness. In Mancall EL, ed. *Continuum: Lifelong Learning in Neurology.* Cleveland, OH: Advanstar Communication; 1996:25-36 and Flint PW, Haughey BH, Lund VJ, et al. *Cummings Otolaryngology—Head and Neck Surgery.* 6th ed. Philadelphia, PA: Saunders; 2015, fig. 164-4.)

7. Posturography: measures interaction of vision, proprioception, and vestibular systems for balance
   a. Helps identify malingerers

PERIPHERAL VESTIBULAR DISORDERS

1. Benign paroxysmal positional vertigo (BPPV)
   a. Posterior canal most 85-90%
      i. Canalithiasis: Rx, Epley/Brandt Daroff
      ii. Cupulolithiasis: Rx, possibly Semont liberatory maneuver
   b. Lateral canal second most common
      i. Canalothiasis: geotropic nystagmus; Rx, logroll
      ii. Cupulothiasis: ageotropic nystagmus; Rx is not well determined
   c. Superior canal: very uncommon; can have pure downbeat nystagmus; Rx, deep head hang
2. Meniere disease
   a. Low-salt diet and diuretics
   b. Vasodilators (Betahistine)
   c. Low intermittent pressure therapy to affected ear
   d. Transtympanic steroids
   e. Transtympanic gentamicin
   f. Oral steroids for exacerbations
   g. Supportive care for acute attacks
3. Vestibular neuronitis: Rx, supportive care, possibly steroids early in onset, vestibular exercises, or therapy to speed up compensation

4. Superior canal dehiscence syndrome
   a. Dehiscence of the superior canal along the floor of the middle cranial fossa creates a 'third window affect'
   b. *Hennebert's sign*- pressure induced vertigo caused by straining or external pressure applied on examination
   c. *Tullio's phenomenon*- sound induced vertigo
   d. Diagnose by history, CT of temporal bones, low frequency mild conductive hearing loss, VEMP (increase amplitude and decreased thresholds)
   e. Treat with surgery (see below)
5. Perilymphatic fistula: Rx, fistula repair for dizziness that does not respond to bed rest and conservative measures
6. Cogan's: Rx, steroids and immunosuppressants
7. Otosyphilis: Rx, antibiotics (penicillin) and corticosteroids
8. Labyrinthine concussion: Rx, supportive care
9. Enlarged vestibular aqueduct: Rx, supportive care for attacks
10. Familial vestibulopathy autosomal dominant, migraine headaches: Rx, acetazolamide and supportive care
11. Bilateral vestibulopathy (Dandy/oscillopsia): Rx, vestibular therapy; substitution exercises

CENTRAL VESTIBULAR DISORDERS

1. Vestibular migraine
   a. Comorbid with
      i. Meniere disease
      ii. BPPV
      iii. Anxiety

b. Treatment
  i. Diet changes, stress modification, and sleep hygiene
  ii. Tricyclic antidepressants
    (1) Amitryptiline
    (2) Nortryptiline
  iii. Calcium channel blockers
    (1) Verapamil
  iv. Antiseizure medications
    (1) Topiramate
    (2) Gabapentin
  v. Beta blockers
    (1) Propranolol
    (2) Atenolol (off label)
  vi. Other antidepressants
    (1) Venlafaxine
  vii. Supportive measures for acute attacks
c. Benign paroxysmal vertigo of childhood likely a migraine equivalent
2. Chronic subjective dizziness
  a. Treatment with selective serotonin reuptake inhibitors
3. Vertebrobasilar insufficiency; likely has other neurologic findings
  a. HINTS test: *h*ead *i*mpulse *n*ystagmus, *t*est of *s*kew
    i. Head impulse usually normal if central
    ii. Nystagmus vertical, direction changing, purely torsional, and/or independent of gaze direction if central
    iii. Skew deviation/abnormal vertical smooth pursuit is central
  b. Lateral medullary syndrome (Wallenberg) (ipsilateral vertebral artery, rarely posterior inferior cerebellar artery occlusion)
  c. Lateral pontomedullary syndrome (anterior inferior cerebellar artery occlusion and, therefore, labyrinthine artery occlusion)
  d. Cerebellar infarction
  e. Nodular infarction (central paroxysmal positional vertigo)
    i. Short latency nystagmus, atypical direction, no fatigability, and no response to Epley
  f. Cerebellar hemorrhage: emergency!
  g. Vertebral artery dissection
4. Tumors of posterior fossa
5. Cervical vertigo: controversial. Rx, neck PT
6. Disorders of the craniovertebral junction
  a. Basilar impression (clivus compresses medulla)
  b. Assimilation of the atlas
  c. Atlantoaxial dislocation
  d. Chiari malformation
    i. Upper-extremity weakness, sensory loss, and pain
    ii. Occipital headaches with straining
    iii. Ataxia and nystagmus
    iv. Lower cranial nerve dysfunction
7. Multiple sclerosis
8. Cerebellar ataxia syndromes
  a. Friedreich (#1), autosomal recessive
  b. Spinocerebellar atrophy
  c. Cerebellar atrophy
  d. Familial episodic ataxia (Rx, acetazolamide)
  e. Paraneoplastic cerebellar degeneration
    i. Anti-Purkinje cell antibodies: small cell cancer lung, breast, ovary, and Hodgkin
9. Focal seizures
10. Normal pressure hydrocephalus
  a. Dementia, gait disturbance, and urinary incontinence
  b. Rx: shunt
11. Motion intolerance
12. Mal de Debarquement syndrome

SURGERY FOR VERTIGO

1. BPPV treatment
  a. Singular neurectomy (rarely done)
  b. Posterior canal occlusion
2. Superior canal dehiscence
  a. Middle fossa plugging or resurfacing
  b. Transmastoid plugging or resurfacing
  c. Round window reinforcement (controversial)
3. Perilymphatic fistula
  a. Support oval and round windows with tissue (not loose, areolar tissue)
4. Meniere disease
  a. Nonablative
    i. Middle ear tenotomy (cut tendons in the middle ear; allow lateral expansion of the oval window; done in Europe)
    ii. Endolymphatic sac surgery
      (1) Decompression
      (2) Shunting (endolymphatic to mastoid)
      (3) Duct plugging (a relatively new procedure)
  b. Ablative
    i. Cochleosacculotomy (can be done under local anesthetic, utilized in older patients who can't tolerate general anesthesia)
      (1) 3-mm hook into the round window toward the oval window
    ii. Labyrinthectomy (sacrifice hearing)
      (1) Transcanal: increased possibility of leaving behind neuroepithelium
      (2) Transmastoid: greater exposure of five organs (saccule, utricle, and ampullae of superior, lateral, and posterior canal)
        (a) Failure possibly because of traumatic neuromas of vestibular nerve branches
        (b) Posterior canal ampulla is most commonly left behind because the facial nerve is located lateral to it
    iii. Vestibular nerve section
      (1) Retrolabyrinthine
      (2) Retrosigmoid
      (3) Middle fossa
      (4) Translabyrinthine

VESTIBULAR REHABILITATION THERAPY

- Peripheral vestibular insult leads to static compensation (central response to decreased asymmetric vestibular input) followed by dynamic compensation (compensates for asymmetric responses with head movement)
- How dynamic compensation occurs (best to have a static insult to the vestibular system):
  1. Adaptation: central neuronal compensation for insult to the vestibular system
  2. Habituation: repeated maneuvers to decrease noxious response/symptoms from maneuvers
  3. Sensory substitution: use of vision and proprioception to compensate for a decrease in vestibular function
- Other terms
  1. Gait exercises: improve ambulation
  2. Canalith repositioning (for BPPV)
  3. General conditioning: improve fitness overall and decrease fatigability
  4. Maintenance: maintain gains in posture and gait stability

TESTS OF FACIAL NERVE FUNCTION
(Fig. 2.21; Table 2.3)

TOPODIAGNOSTIC TESTS (HISTORICAL VALUE ONLY)

1. Schirmer test
2. Taste test
3. Salivary pH
4. Salivary flow (via the submandibular gland)
5. Acoustic reflex

ELECTROPHYSIOLOGIC TESTS

1. Nerve excitability test: thresholds for facial nerve stimulation at the stylomastoid foramen are compared (normal to abnormal)
2. Maximal stimulation test: test unaffected side for threshold that stimulates the facial nerve maximally, apply that stimulus level to the affected side, and measure percent response

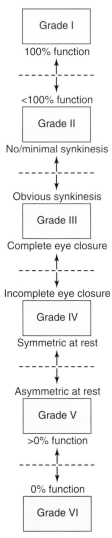

FIGURE 2.21 Schematic diagram of a modified House-Brackmann grading scale using the major functional criteria of absolute movement, synkinesis, eye closure, asymmetry at rest, and absolute paralysis in assigning unambiguous and nonoverlapping degrees of facial paralysis. (From Flint PW, Haughey BH, Lund VJ, et al. *Cummings Otolaryngology—Head and Neck Surgery.* 6th ed. Philadelphia, PA: Saunders; 2015, fig. 169-1.)

3. Electroneurography (evoked electromyography [EMG]): uses surface electrodes maximally to stimulate both sides and measure resulting EMG bilaterally; compare percentage of response as a percentage (affected/unaffected); best between 3 and 21 days (Wallerian degeneration needs to occur because stimulation is at the stylomastoid foramen, distal to the site of injury in the temporal bone; at more than 21 days, dyssynchrony may occur, and therefore degeneration may be overestimated)
4. EMG is useful for prognosis
    a. Best after 14 days
    b. Fibrillation potentials: degeneration
    c. Polyphasic potentials: nerve regrowth
    d. Determination of return of nerve function months after insult to nerve is useful in deciding on transposition surgery

CLINICAL DISORDERS OF THE FACIAL NERVE

ACUTE FACIAL PALSY (Fig. 2.22)

1. Bell palsy: "idiopathic" but likely secondary to herpes simplex viral activation 85% regeneration to HB 1-2
2. Herpes Zoster (Ramsay Hunt): worse prognosis (70% regeneration to HB 1-2); typically not decompressed; treat with steroids and antivirals
3. Guillain-Barré
4. Autoimmune
5. Lyme (especially if bilateral, bilateral 10%)
6. Human immunodeficiency virus
7. Sarcoidosis
8. Melkersson-Rosenthal
9. Kawasaki
10. Trauma
11. OM, acute or chronic
12. Cerebrovascular disorders

CHRONIC FACIAL PALSY

1. Neoplasm: parotid, temporal bone, cutaneous/facial, CPA, and brainstem
2. Cholesteatoma

CONGENITAL PALSY

1. Mobius: bilateral sixth and seventh nerve palsy
2. CULLP: congenital unilateral lower-lip paralysis
3. Oculoauriculovertebral
4. Mononeural agenesis
5. Hemifacial microsomia
6. Teratogens: thalidomide and rubella
7. CHARGE syndrome
8. Poland syndrome: agenesis of pectoralis major muscle

OTHER NOTABLE TYPE OF FACIAL PARALYSIS

1. Familial
2. Recurrent (check for tumor)
3. Bilateral: lumbar puncture, lyme titer, complete blood count, fluorescent treponemal antibody, and MRI for workup

LATERAL SKULL-BASE SURGERY

MOST COMMONS

1. Temporal bone tumor: paraganglioma
2. Adult temporal bone malignancy: squamous cell carcinoma
3. Childhood temporal bone malignancy: rhabdomyosarcoma

Table 2.3   House-Brackmann Facial Nerve Grading System

Grade	Description	Characteristics
I	Normal	Normal facial function in all areas
II	Mild dysfunction	Gross: slight weakness noticeable on close inspection; may have very slight synkinesis At rest: normal symmetry and tone Forehead motion: Moderate to good function Eye motion: complete closure with minimum effort Mouth motion: slight asymmetry
III	Moderate dysfunction	Gross: obvious but not disfiguring difference between two sides; noticeable but not severe synkinesis, contracture, or hemifacial spasm At rest: normal symmetry and tone Forehead motion: slight to moderate movement Eye motion: complete closure with effort Mouth motion: slightly weak with maximum effort
IV	Moderately severe dysfunction	Gross: obvious weakness and/or disfiguring asymmetry At rest: normal symmetry and tone Forehead motion: none Eye motion: incomplete closure Mouth motion: asymmetric with maximum effort
V	Severe dysfunction	Gross: only barely perceptible motion At rest: asymmetry Forehead motion: none Eye motion: incomplete closure Mouth motion: slight movement
VI	Total paralysis	No movement

From Flint PW, Haughey BH, Lund VJ, et al. *Cummings Otolaryngology—Head and Neck Surgery*. 6th ed. Philadelphia, PA: Saunders; 2015, table 169-1.

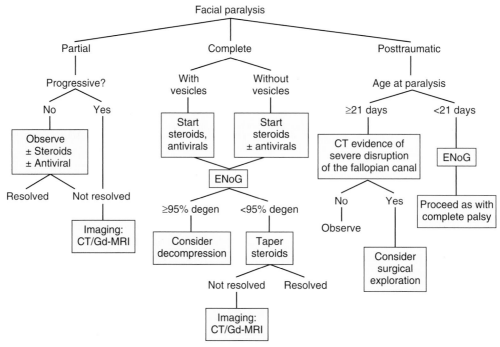

FIGURE 2.22 Management Algorithm for Facial Paralysis. *degen*, Degeneration; *Gd*, gadolinium enhanced. (Modified from Flint PW, Haughey BH, Lund VJ, et al. *Cummings Otolaryngology—Head and Neck Surgery*. 6th ed. Philadelphia, PA: Saunders; 2015, fig. 170-1.)

MORE ENTITIES LISTS

1. Primary benign
   a. Paraganglioma
   b. Meningioma
   c. Schwannoma/neurofibroma
   d. Adnexal tumors
      i. Ceruminous adenoma
      ii. Eccrine cylindroma
      iii. Pleomorphic adenoma
2. Mesenchymal neoplasms

   a. Chondroma
   b. Chondroblastoma
   c. Chondromyxoid fibroma
   d. Lipoma
   e. Myxoma
   f. Fibro-osseous lesions
      i. Fibrous dysplasia
      ii. Ossifying fibroma
   g. Giant cell granuloma
   h. Aneurysmal bone cyst
   i. Osteoblastoma

j. Osteoma/exostosis
k. Unicameral bone cyst
l. Teratoma
3. Dysontogenic tissue
   a. Choristoma
   b. Inverting papilloma
   c. Glioma
4. Metastatic disease
   a. Prostate
   b. Breast
   c. Lung
   d. Gastrointestinal
   e. Renal cell
   f. Myeloma
   g. Lymphoma
   h. Leukemia (granulocytic sarcoma/chloroma)
5. Primary malignant tumor
   a. Epidermal
      i. Squamous cell carcinoma
      ii. Verrucous carcinoma
      iii. Basal cell carcinoma
      iv. Melanoma
      v. Ceruminous adenocarcinoma
      vi. Adenoid cystic
      vii. Mucoepidermoic carcinoma
      viii. Sebaceous cell carcinoma
      ix. Papillary cystadenocarcinoma (endolymphatic sac tumor)
   b. Mesenchymal malignancies
      i. Rhabdomyosarcoma
      ii. Fibrosarcoma
      iii. Osteosarcoma
      iv. Chondrosarcoma
      v. Liposarcoma
      vi. Dermatofibrosarcoma protuberans
      vii. Fibrohistiosarcoma
      viii. Angiosarcoma
      ix. Osteoclastoma
      x. Chordoma
      xi. Plasmacytoma (extramedullary, solitary)
   c. Contiguous tumor invasion
      i. Neuroma
      ii. Glioma
      iii. Meningioma
      iv. Choroid plexus papilloma
      v. Primary parotid malignancy
      vi. Primary cutaneous malignancy
      vii. Pituitary
      viii. Craniopharyngioma
      ix. Nasopharyngeal carcinoma
6. Idiopathic
   a. Langerhans Cell Histiocytosis
   b. Inflammatory myofibroblastic tumor

QUANTITATIVE CEREBRAL BLOOD-FLOW ANALYSIS

1. Xenon CT (most studied)
2. Positron emission tomography
3. MRI perfusion study
4. Cerebral perfusion CT

APPROACHES TO THE INTERNAL AUDITORY CANAL AND CEREBELLOPONTINE ANGLE TUMORS

1. Middle fossa craniotomy
   a. Utilized for IAC tumors with minimal CPA extension, age <65yrs and serviceable hearing (PTA <50 and SDS>50%)

2. Translabyrinthine craniotomy
   a. Utilized when hearing is not serviceable, or large CPA tumors where hearing preservation is less likely
3. Suboccipital/Retrosigmoid craniotomy
   a. Utilized when hearing is serviceable and the tumor is primarily in the CPA with minimal IAC extension
4. Far lateral craniotomy
   a. Utilized for tumors that extend inferiorly to the foramen magnum

SKULL-BASE APPROACHES

The carotid artery is always an important consideration (Fig. 2.23).

Temporal bone resections: Definitions may vary!

Algorithm for EAC carcinoma (Fig. 2.24): sleeve resection is controversial

1. Lateral temporal bone resection (primary tumor in the ear canal without involvement of the mucosa in the middle ear and mastoid)
   a. With or without a parotidectomy
   b. With or without neck dissection
   c. If postoperative radiation therapy is required: do not leave an open cavity; obliterate with vascular tissue (temporalis flap)
2. Subtotal temporal bone resection (for mucosal extension, perform a labyrinthectomy, using middle and posterior fossa bony plates as margins, removing the cochlea and skeletonizing the petrous carotid)
   a. Neck dissection with or without a parotidectomy
   b. With or without facial nerve rerouting or sacrifice
3. Total temporal bone resection (rarely indicated, involves carotid artery sacrifice)

INFRATEMPORAL FOSSA APPROACHES (FOR PARAGANGLIOMA)

1. Transcanal: for glomus tympanicum in the mesotympanum not beyond the annulus
2. Mastoid extended facial recess: glomus tympanicum beyond the annulus
3. Mastoid/extended facial recess/neck: glomus tumor with extension into the jugular bulb; extracranial and not involving the carotid artery (leaves ear canal intact); identify internal carotid artery (ICA) jugular vein, CN 9-12 in neck; with or without "fallopian bridge"
4. Fisch A: glomus jugulare in the middle ear, jugular bulb (same as #3 except for the closed-off ear canal; *classically* reroute facial nerve out of the descending fallopian bridge = facial weakness because of devascularization; sigmoid is packed off proximally, and the jugular vein is taken inferiorly; jugular bulb is removed with the tumor, off of the vertical carotid if necessary; the Eustachian tube, middle ear, mastoid are obliterated)
   a. With or without fallopian bridge
   b. With or without drilling out the inner ear
   c. With or without temporal craniotomy to better isolate the middle fossa floor/skull base
   d. Bleeding along the medial wall of the jugular vein via the inferior petrosal sinus and condylar vein
   e. Lower cranial nerves through the pars nervosa along the medial wall of the jugular bulb
   f. Can also get out through the intracranial extension with ligation of the sigmoid and dural opening
5. Fisch B: same as #4, but for more anterior lesions typically (subtemporal region); *classically*, does not require transposition of the facial nerve. Add detachment of the zygomatic arch and temporalis origin with reflection downward,

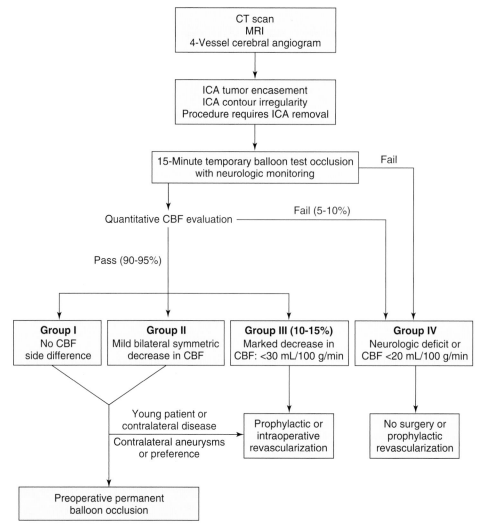

FIGURE 2.23 Algorithm for Preoperative Internal Carotid Artery/Cerebral Blood Flow Evaluation. (From Flint PW, Haughey BH, Lund VJ, et al. *Cummings Otolaryngology—Head and Neck Surgery*. 6th ed. Philadelphia, PA: Saunders; 2015, fig. 176-1.)

as well as downward displacement of the condyle; also typically includes downward reflection of the skull-base periosteum
   a. With or without skeletonizing the horizontal carotid and possible transposition
   b. With or without drilling away the middle cranial fossa floor
   c. With or without sacrificing the middle meningeal and transection of V3 at the foramen ovale
6. Fisch C: same as #5, but for further anterior exposure to the nasopharynx, sphenoid sinus, pterygoids, and posterior maxillary sinus
7. Fisch D: preauricular infratemporal fossa; middle ear and ear canal are not entered; the Eustachian tube is obliterated (serous OM); the condyle is resected; typically, the temporalis and zygomatic arch are swung inferiorly

APPROACHES TO THE JUGULAR FORAMEN

1. Retrosigmoid craniotomy (no sacrifice of hearing or venous drainage)
2. Petrooccipital transsigmoid (sacrifices the sigmoid sinus, presumably for already occluded drainage): retrolabyrinthine and retrosigmoid craniotomy with opening of the posterior fossa dura across the sigmoid with skeletonizing facial nerve; posteriorly based, and therefore can work medially to facial nerve. Does not provide good exposure of the ICA; is better suited for jugular foramen schwannomas and meningiomas
3. Fisch type A approach: more laterally based; it involves working around or transposing the facial nerve; provides better exposure of the ICA; better suited for glomus tumors

FISCH CLASSIFICATION OF GLOMUS TUMORS

- Type A tumor: tumor limited to the middle ear cleft (glomus tympanicum)
- Type B tumor: tumor limited to the tympanomastoid area with no infralabyrinthine compartment involvement
- Type C tumor: tumor involving the infralabyrinthine compartment of the temporal bone and extending into the petrous apex
  - Type C1 tumor: with limited involvement of the vertical portion of the carotid canal
  - Type C2 tumor: invading the vertical portion of the carotid canal
  - Type C3 tumor: invasion of the horizontal portion of the carotid canal

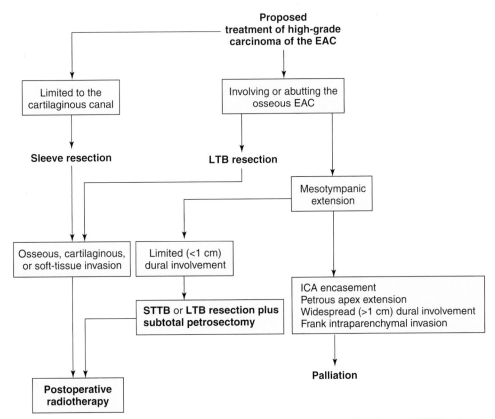

FIGURE 2.24 Algorithm for management of high-grade malignancies of the external auditory canal (EAC) and temporal bone. *ICA*, Internal carotid artery; *LTB*, lateral temporal bone; *STTB*, subtotal temporal bone. (From Flint PW, Haughey BH, Lund VJ, et al. *Cummings Otolaryngology—Head and Neck Surgery.* 6th ed. Philadelphia, PA: Saunders; 2015, fig. 176-25.)

- Type D1 tumor: with an intracranial extension <2 cm in diameter
- Type D2 tumor: with an intracranial extension >2 cm in diameter

STAGING TUMORS OF THE EXTERNAL AUDITORY CANAL (PITTSBURGH SYSTEM)

T Status
- T_1: tumor limited to the EAC without bony erosion or evidence of soft-tissue extension
- T_2: tumor with limited EAC bony erosion (not full thickness) or radiographic finding consistent with limited (<0.5 cm) soft-tissue involvement
- T_3: tumor erodes the osseous EAC (full thickness) with limited (<0.5 cm) soft-tissue involvement or tumor involves the middle ear or mastoid
- T_4: tumor erodes the cochlea, petrous apex, medial wall of the middle ear, carotid canal, jugular foramen, or dura or shows extensive (>0.5 cm) soft-tissue involvement or evidence of facial paralysis

Nodal Status
Involvement of lymph nodes is a poor prognostic finding and automatically places the patient in an advanced stage (ie, stage III [T_1, N_1] or stage IV [T_2, T_3, and $T_4 N_1$] disease).

Metastatic Status
Distant metastasis indicates a poor prognosis and immediately places the patient in the stage IV category.

STEREOTACTIC RADIATION FOR BENIGN SKULL-BASE LESIONS

Goal: devascularize the tumor and decrease growth; *control rates 74-100%* (typically at least 90%) and studies have variable follow-up

DEFINITIONS

1. Stereotactic radiation: image-guided focus of radiation therapy with high precision to a lesion and a minimal dose to the adjacent tissues
2. Stereotactic radiosurgery: not surgery but rather stereotactically applied radiation in one to five shots
3. Fractionated stereotactic radiation (FSR): as its name implies; goal is to fractionate to allow normal tissue recovery and possibly improve hearing preservation

MODALITIES

1. Gamma knife: typical "radiosurgical tool" (201 cobalt-60 sources pointing to center of the tumor; a rigid frame is applied to the patient's head and adjusted to keep the center of the sphere aimed at the tumor)
2. Requires brief anesthetic to pin the frame into the head (rigid frame likely increases accuracy/precision)
3. 50% Isodose levels currently 14 Gy: has been lowered (typically 12.5 Gy) to decrease the complication rate (below), and likely will lose some degree of tumor control in doing so

4. Linear accelerator based can be used for FSR or radiosurgery
5. Mask is applied to the patient; radiation source is moved in arcs around the patient
6. More comfortable in general, but may lose accuracy

COMPLICATIONS

1. Hearing loss
2. Worse vestibulopathy
3. Facial weakness
4. Trigeminal weakness
5. Hydrocephalus
6. Malignant transformation of tumor (1/1000)
7. Failure of control may make surgical salvage more difficult

Facial Plastic and Reconstructive Surgery

EVALUATION

HISTORY QUESTIONS FOR ALL PATIENTS

1. Motivations
2. Expectations
3. Sun exposure
4. Skin cancer
5. Radiation
6. Previous facial procedures (surgery, resurfacing, and injections)
7. Facial trauma
8. Poor wound healing, hypertrophic scarring or keloid formation
9. Connective tissue disorder
10. Bleeding or easy bruising/anticoagulant use
11. Vitamin or herbal supplement use
12. Tobacco, alcohol, or recreational drug use

HISTORY QUESTIONS FOR FACIAL RESURFACING

1. Topical medications
2. Isotretinoin use in last 12 months
3. Cold sores

HISTORY QUESTIONS FOR BLEPHAROPLASTY

1. Periorbital trauma or surgery
2. Xerophthalmia
3. Ocular disorders or visual acuity/field deficits
4. Grave's disease

HISTORY QUESTIONS FOR NASAL SURGERY

1. Nasal trauma or surgery: use of auricular/costal cartilage or implant
2. Nasal sprays
3. Effect of Breathe Right strips or nose cones
4. Fixed vs variable obstruction

HISTORY QUESTIONS FOR TRAUMA PATIENTS

1. Mechanism of injury
2. Other injuries, especially cervical spine
3. Loss of consciousness
4. Neurological symptoms, vision, and hearing
5. Rhinorrhea or salty taste in the mouth
6. Occlusion and loose or missing teeth

FACIAL ANALYSIS

1. Quality of photographs
2. Skin assessment
3. Frontal view
   - Overall symmetry
   - Brow-tip aesthetic line (also assessed in 3/4 view)
   - Facial fifths (Fig. 3.1)
   - Facial thirds (Fig. 3.2)
4. Lateral view
   - Nasofrontal angle
   - Nasion position
   - Straightness of dorsum
   - Nasal length
   - Nasal projection
   - Nasal rotation
   - Columella-alar relationship
   - Nasolabial angle
   - Chin positioning
5. Base view
   - Base shape
   - Tip bulbosity
   - Base width
   - Columella-lobule ratio

PHOTOGRAPH CHARACTERISTICS

1. Intensity and symmetry of lighting
2. Focus
3. Exposure
4. Orientation in the Frankfort horizontal plane: line from the porion/superiormost aspect of the external auditory canal to the orbitale/inferiormost aspect of the orbital rim should be parallel to the floor

FACIAL FIFTHS

- Horizontal width of the face divided evenly into five vertical segments, each the width of one eye
- Helix to lateral canthus, lateral canthus to medial canthus, medial canthus to medial canthus, medial canthus to lateral canthus, and lateral canthus to helix

FACIAL THIRDS

- Vertical height of the face divided evenly into three horizontal segments
- Trichion (midpoint of the frontal hairline) to the glabella (midpoint between the brows), glabella to the subnasale (point where the nasal septum and upper lip meet), and subnasale to the menton (inferiormost point of chin)

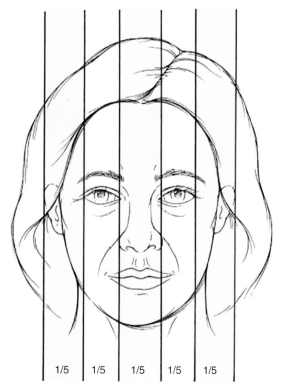

FIGURE 3.1 Facial Fifths. (From Flint PW, Haughey BH, Lund VJ, et al. *Cummings Otolaryngology—Head and Neck Surgery*. 6th ed. Philadelphia, PA: Saunders; 2015, fig. 19-7.)

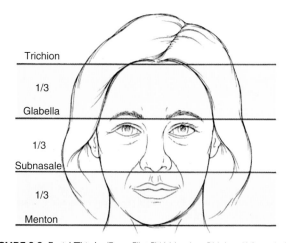

FIGURE 3.2 Facial Thirds. (From Flint PW, Haughey BH, Lund VJ, et al. *Cummings Otolaryngology—Head and Neck Surgery*. 6th ed. Philadelphia, PA: Saunders; 2015, fig. 19-8.)

- When measured from the nasion (frontonasal suture) to subnasale, midface should account for 43% of height when compared to 57% for lower face

AESTHETIC UNITS OF THE FACE

1. Forehead
2. Eyes
3. Nose
4. Lips
5. Chin
6. Ears
7. Neck

GLOGAU PHOTOAGING CLASSIFICATION[1]

- Type 1: no wrinkles, mild pigmentary changes, and no keratoses, minimal wrinkles, and age in the 20s and 30s
- Type 2: hyperkinetic wrinkles, early solar lentigines and palpable keratoses, parallel smile lines, and age in the 40s
- Type 3: static wrinkles, dyschromia, telangiectasias, visible keratosis, and age in the 50s
- Type 4: only wrinkles, yellow-gray skin with neoplasia, and age in the 60s and older

FITZPATRICK SKIN PIGMENTATION CLASSIFICATION[2]

- Based on first 60-minute unprotected exposure to midday sun at the beginning of spring
- Type 1: white, always burns, and never tans (typically redheaded)
- Type 2: white, usually burns, and tans with difficulty (typically blonde)
- Type 3: white, sometimes mildly burns, and on average, tans (typically brunette)
- Type 4: brown, rarely burns, and tans with ease (Mediterranean, Hispanic, East Asian)
- Type 5: dark brown, very rarely burns, tans very easily (South Asian)
- Type 6: black, never burns, tans very easily (African, Caribbean)

NORWOOD-HAMILTON MALE HAIR-LOSS CLASSIFICATION[3]

- Type 1: adolescent or juvenile hairline with no recession; rests at upper brow crease
- Type 2: minimal frontotemporal recession, ≤1.5 cm above the upper brow crease
  - Type 2A: additional recession in the central anterior region
- Type 3: deepening temporal recession, the first stage of balding
  - Type 3A: additional recession in the central anterior region
  - Type 3V: additional hair loss at the vertex
- Type 4: further frontotemporal recession with hair loss from the vertex; areas of recession are separated by a solid band of hair
  - Type 4A: frontotemporal hair loss beyond type 3A, but without loss at vertex
- Type 5: vertex loss is separated from the frontotemporal hairline by a narrow band of hair
  - Type 5A: severe thinning of the central anterior hairline in continuity with thinning at the vertex
  - Type 5V: additional loss at the vertex further thins the band separating it from the frontotemporal hairline
- Type 6: frontal and vertex regions of hair loss are joined, and hairline is relatively high temporally
- Type 7: a narrow band of hair remains in a horseshoe shape, connecting the sides and back of the scalp

DEDO AGING NECK CLASSIFICATION[4]

- Type 1: normal cervicomental angle, good muscle tone, and no submental fat
- Type 2: cervical skin laxity and obtuse cervicomental angle
- Type 3: submental adiposity; rejuvenation will require submental lipectomy
- Type 4: platysmal banding; rejuvenation will require imbrication or plication

- Type 5: retrognathia/microgenia; rejuvenation will require genioplasty or orthognathic surgery
- Type 6: low-lying hyoid; manage by setting appropriate expectations
  - Cervicomental angle: 80-95 degrees

UPPER LIP SUBUNITS

1. Philtrum dimple
2. Philtrum columns
3. Melolabial folds
4. Cupid's bow
5. Vermilion border

PERIORAL PROPORTIONS

- Upper to lower-lip height 1:2
- Line drawn from the menton to the nasal tip: upper lip lies 4 mm posterior; lower lip lies 2 mm posterior
- Zero meridian of Gonzalez-Ulloa (perpendicular to the Frankfort plane; runs from the nasion to the pogonion): the mentolabial sulcus lies 4 mm posterior

PERIORAL ABNORMALITIES

- Types of lip clefts
  - Bilateral and unilateral
  - Complete (through the nasal sill) and incomplete (Simonart's band is intact at the sill)
- More common on the left than on the right, 2:1
- More common in males than in females
- Risk of second child with a cleft lip/palate after the first is affected: 4%
- Most common syndrome with cleft lip/palate: Van der Woude; characterized by lower-lip pits

AURICULAR SUBUNITS

1. Helix
   a. Crus helicis (divides the cymba and the cavum conchae)
2. Antihelix
   a. Superior/posterior crus
   b. Anterior/inferior crus
3. Darwin's tubercle
4. Fossa triangularis (bounded by the antihelical crura and the helix)
5. Tragus
6. Antitragus
7. Intertragal incisura (divides the tragus and the antitragus)
8. Scapha (scaphoid fossa)
9. Conchal bowl
   a. Cymba concha; superior to the crus helicis
   b. Cavum concha; inferior to the crus helicis, contiguous with the external auditory meatus
10. Lobule

AURICULAR PROPORTIONS

- Ratio of auricular width to height: 1:2
- Auricular height 60-65 mm
  - Height roughly equal to nasal height
- Superior margin of the helical rim at the brow level
- Inferior margin of the lobule at the nasal ala level
- Superior pole rotated posteriorly 15 degrees
- Auriculocephalic angle, 20-30 degrees
  - 10-12 mm from the helix to the mastoid at the superior pole
  - 16-18 mm from the helix to the mastoid at the midauricle
  - 20 mm from the lobule to the mastoid at the superior lobule

AURICULAR ABNORMALITIES

1. Prominauris
   a. "Lop ear" deformity resulting from antihelical-fold deficiency
   b. "Cup ear" deformity because of conchal bowl excess
2. Stahl's ear
   a. Third, more superoposterior antihelical crus causes pointed, unfurled superior helix
3. Outstanding lobule
   a. Prominent cauda helicis
4. Cryptotia
   a. Superior aspect of auricular cartilage buried under skin
5. Microtia
   a. Grade 1: most subunits present, although decreased in size
   b. Grade 2: lobule and helical remnant is present
   c. Grade 3: "Peanut ear," with lobule and cartilage remnant present (most common)
   d. Grade 4: anotia, no external structures present
   e. Microtia more common on the right side
   f. May be associated with hemifacial microsomia, Goldenhar syndrome

EYELID PROPORTIONS

- Palpebral fissure width/intercanthal distance
  - Males: 26.5-38.7 mm
  - Females: 25.5-37.5 mm
- Palpebral fissure height
  - 10-12 mm
- Margin-reflex distance (MRD)
  - MRD1 from light reflex to upper-lid margin: 4-5 mm
  - MRD2 from light reflex to lower-lid margin: 5-6 mm
- Tarsal crease 7-15 mm above the lash line; higher in females
- Upper lid should cover a small portion of the iris; inferior limbus should be within 1-2 mm of the lower lid
- Lateral canthus should be 2 mm higher than the medial canthus

BLEPHAROPLASTY TESTS

- Schirmer test: strip of filter paper is inserted at the lower-eyelid margin (both eyes are measured at once) and left in place for 5 minutes with eyes closed; degree of wetting read as a linear measurement on the filter paper (normal ≥10 mm)
- Snap test: measures how quickly the lid margin snaps back against the globe after being distracted; longer than 1-2 seconds indicates lid margin laxity

NASAL SUBUNITS

1. Tip
2. Columella
3. Dorsum
4. Sidewalls ×2
5. Alae ×2
6. Soft-tissue facets/triangles ×2

NASAL SURGERY CONSIDERATIONS

1. Thickness of skin soft-tissue envelope
2. Straightness of dorsum: smooth brow-dorsum-tip aesthetic line is best assessed in a three-fourths view photograph

3. Tip support
4. Tip projection
5. Tip light reflex/symmetry of the nasal tip defining points
6. Tip tension with smile
7. Dynamic collapse
8. Modified Cottle maneuver to assess obstruction at the internal and external valves
9. Columellar show: 2-4 mm; differentiate hanging columella from alar retraction
10. Ala-to-tip ratio 1:1 when viewed from the side
11. Basal view should be triangular, not trapezoid; ratio of the infratip lobule length to the nostril length should be 1:2
12. Nasofacial relationships (Fig. 3.3)

TIP PROJECTION ANALYSIS METHODS

1. Simons method: tip projection to upper-lip length 1:1 ratio
2. Goode method: tip projection to nasal length 0.55-0.6:1 ratio
3. Crumley method: tip projection, nasal height, and nasal length make a 3-4-5 triangle

NASOFACIAL RELATIONSHIPS (Fig. 3.3)

- Nasofrontal angle: 115-135 degrees
- Nasofacial angle: 30-40 degrees, ideally 36 degrees
- Nasolabial angle
  - Males: 90-95 degrees
  - Females: 95-110 degrees; greater rotation acceptable in shorter women
- Nasomental angle: 120-132 degrees

CRANIOMAXILLOFACIAL TRAUMA PRIMARY EVALUATION

1. Airway, breathing, circulation, disability, exposure
   - Orotracheal versus nasotracheal intubation versus tracheostomy
2. Vital signs
3. Neurological exam
   - Cranial nerves with visual acuity and tuning forks
   - Assess for intracranial injury
   - Cervical spine injury occurs in 10% of maxillofacial trauma cases
4. Inspect for lacerations, bleeding, and ecchymosis
   - Periorbital or postauricular ecchymosis may indicate skull-base fracture
5. Evaluate ears for hemotympanum, canal stepoffs, and clear or bloody otorrhea (cerebrospinal fluid [CSF] leak)
6. Evaluate the neck for tracheal deviation, subcutaneous emphysema, and bulging veins (tension pneumothorax or cardiac tamponade)

CRANIOMAXILLOFACIAL TRAUMA SECONDARY EVALUATION (TOP DOWN)

1. Upper face: scalp lacerations, skull deformities, frontal sinus/nasofrontal outflow tract injury, and CSF leak
2. Midface
   - Orbit
     - Periorbital edema and ecchymosis
     - Bony stepoffs at orbital rim

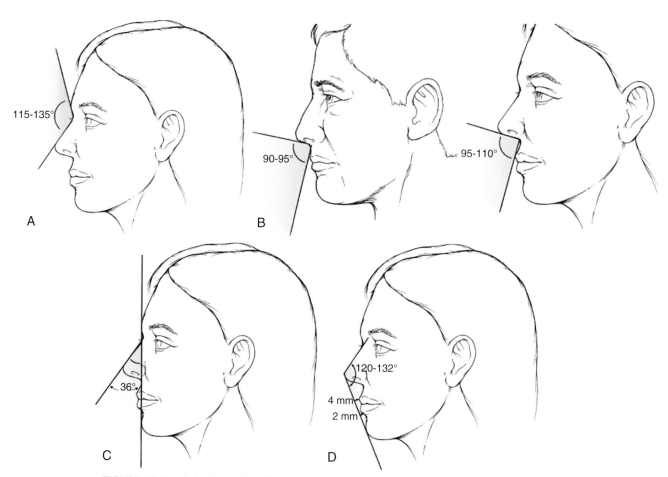

FIGURE 3.3 Nasofacial relationships: (**A**) nasofrontal angle, (**B**) nasolabial angle in men and women, (**C**) nasofacial angle, and (**D**) nasomental angle. (From Flint PW, Haughey BH, Lund VJ, et al. *Cummings Otolaryngology—Head and Neck Surgery.* 6th ed. Philadelphia, PA: Saunders; 2015, figs. 19-12, 19-16, 19-17, 19-18.)

- Assess pupillary response to light
    - Marcus-Gunn pupil = afferent pupillary defect
  - Assess extraocular muscle movement (forced ductions if patient is unresponsive)
  - Assess for eyelid and lacrimal system injuries
  - Ophthalmology consultation to rule out globe injury
- Zygoma
  - Assess for widening of the midface, trismus, and malar depression
  - Infraorbital paresthesia common
- Maxilla
  - Assess for bony stepoffs and mobility of the palate or midface
- Nasal
  - Most common facial fracture
  - Assess for mobility, crepitus, tenderness, and swelling
  - Check for clear or bloody rhinorrhea (CSF leak)
  - Check for septal hematoma
    - May cause septal necrosis and buckling or saddle deformity if untreated
    - Incise and leave a drain
3. Lower face
  - Oral cavity: assess for dental injuries, lacerations, ecchymosis, and trismus
  - Occlusion: assess for open bite, crossbite, inability to close mouth, and missing teeth
    - Angle dental occlusion classification[5]
      - Class 1: the mesiobuccal cusp of the first maxillary molar fits in the buccal groove of the first mandibular molar
      - Class 2 (overjet): the mesiobuccal cusp of the first maxillary molar contacts the mesial to the buccal groove of the first mandibular molar
      - Class 3 (underjet): the mesiobuccal cusp of the first maxillary molar contacts the distal to the buccal groove of the first mandibular molar
  - Mandible
    - Assess for stepoffs and mobility of fractured segments
    - Evaluate maximal incisal opening
    - Assess for deviation of the mandible on opening, premature contact of the molars, loss of mandibular height, and anterior open bite
      - All are signs of ipsilateral subcondylar fracture
    - Look for floor-of-the-mouth hematoma
    - Assess sensation of the mental nerve

FACIAL RESURFACING

INDICATIONS FOR FACIAL RESURFACING
(See *Cummings Otolaryngology*, 6th ed., Chapter 26)

1. Advanced-to-severe skin damage with wrinkles at rest
2. Fine and deep rhytides
3. Uncontrollable acne
4. Acne scars
5. Ephelides
6. Lentigines
7. Actinic keratosis
8. Some skin cancers

ABSOLUTE CONTRAINDICATIONS FOR FACIAL RESURFACING

1. Significant hepatorenal disease
2. Human immunodeficiency virus (HIV)
3. Immunosuppression
4. Emotional instability or mental illness

5. Ehlers-Danlos syndrome
6. Scleroderma or collagen vascular diseases
7. Recent isotretinoin treatment (within 6-12 months before)

RELATIVE CONTRAINDICATIONS FOR FACIAL RESURFACING

1. Darker skin type (Fitzpatrick IV, V, and VI)
2. History of keloid formation
3. History of cold sores
4. Cardiac abnormalities
5. History of previous facial irradiation
6. Unrealistic expectations
7. Physical inability to perform quality postoperative care
8. Anticipation of inadequate photo protection because of job, vocation, or recreation

HERPES SIMPLEX VIRUS PROPHYLAXIS BEFORE PERIORAL OR FULL-FACE RESURFACING[6]

- Valacyclovir 500 mg orally twice a day for 14 days, starting the day of the procedure.

SEQUELAE OF FACIAL RESURFACING

- Pigmentary changes
  - Hyperpigmentation with darker-skinned patients, usually temporary (give 4-8% hydroquinone gel before surgery and sun protection factor [SPF] 30 sunblock after surgery, withhold systemic estrogens)
  - Hypopigmentation is most common; can be permanent
  - Depigmentation (rarely, and in isolated areas)
- Persistence of rhytides
- Prolonged erythema
- Persistent texture change of skin
- Hypertrophic subepidermal healing
- Milia
- Skin pore prominence
- Increased prominence of telangiectasias
- Darkening and growth of preexisting nevi

COMPLICATIONS OF FACIAL RESURFACING

1. Skin infection
   - HSV outbreak
   - *Pseudomonas*, *Staphylococcus*, and *Streptococcus*
   - *Candida*
2. Lower-eyelid ectropion
3. Cardiac arrhythmias
4. Renal failure
5. Laryngeal edema
6. Toxic shock syndrome
7. Facial scarring
8. Telangiectasias

TOPICAL FACIAL RESURFACING THERAPIES

- Retinoids (tretinoin)
- Bleaching agents (hydroquinone)
- Sunscreen
- Moisturizers
- Pretreat skin with the abovementioned products before resurfacing, which may improve resurfacing results; some patients will not need resurfacing after the topical regimen

CHEMICAL PEELS

- Superficial chemical peels act on the epidermis and have no effect on the dermis
  - Salicylic acid 5-15%
  - Glycolic acid 40-70%; must be rinsed off w/H_2O or neutralized w/$NaHCO_3$
  - Jessner solution (resorcinol, salicylic acid, lactic acid, and EtOH)
  - Trichloroacetic acid (TCA) 10-25%
- Medium peels penetrate down to the superficial reticular dermis
  - TCA 50% alone can cause scarring
  - TCA 35% in combination with dry ice pretreatment or Jessner or glycolic acid 70%
- Deep peels penetrate to the midreticular dermis and are often required for Glogau III-IV
  - Baker solution (phenol, septisol, croton oil, and distilled water); phenol penetrates further with decreasing concentrations

DERMABRASION

- Addresses deep scarring, deep rhytides, and acne-related pits/scars
- Variable depth of resurfacing
- Pinpoint bleeding in chamois-colored tissue indicates level of papillary dermis
- Use freezing spray before mechanical abrasion to decrease tissue spatter
- Good for decreasing height of thick scars
- Decreased postoperative erythema
- Microdermabrasion is more superficial and requires no anesthesia or physician

LASER WAVE CHARACTERISTICS

1. Collimated (parallel)
2. Monochromatic (same wavelength)
3. Coherent (in phase)

ABLATIVE LASERS FOR SCAR REVISION AND SKIN RESURFACING

1. CO_2 10,600 nm (far infrared), chromophore: H_2O
2. Er:YAG (erbium-doped yttrium-aluminum-garnet) 2940 nm (near infrared), chromophore: collagen and dermal proteins
   - Either can be used as a fractionated treatment, which is safer for patients with darker skin
   - CO_2 and Er:YAG can be used in sequence, with Er:YAG removing thermally necrotic tissue after CO_2 treatment.
   - Ablative depth can be varied, typically deeper in fractionated treatments (150-300 μm)

NONABLATIVE LASERS FOR VASCULAR ANOMALIES, PIGMENTED LESIONS, AND TATTOO AND HAIR REMOVAL

1. KTP (potassium-titanyl-phosphate) 532 nm (green), chromophore: oxyhemoglobin and red tattoos
2. Pulsed-dye 585-595 nm (yellow), chromophore: oxyhemoglobin (may also be used for scar revision)
3. Alexandrite 755 nm (red), chromophore: melanin, blue, green, and black tattoos
4. Nd:YAG (neodymium-doped yttrium-aluminum-garnet) 1064 nm (near infrared), chromophore: oxyhemoglobin, melanin (in hair follicles), and blue and black tattoos
   - Laser only affects hair follicles in anagen
   - Takes 3-5 treatments, separated by 4-6 weeks, to ensure that all hair follicles are treated during the anagen phase
   - Works poorly on light-colored or vellus hair because of lack of chromophore for laser
5. Intense pulsed light/broadband light (515-1200 nm)—not a true laser—used for melasma, erythema and other hyperpigmentation, hair removal, and skin tightening
   - Requires multiple treatments, maintenance therapy

INJECTABLES

DERMAL FILLER INDICATIONS[7]

1. Static rhytides
2. May help fill in dynamic rhytides after chemodenervation

DERMAL FILLERS

1. Hyaluronic acid
   - Restylane, Perlane, Juvederm, and others
   - Inject into dermis
   - 6-12 months' duration
   - Hyaluronidase to correct excess injections
2. Calcium hydroxylapatite
   - Radiesse
   - Inject into dermis or subdermally
   - ≥12 months' duration
   - Do not inject into lips
3. Poly-L-lactic acid
   - Sculptra
   - Inject subdermally
   - Results take 4 weeks to appear, as new collagen forms
   - Lasts 12 months, but some permanent effect after normal course of two to three injections
   - Indicated for HIV lipoatrophy
4. Autologous fat
   - Harvested from the belly or thigh and centrifuged to concentrate adipocytes
   - Must be transferred atraumatically to improve cell viability
   - Inject at multiple levels, subdermally and deeper
5. Collagen
   - Zyderm and Zyplast
   - Rarely used anymore; requires allergy to bovine collagen testing before injection

CHEMODENERVATION CHARACTERISTICS

1. Most useful for dynamic rhytides
2. Takes 1-2 weeks to reach maximum effect
3. Lasts 3-4 months
4. Shorter duration of action and smaller effect may result from development of antibodies
5. With repeated facial cosmetic doses, patients often require less toxin or have a longer period between injections with the same effect
6. Acts by preventing release of acetylcholine in the neuromuscular junction
7. Recovery occurs first by development of new synapses, followed by recovery of function at the original synapse

CHEMODENERVATION AGENTS

- Botulinum toxin comes in seven varieties: A-G
  - A and E cleave SNAP-25
  - B, D, and F cleave synaptobrevin (VAMP)
  - C cleaves syntaxin
- OnabotulinumtoxinA (Botox)
- AbobotulinumtoxinA (Dysport)

- IncobotulinumtoxinA (Xeomin)
- RimabotulinumtoxinB (Myobloc)

BROW LIFT

IDEAL BROW POSITION (Fig. 3.4)

- Women: begins medially at a vertical line from the ala of the nose; terminates at an oblique line drawn through the ala of the nose and extending past the lateral canthus; apex of brow arc between the lateral limbus and lateral canthus
- Men: lies at the supraorbital rim and does not arch as high as in women

BROW LIFT CONSIDERATIONS

- Glabellar creases
  - Transverse creases caused by procerus, most superficial muscle of the glabella
  - Vertical creases caused by corrugator supercilii, superficial to frontalis, and deep to procerus
  - Division of the corrugator has a similar effect as permanent chemodenervation, but may lateralize the medial brows
- Frontal branch of the facial nerve
  - Within 2 mm of zygomaticotemporal "sentinel" vein between the superficial temporal fascia above and the deep temporal fascia below

INDICATIONS FOR BROW LIFT

- Brow ptosis, especially when it contributes to an upper visual field deficit with dermatochalasis
- Corrugator and procerus hyperactivity are indications for endoscopic forehead lift
- Baldness is not a contraindication

BROW LIFT APPROACHES

1. Endoscopic
2. Coronal
3. Midforehead
4. Direct

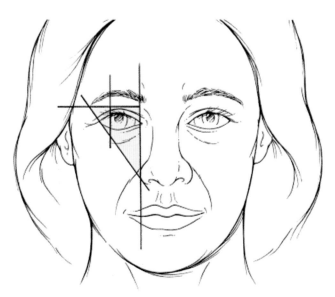

FIGURE 3.4 Ideal Brow Position. (From Flint PW, Haughey BH, Lund VJ, et al. *Cummings Otolaryngology—Head and Neck Surgery.* 6th ed. Philadelphia, PA: Saunders; 2015, fig. 19-13.)

ENDOSCOPIC BROW LIFT[8]

- Patients with short foreheads (<6 cm from brow to hairline), brow ptosis, or corrugator and procerus hyperactivity
- Subperiosteal dissection
- Avoid supratrochlear and supraorbital neurovascular bundles when releasing the periosteum from the supraorbital rim
- Release the periosteum all along the lateral orbital rim to permit temporal lifting and relief of lateral periocular hooding
- 1.5 cm longitudinal incisions placed behind the hairline in median and paramedian positions (superior to the lateral limbus), and longer incisions placed behind the temporal hair tufts
- Periosteum secured in the elevated position with absorbable anchors, or sutures through bone bridges placed under paramedian incisions, or with fibrin glue
- Decreased scarring, alopecia, and numbness of the scalp compared with an open procedure

CORONAL APPROACH TO BROW LIFT

- Subgaleal dissection
- May elevate hairline; pretrichial or trichophytic (just behind hairline) approaches minimize hairline elevation
- Scar may become visible with time as hair thins, particularly in male patients
- Male pattern baldness best predicted by hair pattern of maternal grandfather

MIDFOREHEAD APPROACH TO BROW LIFT

- Excise and elevate via an incision in a transverse forehead rhytid
- More common approach in men

DIRECT APPROACH TO BROW LIFT

- Incisions made along the superior margin of brows
- Most effective for correcting lateral brow ptosis and hooding

BROW LIFT COMPLICATIONS

1. Forehead itching (25%)
2. Diffuse alopecia (5%)
3. Patchy areas of permanent numbness (1%)
4. Excessive brow elevation (0.3%)

BLEPHAROPLASTY

EYELID ANATOMY (See *Cummings Otolaryngology*, 6th ed., Chapter 29)

- Orbicularis oculi forms the transition from the brow into the upper eyelid and surrounds the eye
  - Orbital portion overlies the bony orbit
  - Palpebral portion overlies the eyelid: pretarsal and preseptal portions
  - Tarsal plate and orbital septum lie deep to palpebral orbicularis
- Orbital septum divides the lid into the anterior and posterior lamellae
  - Anterior lamella: skin and orbicularis oculi
  - Posterior lamella: conjunctiva, eyelid retractor, and upper or lower tarsal plate
  - Orbital septum and tarsal plate constitute "middle lamella"

- Septum originates at the arcus marginalis, a confluence of the periosteum of the facial skeleton and the periorbita at the bony orbital rims
- In the upper lid, the septum does not extend over the upper surface of the tarsal plate, but is found as a thin membrane 10 mm or more above the lid margin, inserting on the upper lid retractors
- In the lower lid, the septum is attached to the inferior edge of the tarsal plate
- Tarsal plate is 8-10-mm tall in the upper lid
- Tarsal plate is 4-5-mm tall in the lower lid

PREAPONEUROTIC FAT

- Deep to the septum, superficial to the levator aponeurosis
- Dissection through the septum more superiorly avoids injury to the levator aponeurosis and Müller's muscle, which will result in ptosis
- Upper lid has two fat pads
  - Nasal (medial) and middle (largest), with the temporal (lateral) compartment being occupied by the lacrimal gland
- Lower lid has three fat pads
  - Medial (nasal), central, and lateral (temporal)
  - Inferior oblique muscle separates the medial and central compartments
- Medial compartment in both the upper and lower lids contains denser, whiter fat

LID RETRACTORS

- Upper eyelid
  - Retracted by levator palpebrae superioris and Müller's muscle
  - Primary retractor is the levator muscle, originating in the orbital apex; lies immediately superior to the superior rectus; at the orbital aperture, it is supported by Whitnall's ligament
  - Levator palpebrae superioris splits into the levator aponeurosis anteriorly and Müller's muscle posteriorly
  - Müller's muscle travels inferiorly, closely adherent to the conjunctiva, and inserts on top of the tarsal plate
  - Levator aponeurosis inserts laterally and medially into the canthal tendons, and fuses with the orbital septum and dermis at the upper-eyelid crease; inferiorly, fibers travel anteriorly and posteriorly, attaching to the orbicularis oculi and tarsal plate, respectively
- Lower eyelid
  - Capsulopalpebral fascia of the lower eyelid is analogous to the levator aponeurosis of the upper lid, an extension of the inferior rectus muscle, which depresses the lower lid on downward gaze
  - Densely adherent to the conjunctiva and is routinely transected in lower-lid transconjunctival approaches

BLEPHAROCHALASIS

- Rare variant of angioedema
- Recurrent, painless periorbital edema leading to chronic changes in eyelid skin elasticity, atrophy, hyperpigmentation, and upper lid ptosis
- Can lead to lacrimal gland and fat prolapse

DERMATOCHALASIS

- Redundancy and draping of the eyelid skin in the aged face
- Called "pseudoptosis" when it progresses to the point that skin drapes over the upper eyelashes and causes visual field defects

FESTOONS

- Redundant folds of lax skin and orbicularis muscle
- Usually on the lower lid

UPPER-LID INCISION CONSIDERATIONS

- When deciding how much skin to take, pinch with forceps until slight lid eversion is evident; this will lead to slight postoperative lagophthalmos, which will resolve
- Plan to leave ≥15 mm of skin between the lash margin and the inferior aspect of the brow
- Do not carry the incision medially to the medial canthus or webbing may ensue
- Do not excise orbicularis oculi muscle in patients with history of dry eyes

LOWER-LID BLEPHAROPLASTY APPROACHES

1. Transconjunctival
2. Subciliary skin flap
3. Subciliary skin pinch excision

TRANSCONJUNCTIVAL APPROACH TO LOWER-LID BLEPHAROPLASTY CONSIDERATIONS

- For older patients w/pseudoherniation of orbital fat, limited amount of skin excess
- Young patients w/familial hereditary pseudoherniation of orbital fat and no excess skin
- Revision blepharoplasty patients, patients who do not want to have an external scar or have a history of keloid or dark-skinned individuals because of the possibility of hypopigmentation of an external scar
- Does not disrupt the orbicularis oculi, minimizing the incidence of ectropion
- Avoid damage to the inferior oblique muscle
- Do not pull fat out of the orbit; coax it out gently and cauterize carefully to avoid intraorbital hematoma

PRESEPTAL APPROACH TO TRANSCONJUNCTIVAL BLEPHAROPLASTY

- Conjunctival incision made 2 mm posterior to the inferior border of the inferior tarsal plate
- Dissect along the anterior face of the septum and then open the septum to access orbital fat
- Preferred approach for orbital floor fractures; allows elevation of the orbital floor periosteum

POSTSEPTAL APPROACH TO TRANSCONJUNCTIVAL BLEPHAROPLASTY

- Conjunctival incision made 4 mm posterior to the inferior border of the inferior tarsal plate
- Accesses orbital fat compartments directly
- Septum remains intact; decreased risk of ectropion

SUBCILIARY APPROACH TO LOWER-LID BLEPHAROPLASTY

- For large amounts of excess skin and orbicularis oculi
- Safely and easily dissect in a relatively avascular submuscular plane
- Ability to remove redundant lower-eyelid skin

- Additional tightening of skin and muscle with lateral suspension sutures
- Do not carry incision past the inferior punctum
- Skin-muscle flap procedure: subciliary incision with elevation of skin-muscle flap, fat resection, and skin-muscle flap resection
- May be combined with transconjunctival approach to address skin, muscle, and fat

ASIAN EYELID CONSIDERATIONS

- Defined by the epicanthal fold and absence of upper-eyelid tarsal crease
- 50% of Asians have a tarsal crease ("double eyelid")
- If the crease is absent, the orbital septum and levator aponeurosis attach to the skin farther inferiorly, anterior to tarsal plate
- Orbital fat prolapses anteriorly, preventing the formation of a prominent upper-eyelid crease and creating fullness of the upper eyelid

BLEPHAROPLASTY COMPLICATIONS

1. Milia
2. Hematoma/blindness
3. Lagopthalmos
4. Ectropion: eversion from excessive lower-lid skin or muscle excision, lid contracture, or lateral laxity
5. Ptosis
6. Epiphoria
7. Diplopia
8. Conjunctival chemosis/ecchymosis

ECTROPION MANAGEMENT

- Lower-lip tape splinting or forceful eye closure
- Gentle massage + corneal protection
- Surgical correction after 3 months
  - Full-thickness skin graft (FTSG) from the upper lid
  - If from lateral lid laxity
    - Horizontal lid shortening
    - Z-plasty
    - Muscle suspension

FACE LIFT

MIDFACE LIFT CONSIDERATIONS
(See *Cummings Otolaryngology*, 6th ed., Chapter 27)

- Elevates malar fat pad and suborbicularis oculi fat (SOOF)
- Effaces deep nasolabial folds
- Often combined with lower-lid blepharoplasty to avoid redundant lower-lid skin after lift
  - SOOF may be transferred inferiorly to augment malar eminence
  - May augment effect with fillers and/or cheek implants

MIDFACE LIFT APPROACHES

- Endoscopic access
  - Similar to the lateral aspect of the endoscopic brow lift but periosteal elevation and release are carried around the infraorbital rim
  - Periosteum suture is suspended to the temporalis fascia
- Intraoral access
  - Subperiosteal dissection of midface via a gingivobuccal sulcus incision

- Absorbable implant suspends the midface periosteum to the temporalis fascia
- Implant anchored to the temporalis fascia via a temporal hair-tuft incision

RHYTIDECTOMY ANATOMY BY LAYERS
(See *Cummings Otolaryngology*, 6th ed., Chapter 27)

1. Skin
2. Subcutaneous fat contains hair follicles
3. Galea aponeurotica/frontalis muscle/temporoparietal fascia (TPF) superiorly, contiguous with superficial musculoaponeurotic system (SMAS) in the mid and lower face and then platysma in the lower face and neck[9]
4. Parotidomasseteric fascia surrounds the parotid posteriorly and the masseter anteriorly, contiguous with the periosteum of zygomatic arch and temporalis fascia

RHYTIDECTOMY INCISIONS

- Female: typically posttragal to break up the scar
- Male: typically preauricular to avoid pulling hair-bearing beard skin closer to the auricle or onto the tragus; there is usually a <1-cm-wide vertical band of non–hair-bearing skin anterior to the auricle that should remain intact

RHYTIDECTOMY APPROACHES

1. Subcutaneous lift
2. SMAS lift
3. Deep-plane lift
4. Composite lift
5. Minimal-access cranial-suspension (MACS) lift

SUBCUTANEOUS LIFT

- Original facelift operation
- Short-lived results
- No longer performed

SMAS LIFT

- Subcutaneous flap raised in the face and neck
- SMAS incised overlying parotid and plicated to bear tension of the lift
- Facial nerve branches are not ordinarily visualized

DEEP-PLANE LIFT[10]

- Subcutaneous flap raised until the line between the zygoma and the angle of mandible is reached; SMAS is incised, and dissection is carried anteriorly along the plane of the zygomaticus major muscle, elevating the malar fat pad into the flap
- Facial nerve branches visualized and avoided
- Entire flap bears tension; excellent vascularity medially because of the thickness of the flap
- Neck is addressed as for SMAS flap rhytidectomy, leaving face and neck dissections in different planes, separated by the platysmal insertion at the level of the mandible
- May help efface nasolabial folds

COMPOSITE LIFT

- Deep-plane lift with repositioning of SOOF via transconjunctival lower-lid blepharoplasty

MINIMAL-ACCESS CRANIAL-SUSPENSION LIFT

- Three purse-string loops of suture plicate SMAS to elevate the face in a vertical vector
  - Vertical loop elevates the neck
  - Oblique loop elevates the jowl
  - Malar loop elevates the midface
- Short incision with no postauricular component

PLATYSMAPLASTY

- Addresses platysmal banding
- Done with submental liposuction and/or direct lipectomy
- Medial borders of the platysma are sutured together down to the hyoid level
- May also divide platysma transversely
- Provides additional cervical soft-tissue support before lateral suspension

RHYTIDECTOMY COMPLICATIONS

1. Great auricular nerve injury: most common nerve to be injured
2. Frontal branch and marginal mandibular branch injury: most common facial nerve branches injured
3. Hematoma: generally within 24 hours of surgery, and more common in males because of increased blood flow to hair follicles
4. Pixie (satyr) ear lobe: because of tension on the lobule of the auricle at the closure secondary to excessive skin resection
5. Cobra neck deformity: because of excessive central neck adipose tissue removal with insufficient removal laterally
6. Parotid injury
7. Alopecia
8. Widened scar

HAIR RESTORATION

HAIR ANATOMY AND GROWTH CYCLE
(See *Cummings Otolaryngology*, 6th ed., Chapter 25)

- Scalp contains 100,000 to 150,000 hairs
- ~90% of follicles are in the growth (anagen) phase
- Next stage is involutional (catagen); <1% of the hair follicles are in this phase
- 5-10% of hair follicles are in the resting (telogen) phase

MALE PATTERN BALDNESS (ANDROGENIC ALOPECIA)

- Mediated by increased 5α-reductase activity and by lack of aromatase enzyme in specific regions of the scalp, thereby resulting in higher levels of dihydrotestosterone (DHT)
- Most common in Caucasians and then Asians and then Blacks
- Incidence increases with age, ~30% at 30 years of age in Caucasian males; 50-60% at 50 years of age
- Bitemporal recession occurs first and then balding of the vertex

MEDICAL MANAGEMENT OF ALOPECIA

- Minoxidil (Rogaine)
  - Causes vellus hairs to develop into terminal hairs; miniaturized hair follicles revert to normal morphology, and the number of hair follicles in anagen increases

- Finasteride (Propecia)
  - Inhibits action of 5α-reductase type 2, blocking conversion of testosterone to DHT
  - Cannot be safely used in women of reproductive age because 5α-reductase inhibition during pregnancy may lead to genital abnormalities in male fetus
- Results are seen only after several months of therapy and are rapidly reversed upon discontinuing therapy

HAIR REPLACEMENT CONSIDERATIONS

- Goals of surgery are to create a natural-appearing hairline and to increase scalp coverage
- Prediction of future hair loss needs to be factored into the surgical planning
- Frontal hairline is most important
- Patient must have adequate donor hair available

HAIR REPLACEMENT APPROACHES

1. Punch method
2. Strip grafting
3. Follicular-unit transplantation
4. Scalp reduction

PUNCH METHOD

- 4-5 mm; sharp, round punches to harvest from the parietal and occipital scalp with 10-20 hairs per punch
- Recipient sites are slightly smaller than donor site are and are spaced so as not to compromise blood supply
- 6 weeks between sessions, usually at least four sessions are required

STRIP GRAFTING

- 5-8 mm in width, typically in two sessions to recreate frontal hairline
- Donor site incised to the galea level and then elevated and closed primarily
- Graft inset to angle hairs anteriorly

FOLLICULAR-UNIT TRANSPLANTATION

- Most commonly used method
- Multiple minigrafts (three to four hairs per graft) and micrografts (one to two hairs per graft) are used
- Donor hair is harvested from the occipital scalp in one large ellipse
- Donor tissue is first cut into 2-mm segments, aligning all incisions in the direction of follicle growth and then further dissected into micro- and minigrafts, taking care to preserve natural groupings of hair follicles
- Slits are created in the recipient scalp 4-5 mm apart; a second and sometimes third pass over the area may be performed to obtain the desired density

SCALP REDUCTION

- Serial excisions to remove bald areas
- Limited by amount of available hair-bearing scalp and wound tension
- Can use tissue expanders to increase hair-bearing area or use silastic sutures to support incision closure and decrease tension
- Juri temporoparietal transposition flaps based on superficial temporal arteries can be rotated to address frontal baldness

RHINOPLASTY

RHINOPLASTY LANDMARKS (See *Cummings Otolaryngology*, 6th ed., Chapters 34-37)

1. Tip defining points: light reflection from the skin overlying the domes of alar cartilages; excessive distance between points causes boxy/trapezoidal tip
2. Gull-in-flight: ideal appearance of the nasal tip on frontal view, with columella hanging just inferior to the alar rims
3. Supratip break: just superior to the domal region; helps distinguish the dorsum from the tip; absent in "polly beak" deformity
4. Skin: thinnest at the rhinion/middle one-third and thickest in the tip/lower one-third and glabellar region/upper one-third
   - Thin skin at the rhinion means that hump reduction must consider skin thickness and not completely remove the hump, or the appearance of a saddle will result once the skin and soft tissue are replaced
5. Double-break: first break where the tip turns posteroinferiorly onto the infratip lobule; second break at the midcolumella, where the columella takes a more horizontal course and extends posteriorly to the subnasale

MAJOR NASAL TIP SUPPORT ELEMENTS

1. Size, shape, and resiliency of the medial/lateral crura of the lower lateral cartilages
2. Attachment of medial crural footplates to the caudal margin of the cartilaginous septum
3. Attachment of the cephalic margins of the lower lateral cartilages to the caudal portions of the upper lateral cartilages (scroll region)

MINOR NASAL TIP SUPPORT ELEMENTS

1. Interdomal ligaments
2. Dorsal cartilaginous septum
3. Membranous septum
4. Skin and subcutaneous tissue
5. Sesamoid cartilages
6. Nasal spine

TRIPOD MODEL

- Conjoined medial crura of the lower lateral cartilages act as the central leg of the tripod and the lateral crura act as the other two legs
- Manipulating one leg of the tripod will affect the other two legs

INTERNAL NASAL VALVE CHARACTERISTICS

- Bordered by the nasal septum, caudal margin of the upper lateral cartilage, piriform aperture, and face of the inferior turbinate
- Angle of the internal nasal valve is ~15 degrees
- Evaluate with Cottle maneuver

SURGICAL APPROACHES TO CORRECT NARROW INTERNAL NASAL VALVE

1. Spreader grafts[11]
2. Flaring sutures
3. Butterfly grafts
4. Orbital suspension suture
5. Lateral batten grafts
6. Lateral crural "flip-flop"

EXTERNAL NASAL VALVE CHARACTERISTICS

- Bordered by the caudal edge of the lateral crus of the alar cartilage, the soft-tissue alae, the membranous septum, and the sill of the nostril
- Evaluate by looking for alar collapse with inspiration

SURGICAL APPROACHES TO CORRECT NARROW EXTERNAL NASAL VALVE

1. Alar batten/lateral crural strut grafts
2. Narrow columella
3. Septoplasty
4. Spreading suture
5. Nasal-floor cartilage graft

METHODS TO INCREASE NASAL TIP PROJECTION

1. Transdomal suturing: mild increase in projection and no increase to tip support
2. Lateral crural steal: suture more lateral than transdomal; greater increase in projection and no added tip support
3. Tip grafting: shield-shaped onlay graft of autologous cartilage adds more tip definition
4. Columellar strut: cartilage graft placed in a pocket between the medial crura; gives the most tip support of all techniques and is often used in combination with one or more of the other for support; does not need to contact the nasal spine
5. Septocolumellar suture: suspend the medial crura high on the caudal septum, best performed with either a columellar strut or a septal extension graft

METHODS TO DECREASE NASAL TIP PROJECTION

1. Full transfixion incision
2. Shortening of the medial crura
3. Dome division
4. Medial crural steal
5. Shaving of the dorsal and caudal septum if the cartilaginous septum is excessive on physical examination
6. Septocolumellar suture: suspend medial crura low on the caudal septum

METHODS TO INCREASE NASAL TIP ROTATION

1. Cephalic trims of the lower lateral cartilages
   - Excise a portion of the bilateral cephalic margins of the lateral crura of the alar cartilages
   - 6-8-mm residual strip should be left for tip and alar support
   - Incomplete remaining strips of the lateral crura will further increase tip rotation
2. Tongue-in-groove suture the caudal septum between medial crura
3. Suspend the cephalic margins of the lateral crura of the lower lateral cartilages onto the upper lateral cartilages in a more cephalad position than that of the natural scroll region

METHODS TO NARROW NASAL TIP

1. Transdomal sutures
2. Dome division
3. Excision of subcutaneous tissue

METHODS TO CORRECT CAUDAL SEPTAL DEFLECTION

1. Excise deviated portion if quadrangular cartilage is too long
2. Replace the caudal septum with a septal extension graft
3. Tongue-in-groove technique with or without cartilage scoring
4. Swinging-door technique
5. Extended spreader grafts/septal batten grafts

METHODS TO ADDRESS CROOKED NOSE

1. Vertical spreader grafts if midvault/internal valve obstruction is present
2. Onlay camouflage graft for solely cosmetic purposes
3. Osteotomies to straighten or narrow the upper one-third

OSTEOTOMY CONSIDERATIONS[12]

- Begin with lateral osteotomy on the concave side and then ipsilateral medial osteotomy, contralateral medial osteotomy, and contralateral lateral osteotomy
- If the dorsal hump has been removed, no medial osteotomies are necessary
- To mobilize bones with the upper vault intact (no narrowing or widening required), perform lateral osteotomies and transverse root osteotomy
- Intermediate osteotomy may be required if one nasal bone is significantly wider than the other
- Intranasal approach requires no external incisions and can be used to push out concave bone segments but causes continuous osteotomies, which may lead to less stable bone fragments
- Percutaneous osteotomies
  - 2-mm osteotome through one or two stab incisions per side permits "postage stamp" lateral, transverse, and intermediate osteotomies that cause minimal periosteal and mucosal trauma, and have an irregular osteotomy line, which helps prevent flail bone fragments

METHODS TO ADDRESS ASYMMETRIC TIP

1. Asymmetric interdomal sutures may recreate symmetry
2. Asymmetric intradomal sutures may help
3. Shield grafting or crushed-cartilage camouflage grafting
4. Lateral crural strut grafting (on deep surface of the lateral crura of the lower lateral cartilages)
5. Cephalic turn-in (cephalic trim but with folding cephalic aspect of the lateral crura underneath the remaining strip rather than removing it; this helps to reinforce the lateral crura and remove irregular curvatures)
6. Lateral crural "flip-flop" division and reversal of lateral crura

RHINOPLASTY APPROACHES

1. Endonasal nondelivery
2. Endonasal delivery
3. Open

ENDONASAL APPROACHES

- Nondelivery
  - Addresses dorsal irregularities, such as a hump
  - Less tip support disruption, more control of healing/scarring
  - Via intercartilaginous incisions, disrupts scroll region
- Delivery
  - Additionally allows for manipulation of the tip
  - Less edema than occurs with an open approach
  - Via intercartilaginous-full transfixion and marginal-lateral columellar incisions

OPEN-APPROACH

- Maximal exposure
- Significant edema
- Disrupts tip support with violation of interdomal ligaments
- Via transcolumellar and marginal incisions

INTRANASAL INCISIONS

1. Hemitransfixion: unilateral septal incision at the junction of skin and mucosa
2. Transfixion: same as hemitransfixion, except it extends all the way through the septum
3. Killian: posterior to hemitransfixion; used to address isolated posterior spurs, often used endoscopically
4. Intercartilaginous: made at the internal nasal valve between the upper and lower lateral cartilages; suboptimal healing may lead to nasal obstruction
5. Intracartilaginous: parallel to the lateral crus cephalic border, 2-6 mm closer to the nostril opening, incising through the lower lateral cartilage and removing a 3-5-mm strip of cartilage; lowers the risk of nasal valve stenosis
6. Marginal: follows the caudal border of the lower lateral cartilage, not the alar rim
7. Transcolumellar: for open approach, use an inverted-V incision and make sure to connect with the marginal incisions at right angles

SADDLE NOSE DEFORMITY CHARACTERISTICS

- Compromise of septal cartilage leading to decreased dorsal nasal structural support
- Surgical correction for patients without obstruction: onlay grafting
- With obstruction: extended spreader grafts with columellar strut to construct an L-shaped strut; may require rib or split calvarial bone
- Aim to restore middle vault function, reverse internal valve narrowing, reinforce nasal tip and dorsal support mechanisms

CAUSES OF SADDLE NOSE DEFORMITIES

1. Traumatic
2. Iatrogenic
3. Wegener granulomatosis
4. Relapsing polychondritis
5. Leprosy (Hansen disease)
6. Syphilis
7. Ectodermal dysplasia
8. Intranasal cocaine

POLLY BEAK DEFORMITY CHARACTERISTICS

- Excessive supratip fullness
- Associated with tip deprojection and ptosis

CAUSES OF POLLY BEAK DEFORMITY

1. Over-resection of the bony dorsum
2. Under-resection of the cartilaginous dorsum
3. High cartilaginous hump at the anterior septal angle
4. Over-resection of alar cartilages, leading to loss of tip support
5. Dead space between the dorsal nasal skin and the nasal skeleton; scar tissue will fill this space and produce supratip fullness

METHODS TO CORRECT WIDE NASAL BASE

1. Weir excisions: wedge excisions in alar-facial grooves
2. Nasal sill excisions: maintain the natural curvature of nostrils, avoid alar-facial webbing, and may cause stepoff deformity in the nasal sill
3. Cinching stitch: permanent suture placed via the gingivobuccal sulcus

GRAFT OPTIONS

1. Septal cartilage
2. Auricular cartilage
3. Autologous rib cartilage (sixth rib): may be calcified in adults and tends to warp; must soak the graft to allow warping to occur before placement; consider cutting the graft into layers and laminating it before placement to reduce warping
4. Split calvarial bone: outer table harvested from nearly flat parietal skull ipsilateral to the dominant hand; inner table is left intact
5. Cadaveric rib cartilage and bone: have a higher potential for resorption than autologous materials
6. Gore-Tex: allows tissue ingrowth and provides support; difficult to obtain now
7. Silicone: forms a capsule, does not allow tissue ingrowth, high rate of extrusion and chronic infection
8. For nonstructural grafts, temporalis fascia and acellular dermis (Alloderm) work well to camouflage contour irregularities

METHODS TO ADDRESS SEPTAL PERFORATION[13]

1. Silastic button
2. Local flaps, bipedicled with cartilage or Alloderm graft interposed between mucoperichondrial flaps
   * Releasing incisions may be made superior and inferior, taking care not to oppose the releasing incisions
   * Tissue expander placement may increase available tissue for advancement
3. Regional flaps, including the inferior turbinate (usually anteriorly pedicled), gingivobuccal sulcus mucosa, and facial artery musculomucosal flap; may require a second stage to take down the interpolated pedicle
4. Free flap, such as a radial forearm: access via an external rhinoplasty approach or midfacial degloving

RHINOPLASTY COMPLICATIONS OF THE UPPER ONE-THIRD OF THE NOSE

1. Rocker deformity: when osteotomies are extended too far superiorly, into the frontal bone
2. Step deformity: stepoff between the nasal bones and maxilla after osteotomy
3. Open-roof deformity: lack of osteotomies to medialize the nasal bones after removal of a dorsal hump

RHINOPLASTY COMPLICATIONS OF THE MIDDLE ONE-THIRD OF THE NOSE

1. Inverted-V deformity: disarticulation of upper lateral cartilages from nasal bones
2. Saddle nose: concave bowing of the midvault because of insufficient strength of the dorsal septal strut or disarticulation of the "keystone" region, where the cartilaginous septum meets the bony septum along the dorsum

3. Parenthesis deformity: cephalic over-rotation of the lateral crura of the lower lateral cartilages
4. Polly beak

RHINOPLASTY COMPLICATIONS OF THE LOWER ONE-THIRD OF THE NOSE

1. Malrotation
2. Malprojection
3. Bossae: knuckling at the domes, showing through skin
4. Pinched tip: overtightening of interdomal sutures distorts tips and eliminates natural tip bifidity
5. Alar retraction: because of excessive cephalic trimming
6. Hanging columella: results from failure to reduce overly long caudal septal cartilage

OTOPLASTY

COMMON INDICATIONS FOR OTOPLASTY (See *Cummings Otolaryngology*, 6th ed., Chapter 31)

1. Antihelical-fold deficiency, "lop ear"
2. Conchal bowl excess, "cup ear"
3. Stahl's ear
4. Outstanding lobule

MUSTARDÉ SUTURES[14]

* Used to create an antihelical fold
* Horizontal mattress sutures 15 mm anteroposteriorly × 10 mm superoinferiorly
* 2 mm between sutures, usually 3 or 4 sutures in total

FURNAS SUTURES[15]

* Shaving or resection of cartilage in the conchal bowl allows retrodisplacement of the auricle and suspension to the mastoid periosteum, usually three sutures
* Medialization without retrodisplacement may stenose external auditory meatus
* Excessive medialization of the middle suture may cause telephone-ear deformity

STAHL'S EAR

* Difficult to correct
* May require wedge or star-shaped resection

OUTSTANDING LOBULE

* Dissection of the cauda helicis as an inferiorly based cartilage flap
* Posterior suture fixation to the conchal bowl may help rotate the lobule inferomedially

MICROTIA REPAIR CONSIDERATIONS (See *Cummings Otolaryngology*, 6th ed., Chapter 193)

* Best undertaken at age 10 or older so that the patient can participate in care and has sufficient costal cartilage to construct an auricular skeleton
* Canal atresia repair undertaken after microtia repair to avoid disruption of blood supply before auricular reconstructive surgery

BRENT TECHNIQUE (FOUR STAGE)[16]

1. Construction and placement of costal cartilage construct: taken from synchondrosis of ribs seven and eight, with the ninth rib cartilage used for the helical rim
2. Lobule transposition: modified Z-plasty used to transfer the "peanut" remnant from the anterior vertical position to the inferior horizontal position; cartilage is removed from the remnant at this time
3. Elevation of auricle: a split-thickness skin graft (STSG) from the groin is used to create the postauricular sulcus
4. Tragal reconstruction: contralateral conchal bowl composite graft and postauricular skin graft taken to create tragus and line conchal bowl

NAGATA TECHNIQUE (TWO STAGE)[17]

1. Construction and placement of costal cartilage construct, which includes a tragus carved from costal cartilage, and simultaneous lobule transposition
2. Elevation of the auricle and placement of a pedicled temporoparietal fascia flap (TPFF) along with STSG, which may be harvested from the shaved parietal scalp, in continuity with the full-thickness skin overlying the costal cartilage construct

POROUS POLYETHYLENE IMPLANTATION

- Implant use avoids costal cartilage harvesting and carving; higher rate of extrusion
- Requires a two-stage procedure: placement and elevation
- TPFF may be used to improve vascularity

AURICULAR PROSTHESIS

- May be secured with adhesive or via osseointegrated implants and magnets
- May require two prostheses if patients have fair skin that changes color significantly between spring/summer and fall/winter

COMPLICATIONS OF MICROTIA REPAIR

1. Skin breakdown and cartilage erosion
   - Typically at the superior helical rim
   - May require multiple revisions
   - TPFF and STSG coverage of exposed cartilage as soon as possible
2. Migration of implant or costal cartilage, particularly antero-inferiorly onto the cheek
3. Facial nerve injury because of lack of predictable anatomical course with a maldeveloped ear
4. Hairy ear because of low hairline and placement of an implant or construct under hair-bearing scalp; treat with laser hair removal

CLEFT LIP

CLEFT LIP ANATOMY (See *Cummings Otolaryngology*, 6th ed., Chapter 187)

- Incomplete orbicularis oris sphincter: muscle parallels cleft margin and inserts into the nasal sill
- Septum deviated toward the cleft
- Nasal tip and base of columella deviate away from the cleft
- Nostril on the cleft side is flattened and stretched inferiorly and laterally

CLEFT LIP RULE OF 10s

1. Repair when child weighs 10 lbs
2. Child is 10 weeks old
3. Child has a hemoglobin of ≥10 mg/dL

CLEFT LIP SURGICAL CONSIDERATIONS

- Preoperative care may improve surgical results
  - Lip adhesion of the superior aspect of the cleft may help narrow the soft-tissue defect
  - Lip taping also acts as a tissue expander to help narrow the cleft preoperatively
  - Presurgical nasoalveolar molding may also improve nasal morphology
- Millard advancement-rotation technique most common for unilateral cleft lip (Fig. 3.5)[18]
  - Reconstructs the philtral column and cupid's bow
  - Rotation of tissue from the noncleft side and advancement from the cleft side
  - Important to reconstruct the orbicularis oris
- Primary rhinoplasty is often performed at time of lip repair
  - Goals are to improve tip projection, narrow the alar base, straighten the caudal septum, and reshape the cleft-side lower lateral cartilage
  - Definitive rhinoplasty may be performed during teenage years
- Bilateral cleft lip repair
  - A narrow central prolabial flap is elevated, and the lateral lip elements are advanced medially

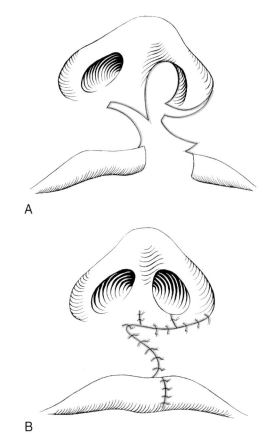

FIGURE 3.5 Millard Advancement-Rotation Technique for Repair of Unilateral Cleft Lip. (**A**) Rotation-advancement technique: flaps incised and elevated. (**B**) Rotation-advancement technique: final suturing. (From Flint PW, Haughey BH, Lund VJ, et al. *Cummings Otolaryngology—Head and Neck Surgery*. 6th ed. Philadelphia, PA: Saunders; 2015, fig. 187-24.)

- Primary rhinoplasty provides tip projection and support via interdomal sutures and suspension of the lower lateral cartilages to the upper lateral cartilages
- Restore complete orbicularis oris sphincter
- Facial symmetry is easier to obtain with bilateral cleft lip repair than with unilateral, although nasal projection is more difficult

SCAR REVISION

SCAR REVISION CONSIDERATIONS
(See *Cummings Otolaryngology*, 6th ed., Chapter 21)

- Scars take ~12 months to mature, but may continue to improve spontaneously for 1-3 years
- Important to protect from sun exposure for the first 12 months
- Can revise as early as 2 months if poor healing is obvious
- Early pulsed-dye laser treatment will help decrease erythema, as early as 3 weeks after injury/surgery

SCAR MANAGEMENT OPTIONS

1. Massage
2. Topical therapy: vitamin E oil, over-the-counter and prescription scar creams with moisturizer, and steroids
3. Silicone sheeting: apply 12 hours/day for 6 months
4. Resurfacing
5. Laser or dermabrasion, as discussed in the section on skin resurfacing
6. Surgical revision

RELAXED SKIN TENSION LINES (Fig. 3.6)

- Relaxed skin tension lines (RSTLs) follow furrows formed when the skin is relaxed
- RSTLs run perpendicular to the direction of underlying muscle contraction

- Incisions made parallel to tension lines heal better than those made tangentially to tension lines

OPERATIVE REVISION

1. Z-plasty
2. W-plasty
3. Geometric broken line closure: a series of geometric shapes to break up the line of a scar
4. M-plasty: allows shortening of the long axis of fusiform excisions
5. V to Y advancement: lengthens the scar without changing orientation
6. A to T-plasty: variant of V to Y advancement that aids restoration of facial subunit boundaries, such as the vermilion border
7. O to Z-plasty

Z-PLASTY (Fig. 3.7)

- Angles
  - 30-degree angle lengthens the scar by 25% and rotates by 30 degrees
  - 45-degree angle lengthens the scar by 50% and rotates by 60 degrees
  - 60-degree angle lengthens the scar by 75% and rotates by 90 degrees
- Combine serial Z-plasties along the scar to interdigitate wound edges and camouflage the scar better
- Z-plasties with angles <30 degrees may have skin necrosis at the tip
- Z-plasties with angles >60 degrees may result in standing cutaneous cone deformities
- If a Z-plasty of >60 degrees is necessary, two 60-degree Z-plasties may be compounded to achieve the effect of 120 degrees without standing cutaneous deformities

W-PLASTY

- Zig-zag excision provides an erratic scar that diffuses light
- Best for scars >2 cm in length
- Allows oblique or curvilinear scars to be broken down into small segments, parallel to RSTLs
- Each limb should not exceed 6 mm
  - <3 mm per limb will cause loss of irregularization as the scar contracts into a straight line
  - ≤90-degree angles

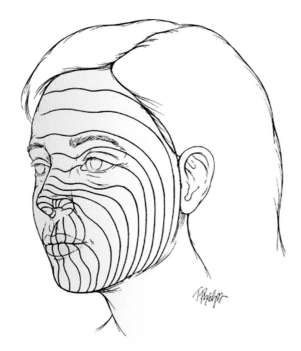

FIGURE 3.6 Relaxed Skin Tension Lines. (From Flint PW, Haughey BH, Lund VJ, et al. *Cummings Otolaryngology—Head and Neck Surgery*. 6th ed. Philadelphia, PA: Saunders; 2015, fig. 19-11.)

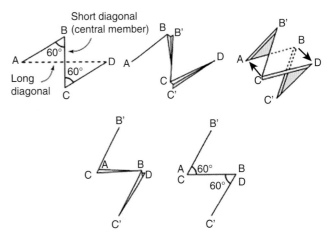

FIGURE 3.7 Z-Plasty. (From Flint PW, Haughey BH, Lund VJ, et al. *Cummings Otolaryngology—Head and Neck Surgery*. 6th ed. Philadelphia, PA: Saunders; 2015, fig. 21-6.)

O TO Z-PLASTY

- Not a true Z-plasty
- Dual advancement-rotation flaps allow closure of a circular defect
- Three flaps may be used if necessary

KELOID TREATMENT CONSIDERATIONS

- Multimodality treatment is preferred
- Preoperative intralesional steroid injection 3 times, separated by 6 weeks
- Subtotal resection with primary closure
  - Subtotal resection with positive margins all around prevents violation of virgin tissue
  - Elevation of overlying skin flaps away from the keloid, rather than resection of the skin and keloid en bloc, allows primary closure and obviates need for and risk associated with skin graft harvest[19]
- Postoperative pressure therapy, particularly in ear lobule keloids, may help
- Silicone sheeting

ADJUNCTIVE KELOID TREATMENT

1. Immediate postoperative electron-beam radiation therapy
2. Laser treatment, such as fractionated Er:YAG
3. Intralesional 5-fluorouracil

RECONSTRUCTIVE OPTIONS
(See *Cummings Otolaryngology*, 6th ed., Chapter 24)

THE RECONSTRUCTIVE LADDER[20]

1. Wound healing by secondary intention: allows granulation tissue to fill a defect
2. Primary closure
3. Delayed primary closure: allows granulation tissue to progress until the area is sufficiently well vascularized to permit operative closure
4. Skin graft
5. Tissue expansion
6. Local flap
7. Regional flap
8. Free flap

FOUR PHASES OF PRIMARY WOUND HEALING

1. Hemostatic: vasoconstriction and coagulation
2. Inflammatory (up to 4 days): infiltration of neutrophils, macrophages, and fibroblasts
3. Proliferative (4 days to 2 weeks)
   - Re-epithelialization
   - Neovascularization
   - Collagen deposition: type III first and then type I
   - Wound contraction: myofibroblast activity
4. Maturation (2 weeks to 2 years)
   - Type I collagen replaces type III, and fibers align in parallel
   - At 3 weeks, 15% of original tensile strength is achieved
   - At 6 weeks, 60% of original tensile strength is achieved
   - At 6 months, 70-80% of original tensile strength is achieved, which is the maximum

FACTORS THAT MAY COMPROMISE WOUND HEALING

1. Local factors
   - Infection, desiccation, hematoma, neoplasm, contamination, and radiation
2. Systemic factors
   - Malnutrition, metabolic derangement, vasculopathy, smoking, connective tissue disorders, and immunodeficiency
3. Medications
   - Steroids, nonsteroidal antiinflammatory drugs, chemotherapy, and immunosuppressive agents
4. Technical errors
   - Traumatic technique, closure under tension, and poor hemostasis

FACTORS THAT MAY IMPROVE WOUND HEALING

1. Hyperbaric oxygen
2. Nutritional supplementation
3. Debridement of contaminants and nonviable tissue
4. Appropriate dressings

THREE PHASES OF SKIN GRAFT HEALING

1. Plasmatic imbibition
2. Capillary inosculation
3. Neovascularization

SPLIT-THICKNESS SKIN GRAFT

- Epidermis and partial-thickness dermis
- Poor color and texture match
- Significant contracture
- More reliable healing than FTSG
- May remain insensate and dry
- Harvested with dermatome: upper thigh and upper arm

FULL-THICKNESS SKIN GRAFT

- Epidermis and full-thickness dermis
- Better color and texture match
- Less contracture
- Lower success rate compared with STSG
- Likely to develop sensory innervation and sebaceous function, possibly hair growth
- Harvested with scalpel: groin, post/preauricular, and supraclavicular

COMPOSITE GRAFTS

- Full-thickness skin and cartilage
- Graft size >1.5 cm leads to vascular compromise and poor healing

HISTOLOGICAL CHANGES FROM TISSUE EXPANDERS

- Increased vascularity leads to potential for increased flap length to width ratio
- Epidermis thickens
- Dermis thins
- Subcutaneous fat thins
- Muscle thins
- Fibrous capsule with vascular network develops
- Underlying bone may resorb

INTERNAL TISSUE EXPANSION

- Silastic balloon with resealable injection port for normal saline; use before tissue is resected
- May be used briefly during surgery (for 20 minutes) to augment skin creep; skin lengthens by stretching collagen fibers and displacing interstitial fluid
- Make incisions for expander placement along the margins of the planned excision
  - Avoid disrupting major blood vessels or cutaneous nerves
  - May leave sutures in place for the duration of the expansion
- Fill 10% of the expander's volume at time of surgery
- Add volume as tolerated 1-2 times per week for 6-8 weeks
  - Pain level and stress relaxation determine frequency of expansion; ability of skin strain to decrease while skin is under constant tension
  - Begin expansion 10-14 days after surgery
  - Wound dehiscence is not an absolute contraindication to further expansion; however, further expansion may serve only to widen the dehiscence
  - Plan to produce 10% more expanded tissue than needed to cover the base of the defect

EXTERNAL TISSUE EXPANSION

- Skin anchors, purse-string line, and tension controller reels apply tension to approximate the wound edge
- Use after tissue is resected and the wound is open
- Tension controller does not require additional patient visits to increase tension

LOCAL FLAPS[21]

1. Random
   a. Advancement
   b. Rotation
   c. Transposition
   d. Interpolated
2. Axial

RANDOM FLAPS (Fig. 3.8)

- Blood supplied via the subdermal plexus
- Length depends on the intravascular resistance of the supplying vessels and the perfusion pressure

ADVANCEMENT FLAP

- Tissue slides to close the defect
- Undermining >4 cm will not further decrease closing tension[22]
- May align incisions in RSTLs
- Unipedicle
- Bipedicle
- V to Y
- Y to V
- A to T
- Subcutaneously pedicled island

ROTATION FLAP

- Tissue pivots around a point
- Increasing arc of rotation to >90 degrees will not further decrease closing tension
- Standing cutaneous deformity will occur at the base of the flap: Burow's triangle excision is required
- Difficult to align in RSTLs
- O to Z: for scalp reconstruction
- Rieger dorsal nasal flap: for reconstruction of midnasal dorsal defects up to 2 cm

- Tenzel semicircular flap: for reconstruction of eyelid defects up to 50% of eyelid width; may require periosteal release for larger defects

TRANSPOSITION FLAP

- Also pivots around a point and creates a standing cutaneous cone
- Length of random transposition flap should not exceed 3 times its width
- Difficult to align in RSTLs
- Flap rotation decreases the effective length
  - Rotating a flap by 45 degrees reduces length by 5%
  - Rotating a flap by 90 degrees reduces length by 15%
  - Rotating a flap by 180 degrees reduces length by 40%
- Rhombic (Fig. 3.9)
  - Limberg
  - Uses a rhombus with 120-degree and 60-degree angles
  - Rotates through 60 degrees
- Dufourmental modification
  - Variable angles within a rhombus
  - Variable arc of rotation
  - Spares more tissue
- Note flap
  - Variant of rhombic flap to close a circular defect
- Bilobe (Fig. 3.10)
  - Zitelli modification[23]
    - Rotation through 90 degrees instead of 180 degrees
    - First lobe is equal to the size of the defect
    - Second lobe may be slightly smaller
    - Good for repair of nasal defects <1.5 cm; base flap laterally on nose when possible
    - Also good for lateral cheek defects up to 6 cm
- Z-plasty

INTERPOLATED FLAP

- Flap is advanced and/or rotated over normal tissue
- Requires a second stage to take down the pedicle and complete the inset of the flap
- Melolabial flap: good for reconstruction of the medial cheek and nasal alar defects
- Hughes tarsoconjunctival flap
  - Tarsal plate and conjunctiva of the upper eyelid are used to reconstruct 50-100% of the defect in the lower lid
  - Requires advancement of skin from cheek
- Cutler-Beard flap: full-thickness advancement of the lower lid into 50-100% of the upper-eyelid defect

AXIAL FLAP

- Blood supplied by named vessel
- Length-to-width ratio of the flap may exceed 4:1
- Paramedian forehead
  - Good for reconstruction of nasal tip defects >1.5 cm
  - Based on the supratrochlear artery: located 15-20 mm lateral to midline
- Facial artery musculomucosal
  - Good for reconstruction of intraoral or nasal defects
  - Mucosa and buccinator muscle pedicled on the facial artery
  - May be based on anterograde or retrograde flow in the facial artery
- TPFF
  - Good for providing bulk or a barrier in the face or auricle: used in microtia and Frey's syndrome
  - Based on the superficial temporal artery
- Temporalis muscle
  - May be used for facial reanimation
  - Based on middle temporal arteries

- Lip switch
  - Based on the labial artery
  - Flap width is 50% of the defect width
  - Rotated through 180 degrees
  - May reconstruct 50% of the lip width
  - Abbé flap: for reconstruction of full-thickness lip defects

- Estlander
  - For defects involving oral commissure
  - Blunts oral commissure
  - Does not require a procedure to take down the pedicle
  - Secondary commissuroplasty may be performed

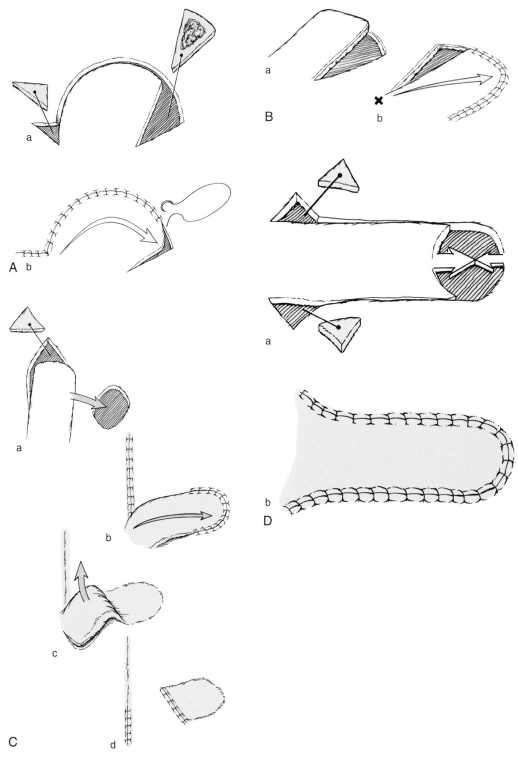

FIGURE 3.8 Types of Local Flaps. (**A**) Rotation flap, (**B**) transposition flap, (**C**) interpolated flap, and (**D**) advancement flap. (From Flint PW, Haughey BH, Lund VJ, et al. *Cummings Otolaryngology—Head and Neck Surgery*. 6th ed. Philadelphia, PA: Saunders; 2015, figs. 24-3, 24-4, 24-5, 24-6). (**A**) From Baker SR, Swanson N. *Local Flaps in Facial Reconstruction*. St. Louis, MO: Mosby; 1995. (**B**) Adapted from Baker SR, Swanson N. *Local Flaps in Facial Reconstruction*. St. Louis, MO: Mosby; 1995. (**C**) From Flint PW, Haughey BH, Lund VJ, et al. *Cummings Otolaryngology—Head and Neck Surgery*. 6th ed. Philadelphia, PA: Saunders; 2015. (**D**) Modified from Baker SR, Swanson N. *Local Flaps in Facial Reconstruction*. St. Louis, MO: Mosby; 1995.

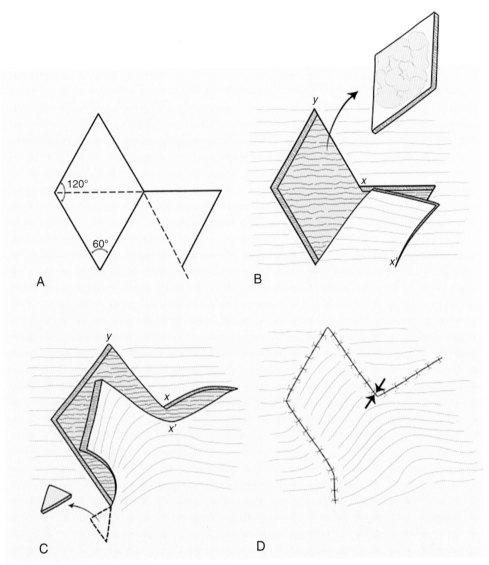

FIGURE 3.9 (A) Limberg flap design; (**B**) defect is modified so configuration is 60-120-degree rhombus; (**C**) flap transposed; standing cutaneous deformity excised; (**D**) primary vector of tension is approximately parallel to the original border of the defect adjacent to the flap (*opposing arrows*); standing cutaneous deformity excised at base of flap. (From Shan R. Baker: *Local Flaps in Facial Reconstruction.* 3rd ed. Philadelphia, PA: Saunders Elsevier; 2014.)

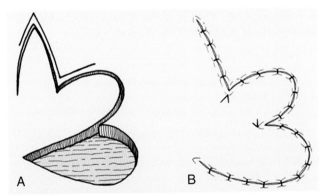

FIGURE 3.10 Bilobe Flap. (**A**) Bilobe flap incisions. Note the acute angle at the left of the defect; this is where the standing cutaneous deformity would occur. (**B**) Flap transposed and defect closed. (From Shan R. Baker: *Local Flaps in Facial Reconstruction.* 3rd ed. Philadelphia, PA: Saunders Elsevier; 2014.)

- Karapandzic flap[24]
  - Based on labial arteries
  - May reconstruct up to two-thirds of the lip width
  - Oral sphincter function is preserved
  - Produces microstomia
- Gillies fan and McGregor flaps
  - Based on labial arteries
  - May reconstruct full lip defects of the lower (Gillies) and upper (McGregor) lips

REGIONAL FLAP EXAMPLES

- Pectoralis myocutaneous
  - Based on the pectoral branch of the thoracoacromial artery
  - Pectoralis major muscle may be taken with overlying fascia with or without skin
- Deltopectoral flap
  - Based on second, third, and fourth perforators off the internal mammary artery
  - Most distal portion may be randomly based and therefore less reliable if harvested over the deltoid

- Submental island flap
  - Based on the submental artery
    - May be harvested with anterograde or retrograde flow, or as a free flap
    - May include platysma or just skin and subcutaneous tissue
- Supraclavicular artery island flap
  - Based on the supraclavicular artery
  - Pliable flap with a 180-degree arc of rotation

FREE FLAP EXAMPLES[25]

- Radial forearm
  - Based on the radial artery
  - May include nearly all of the forearm skin, except for the skin overlying the ulnar artery
  - May include up to 40% of the thickness of the radius, but is poor bone stock for dental implants
  - Sensation through the lateral antebrachial cutaneous nerve
  - Perform preoperative Allen's test to avoid devascularization of the hand
- Anterolateral thigh
  - Based on septocutaneous or musculocutaneous perforators of the lateral circumflex femoral artery
  - Up to 20 × 30 cm of skin
  - Sensation through the lateral femoral cutaneous nerve
- Fibula
  - Based on the peroneal artery
  - Up to 30 cm of bone
    - Leave 6-7 cm of bone intact distally proximally to stabilize the ankle and protect the common peroneal nerve
    - Best for reconstruction of the mandible and placement of dental implants
  - Sensation through the lateral sural cutaneous nerve
  - Injury to the peroneal nerve may cause foot drop
- Iliac crest
  - Based on the deep circumflex iliac artery
  - May include bone stock for dental implants
  - Harvest may cause hernia or gait disturbance
- Scapula
  - Based on the circumflex scapular artery
  - May include bone for palatal or mandibular reconstruction
    - Not usually thick enough for dental implants
  - May be harvested with the latissimus dorsi as a "mega flap" for greater soft-tissue coverage
- Latissimus dorsi
  - Based on the thoracodorsal artery
  - Thoracodorsal nerve may be used to innervate the latissimus dorsi for reanimation
- Deep inferior epigastric perforator
  - Based on deep inferior epigastric perforating vessels
  - Includes skin and subcutaneous tissue but no muscle
- Gracilis
  - Based on the adductor artery
  - Innervated by the obturator nerve
  - May include overlying skin
  - Ideal for facial reanimation

COMPOSITE TISSUE ALLOGRAFTS (FACIAL TRANSPLANTATION)[26]

- Type I: lower central face, including the nose, lips, and chin
- Type II: midface, including the nose, upper lip, and cheeks (soft tissue with or without maxilla)
- Type III: upper face, including the forehead, eyelids, and root of the nose
- Type IV: total facial skin
- Type V: full facial, including complete soft tissue, with or without maxilla and/or mandible

- Entire graft may be perfused via a single facial artery
- Sensory function returns even without trigeminal neurorrhaphy
- Motor coordination is improved (less synkinesis) with distal facial branch neurorrhaphies rather than main trunk neurorrhaphy
- Results are comparable to or better than homograft neural reconstruction, likely because of tacrolimus

FACIAL PARALYSIS (See *Cummings Otolaryngology*, 6th ed., Chapter 172)

DIFFERENTIAL DIAGNOSIS FOR ACUTE FACIAL PALSY[27]

1. Bell's palsy
2. Iatrogenic injury
3. Ramsay Hunt syndrome
4. Temporal bone fracture
5. Soft-tissue injury
6. Lyme disease
7. Central nervous system (CNS) lesion
8. Autoimmune disease (eg, Melkersson-Rosenthal, Guillain-Barré, and sarcoidosis)
9. Otologic disease (acute otitis media and cholesteatoma)
10. Stroke
    - Brainstem stroke presents as hemifacial palsy ipsilateral to stroke because of involvement of the facial nucleus
    - Cortical stroke presents as mid and lower facial palsy contralateral to stroke
11. Neoplasm (usually presents with insidious onset but not always)

HOUSE-BRACKMANN FACIAL NERVE GRADING SYSTEM[28]

1. House-Brackmann (HB) I: normal
2. HB II: mild asymmetry with movement, symmetric at rest, complete eye closure with gentle effort, and slight synkinesis
3. HB III: obvious asymmetry with movement, symmetric at rest, complete eye closure with full effort, and noticeable synkinesis
4. HB IV: obvious asymmetry with movement, symmetric at rest, and incomplete eye closure
5. HB V: minimal movement and asymmetric at rest
6. HB VI: no movement

SUNDERLAND (SEDDON) CLASSIFICATION OF PERIPHERAL NERVE INJURIES[29,30]

1. Class I (neurapraxia): conduction block with anticipated complete recovery
2. Class II (axonotmesis): endoneurium intact with anticipated complete recovery
3. Class III (axonotmesis): perineurium intact with anticipated synkinesis
4. Class IV (axonotmesis): epineurium intact with anticipated synkinesis
5. Class V (neurotmesis): nerve transected; will require neurorrhaphy
6. Class VI (mixed injury): crush and transection components, with variable prognosis

ANATOMY OF THE FACIAL NERVE

- Exits the brainstem at the pontomedullary junction with the cochleovestibular nerve
- Intracanalicular (meatal) segment in the internal auditory canal (8-10 mm in length)

- Labyrinthine segment between the fundus of the internal auditory canal and geniculate ganglion
  - Narrowest portion of the facial nerve: diameter of the fallopian canal decreases from 1.2 to 0.7 mm
  - 2-4 mm in length
  - Segmented inflamed in Bell's palsy
- Tympanic (horizontal) segment 11 mm in length
  - Passes over the oval window/stapes footplate
- Mastoid (vertical) segment 12-14 mm in length
  - Gives off chorda tympani
- Exits the temporal bone via the stylomastoid foramen
- Divides into five main branches within the parotid gland, separating deep and superficial lobes
- Frontal (temporal branch) exits the superior aspect of the parotid and traverses the zygomatic arch
  - Travels on the deep surface of TPF, which is tightly adherent to the periosteum of the zygomatic arch
  - Passes across the brow from inferoposterior to superoanterior to innervate the frontalis muscle
    - Runs along Pitanguy's line from 5 mm inferior to the tragus to 15 mm above the lateral extent of the brow[31]
- Midfacial branches (zygomatic and buccal) exit the anterior surface of the parotid, traveling on the superficial surface of the masseteric fascia
  - Significant redundancy because of neural anastomoses
  - Midfacial branch transection injuries do not need to be repaired if they occur anterior to the lateral canthus
  - Transverse facial vessels course superior to parotid duct, near buccal branches
  - Mimetic muscles are innervated from the deep surface except for the mentalis, levator labii superioris (quadratus labii), and buccinator
- Marginal mandibular and cervical branches exit the inferior aspect of the parotid
  - Marginal mandibular branch crosses into the submandibular space at the gonial notch, along with facial vessels, and follows them back toward the oral commissure anteriorly
    - Closely associated with and often wrapped around the facial vein
    - Innervates the depressor labii inferioris, depressor anguli oris, and mentalis
  - Cervical branch innervates the platysma

BRANCHES OF THE FACIAL NERVE

1. Greater superficial petrosal nerve
2. Nerve to the stapedius muscle
3. Sensory auricular branch of the facial nerve
4. Chorda tympani nerve
5. Branches to auricular muscles
6. Nerve to the posterior belly of the digastric muscle
7. Nerve to the stylohyoid muscle
8. Temporal/frontal branch
9. Zygomatic branch
10. Buccal branch
11. Marginal mandibular branch
12. Cervical branch

SURGICAL METHODS TO FIND THE FACIAL NERVE

1. 1-cm deep, 1-cm inferior, and 1-cm anterior to the tragal pointer
2. Just to the posterior belly of the digastric (use as a depth indicator with the tragal pointer as direction indicator)
3. 1-cm deep to the proximal end of the tympanomastoid suture line
4. Locate a vertical segment in the mastoid and follow it distally
5. Locate a distal branch in the midface and follow it proximally

FACIAL NERVE EXPLORATION AND DECOMPRESSION[32]

- Electrodiagnostic testing should be performed for complete hemifacial paralysis of sudden onset (immediate onset in case of trauma)
  - If electroneuronography (ENoG) shows ≥90% degeneration, perform electromyography (EMG)
  - If EMG shows no voluntary motor units, consider exploration or decompression
- If the nerve is injured across >50% of its diameter, resect the injured segment and repair primarily
- If tension-free neurorrhaphy cannot be performed, place an interposition (cable) graft
  - Harvest from the greater auricular, sural, or medial antebrachial cutaneous nerve
  - Reverse the direction of the graft to minimize axonal loss through the branches

FACIAL REINNERVATION

- Repair of facial nerve injuries must be accomplished early so that axons can regrow before muscle begins to atrophy
  - Axons grow at 1 mm/day
  - Facial muscles atrophy irreversibly after 12-18 months of denervation
- Coapting a donor nerve to the main trunk of the facial nerve will result in severe synkinesis, which may be worse than paralysis
  - Neural coaptation should be done with a specific muscle target in mind, such as the orbicularis oculi or zygomaticus major, to maximize functional recovery
- Cross face nerve grafting
- Cranial nerve transpositions
  - Hypoglossal-facial neurorrhaphy
  - Masseteric-facial neurorrhaphy
  - Deep temporal-facial neurorrhaphy

FACIAL REANIMATION

- First priority is corneal protection
- Static reanimation
  - Brow lift
  - Eyelid weight
  - Tarsal strip, canthopexy, and tarsorrhaphy
  - Fascia lata/Gore-Tex sling
  - Chemodenervation with botulinum toxin may improve symmetry by weakening overactive areas on the unaffected side or by releasing synkinetic muscle spasm on the ipsilateral side
- Dynamic reanimation
  - Gracilis free muscle transfer
    - Innervated by contralateral facial nerve input via the cross face nerve graft
      (1) Not for use in patients with bilateral facial paralysis or potential to develop it; for example, neurofibromatosis type II
      (2) Provides spontaneous smile
    - Innervated by the ipsilateral masseteric nerve
      (1) Requires jaw clenching to smile
  - Latissimus dorsi free muscle transfer
  - Pectoralis minor free muscle transfer

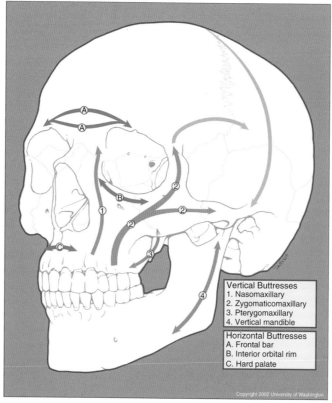

FIGURE 3.11 Buttresses of the Facial Skeleton. (From Som PM, Curtin HD. *Head and Neck Imaging*. 5th ed. St. Louis, MO: Mosby; 2011.)

- Temporalis muscle transfer
  - As a rotational flap with superior aspect is rotated over the zygomatic arch and secured to the oral commissure
  - As an advancement flap with the coronoid process of the mandible is detached and sutured to the oral commissure
  - Provides less oral commissure excursion during smiling compared with free muscle transfer

MAXILLOFACIAL TRAUMA (See *Cummings Otolaryngology*, 6th ed., Chapters 22, 23, and 121)

FACIAL BUTTRESS CHARACTERISTICS

- Pillars of the maxillofacial skeleton that provide structural support (Fig. 3.11)
- Commonly recognized facial fracture patterns in the midface follow the buttresses

VERTICAL BUTTRESSES OF THE FACE

1. Nasomaxillary
2. Zygomaticomaxillary
3. Pterygomaxillary
4. Ramus/condyle unit of mandible

HORIZONTAL BUTTRESSES OF THE FACE

1. Frontal bar
2. Infraorbital rims

3. Maxilla/hard palate
4. Mandibular body

FACIAL SKELETAL PROPORTIONS

- Facial width determined by bizygomatic and intergonial distances
  - Inadequate reduction of zygomatic or mandibular fractures can result in a widened face
- Facial height is determined by vertical buttresses and the mandibular ramus/condyle unit
  - Inadequate reduction of Le Fort injuries and mandibular ramus/condyle fractures can result in abnormal height

FRONTAL SINUS FRACTURE

- Anterior and posterior tables
  - Nondisplaced: no treatment necessary
  - If displaced more than one table width, open reduction is required
- Nasofrontal outflow tract injury
  - May be identified on sagittal or coronal slices on computed tomography (CT)
  - If injured, obliterate the duct
  - Frontal sinus mucocele: may occur if the nasofrontal duct is not obliterated or if the sinus lining is not completely extirpated after injury
- CSF leak
  - Presents with rhinorrhea
  - Evaluate using halo test, glucose level, or β-2 transferrin assay
  - Metrizamide CT detects other sources of CSF leak
  - Observe for 7-10 days to see if the leak resolves in the setting of a nondisplaced fracture

* Consider a lumbar drain
* Cranialization of the frontal sinus with galeal and pericranial flaps, repair of dural tear, and lumbar drain for displaced fracture

NASO-ORBITO-ETHMOID FRACTURE PRESENTING SIGNS

1. Telecanthus
   * Intercanthal distance >40 mm
   * Distinguish from hypertelorism, which is an increased intraorbital distance
2. Saddle nose deformity
3. Epiphora

MARKOWITZ-MANSON NASO-ORBITO-ETHMOID FRACTURE CLASSIFICATION (Fig. 3.12)[33]

1. Type I: single central fragment with the medial canthal tendon attached—treatment is open reduction and internal fixation (ORIF) if displaced, via a coronal incision
2. Type II: comminuted central fragment, medial canthal tendon attached—treatment is ORIF if displaced
3. Type III: comminuted with disruption of medial canthal attachment—treatment is ORIF with an open transnasal medial canthoplasty

ORBITAL FRACTURE–ASSOCIATED INJURIES

* Globe injury
  * Anisocoria, ocular pain, visual acuity changes, and diplopia
* Traumatic optic neuropathy
  * From shear force on the optic nerve
  * Mild injury may present with diminished color perception and afferent pupillary defect
  * Severe injury may cause blindness
  * Steroids: possible orbital canal decompression
* Superior orbital fissure (SOF) versus orbital apex syndrome
  * SOF syndrome: only cranial nerves III, IV, V_1, and VI are affected
  * Orbital apex syndrome: the same nerves affected by SOF syndrome plus the optic nerve are affected

ABSOLUTE INDICATIONS FOR ORBITAL FLOOR FRACTURE REPAIR

1. Entrapment: presents with diplopia, nausea, bradycardia, and pain
2. Loss of >50% of the orbital floor or fracture size >1.5 cm^2
3. Persistent diplopia in the absence of other causes (>2 weeks)
4. Enophthalmos ≥2 mm

ORBITAL FLOOR FRACTURE CONSIDERATIONS

* Relative indication for repair: mild diplopia (within 20-30 degrees of primary gaze)
* Repair is best approached via a transconjunctival incision
  * Preseptal approach facilitates elevation of the floor periorbita
  * Endoscope may improve visualization
* Medial-wall fractures
  * Lamina papyracea of the ethmoid bone fractures easily because of its paper-like thinness
  * Use a transcaruncular approach (superficial to the septum and deep to Horner's muscle) to access the medial orbit

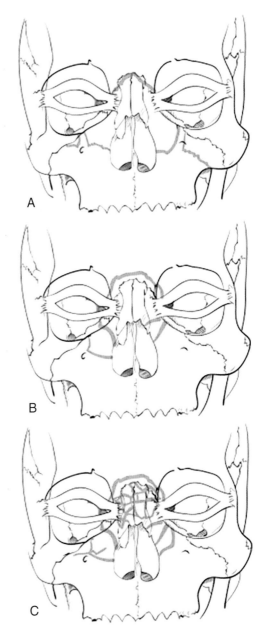

FIGURE 3.12 Markowitz-Manson Classification of Naso-Orbito-Ethmoid Fractures. (**A**) Type I, (**B**) Type II, (**C**) Type III. (From Flint PW, Haughey BH, Lund VJ, et al. *Cummings Otolaryngology—Head and Neck Surgery*. 6th ed. Philadelphia, PA: Saunders; 2015, fig. 23-13. Modified from Markowitz BL, Manson PN, Sargent L, et al. Management of the medial canthal tendon in nasoethmoid orbital fractures: the importance of the central fragment in classification and treatment. *Plast Reconstr Surg*. 1991;87:843-853.)

NASAL FRACTURE

* Management: closed reduction, intranasal packing, and external casting; may require osteotomies with closed reduction if bones have begun to set, usually 7-14 days after injury
* Septal fracture: closed reduction with internal splints
* If unsuccessful, will need definitive rhinoplasty 6-12 months later

ZYGOMATIC FRACTURE

* The zygomatic bone has four articulations
  * Zygomaticofrontal
  * Zygomaticosphenoid
  * Zygomaticotemporal
  * Zygomaticomaxillary

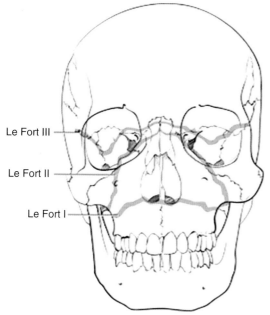

FIGURE 3.13 Le Fort Classification of Midfacial Fractures. (From Flint PW, Haughey BH, Lund VJ, et al. *Cummings Otolaryngology—Head and Neck Surgery.* 6th ed. Philadelphia, PA: Saunders; 2015, fig. 23-12.)

- Zygomaticomaxillary complex (ZMC) (tripod) fracture disrupts all four
- Reduction of a ZMC fracture requires restoration of all four articulations
  - Zygomaticosphenoid alignment is the most reliable method of ensuring adequate reduction
  - Inadequate reduction may cause inappropriate midfacial width, malar flattening, and vertical dystopia
  - Upper and lower eyelid and gingivobuccal sulcus incisions provide access for ORIF; coronal approach can be used to access the arch
  - Zygomatic arch fracture disrupts the zygomaticotemporal joint and may cause trismus from impingement on the temporalis tendon/coronoid process
  - Isolated arch fractures can be approached via an incision in the temporal scalp (Gillies) with placement of an elevator at the depth of the temporalis fascia to avoid frontal branch injury, or by an intraoral approach (Keen)

LE FORT MIDFACIAL FRACTURE CLASSIFICATION (Fig. 3.13)

1. Le Fort I: separates the maxillary dentoalveolar segment and palate from the midface
2. Le Fort II: separates the maxilla and nasal complex from the facial skeleton
3. Le Fort III: separates the facial skeleton from the skull, and includes NOE fracture

LE FORT FRACTURE CHARACTERISTICS

- All three patterns include pterygoid plate fractures
- Present with malocclusion, typically an open bite because of posterosuperior displacement of the maxilla
- Displaced fractures with associated malocclusion should be managed with ORIF
- Incomplete fractures may require osteotomies to mobilize the midface and allow for adequate reduction
- Fractures with a palatal split should be managed with reestablishment of the transverse width and occlusion using a palatal plate or an acrylic dental splint

MANDIBLE FRACTURE

- Often present with malocclusion (prematurity and open bite)
- Management options are based on anticipated patient compliance and fracture type
- Nondisplaced fractures without malocclusion in a reliable patient are often managed with a soft diet
- Displaced fractures in the dentate mandible are managed with 4-6 weeks of maxillomandibular fixation (MMF) or ORIF
  - Rigid fixation requires an inferior border plate with bicortical screws and a tension band on the superior margin of the mandible (miniplate or arch bar)
- Displaced fractures of the mandibular angle are managed with ORIF: a semirigid fixation (Champy) involves a single miniplate along the oblique line,[34] which requires a soft diet unless another plate is placed along the inferior border
- Teeth in the line of the fracture: should be removed when they interfere with reduction or are fractured, loose, or do not have a functional use (ie, no opposing tooth)
- Consider ORIF in patients with seizure disorders, high risk for vomiting, or poor likelihood of follow-up
- Edentulous fractures can be managed with Gunning splints (dentures that allow for MMF); displaced fractures of the atrophic, edentulous mandible may require ORIF with bone grafting
- Generally, consider the shortest possible interval for MMF to allow for adequate mobilization after surgery
  - 7-10 days: intracapsular condylar fractures
  - 2-4 weeks: after ORIF of an angle fracture with a Champy plate
  - 4-6 weeks: fractures managed by closed reduction
  - No MMF is required if ORIF is performed
- Arch bars may be used for placement of guiding elastics and to assist with physical therapy (eg, for subcondylar injuries)

CONDYLAR HEAD FRACTURE

- Intracapsular injuries are managed with 7-10 days of MMF if there is malocclusion
- If no malocclusion, soft diet and early mobilization
- Longer periods of MMF may result in temporomandibular joint ankyloses
- Condylar/subcondylar injuries are managed closed if minimally displaced

ZIDE AND KENT ABSOLUTE INDICATIONS FOR OPEN REDUCTION AND INTERNAL FIXATION OF CONDYLAR/SUBCONDYLAR FRACTURES[35]

1. Condylar displacement into the middle cranial fossa or external auditory canal
2. Inadequate occlusion with closed reduction
3. Lateral extracapsular condylar displacement
4. Intraarticular invasion with a foreign body (eg, bullet)

ZIDE AND KENT RELATIVE INDICATIONS FOR OPEN REDUCTION AND INTERNAL FIXATION OF CONDYLAR/SUBCONDYLAR FRACTURES[35]

1. Bilateral subcondylar fractures with comminuted midface, edentulous patient, or prior malocclusion
2. If splinting is not recommended, ORIF is indicated

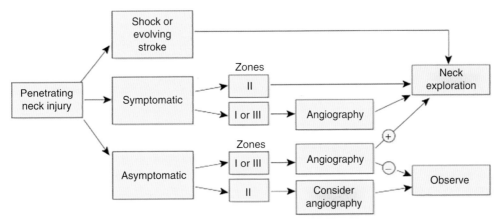

FIGURE 3.14 Algorithm for Management of Penetrating Neck Trauma. (From Flint PW, Haughey BH, Lund VJ, et al. *Cummings Otolaryngology—Head and Neck Surgery*. 6th ed. Philadelphia, PA: Saunders; 2015, fig. 121-4. Modified from McConnell D, Trunkey D. Management of penetrating trauma to the neck. *Adv Surg*. 1994;27:97.)

PENETRATING TRAUMA ZONES OF THE NECK (Fig. 3.14)

1. Zone I: clavicle to cricoid cartilage
   - Includes the lung apices, trachea, great vessels, esophagus, thoracic duct, cervical sympathetic trunks, cervical vertebrae, and spinal cord
   - Surgical exploration for the unstable patient, otherwise consider invasive studies (angiography, bronchoscopy, and esophagoscopy) dictated by suspicion of injury
   - Operative exploration necessary for injury to critical structures
2. Zone II: cricoid cartilage to mandibular angle
   - Includes neck vasculature, trachea/esophagus, spinal cord, and larynx
   - Role of invasive studies is debatable
   - Surgical exploration for the symptomatic or unstable patient, otherwise consider invasive studies
3. Zone III: mandibular angle to the skull base
   - Includes the neck vasculature, pharynx, and facial nerve
   - Surgical exploration for the unstable patient, otherwise consider invasive studies
   - Operative management may require mandibular disarticulation and skull-base access

SOFT-TISSUE TRAUMA

WOUND CLASSIFICATION

1. Class 1: clean (eg, surgical incision on prepped skin)
2. Class 2: clean-contaminated (eg, surgical incision in the pharynx)
3. Class 3: contaminated (eg, gross spillage of gastrointestinal contents into the wound)
4. Class 4: dirty (eg, infected wound)

TETANUS GUIDELINES

- If immunization history is unknown or series is incomplete, give vaccine
- If the wound is dirty, give tetanus immunoglobulin
- If the immunization series was completed or boosted <5 years ago, do nothing
- If the series was completed or boosted ≥5 years ago and the wound is dirty, give vaccine
- If series completed or boosted ≥5 years ago and wound clean, no vaccine required
- If series completed or boosted ≥10 years ago, give vaccine

INDICATIONS FOR ANTIBIOTICS

- Broad spectrum for class 3 and class 4 wounds, commonly human bite wounds
- Debatable for animal bites, but amoxicillin-clavulanate is often used
- Not required for most other lacerations unless debris or foreign bodies are in the wound

WOUNDS NOT TO BE CLOSED

1. Puncture wounds: wound is deeper than it is wide, and the depths are not visible
2. Grossly contaminated wounds (eg, gunshot wounds): because of the introduction of debris and foreign bodies deep into the wound tract and high infection risk
3. Delayed presentation: up to 24 hours it is generally safe to close in the head and neck, because of blood supply

LOCAL AND REGIONAL ANESTHESIA CHARACTERISTICS

- Lidocaine
  - Aminoamide anesthetic
  - Maximum dose: 7 mg/kg with epinephrine; 4 mg/kg without epinephrine
  - Onset: rapid (<1 minute)
  - Duration: 2 hours; up to 4 hours with epinephrine
  - Toxicity: CNS and cardiac
    - CNS excitation at lower doses: anxiety, circumoral paresthesia, and seizures
    - CNS depression at higher doses: lethargy, respiratory depression, and loss of consciousness
    - Cardiac: hypotension, bradycardia, arrhythmia, and cardiac arrest
- Bupivicaine
  - Aminoamide anesthetic
  - Maximum dose: 4 mg/kg (1 mL/kg of 0.25% solution)
  - Onset: slow
  - Duration: 4 hours; up to 8 hours with epinephrine
  - Toxicity: more cardiotoxic than other local anesthetics, but also CNS toxic
  - Overdose: give intralipid for cardiotoxicity

LOCAL INFILTRATION VERSUS REGIONAL BLOCKS

- Large areas: regional blocks are best
  - Avoids toxicity with large doses of locally infiltrated anesthetic
  - Avoids distortion from large volumes of infiltrated solution
  - Drawback: no hemostasis
- Small areas: local infiltration best
  - Hemostasis from epinephrine in anesthetic solution
  - Rapid onset
  - Only anesthetizes area of concern

SUTURE-TECHNIQUE CONSIDERATIONS

- Irrigate copiously before beginning closure
- Remove all foreign bodies
- Debride nonviable tissue
- Reapproximate free margins and subunit borders first (eg, vermilion border)
- Wound eversion to prevent depressed scars: vertical mattress sutures if necessary

PAROTID INJURIES

- Injury to the buccal branch of the facial nerve is common with parotid-duct injury
  - Duct runs along the line from the tragus to the midpoint of the upper lip
- Suture repair over a stent if possible
  - Remove the stent in 2-3 weeks
  - If a large segment of the duct is avulsed, replant into the buccal mucosa
  - If unable to replant because of proximal injury, ligate the duct
- Consider pressure dressing, anticholinergics, botulinum toxin, and nothing by mouth for salivary fistula or sialocele.

BURNS: CLASSIFICATION

1. Superficial/First degree: epidermal injury only; will heal with minimal to no permanent damage
2. Partial thickness/Second degree: injury extends into the dermis; causes blistering. Superficial partial thickness burns are unlikely to scar.
3. Full thickness/Third degree: full thickness through the dermis; may be conceptualized as an avulsion injury from a reconstructive standpoint
4. Fourth degree: extends into deeper structures such as muscle or bone

BURNS: TREATMENT GOALS

- Provide re-epithelialization by 14 days after injury
- Spontaneous healing or debridement/excision with or without skin grafting

ORAL COMMISSURE BURNS

- Usually occur in small children because of biting electrical cords
- Manage conservatively
  - Minimize debridement
  - Consider splinting to prevent microstomia

FROSTBITE

- Rapid rewarming is the most important treatment
- 40°C water bath for 15-30 minutes

REFERENCES

1. Glogau RG. Aesthetic and anatomic analysis of the aging skin. *Semin Cutan Med Surg.* 1996;15(3):134-138.
2. Fitzpatrick TB. The validity and practicality of sun-reactive skin types I-VI. *Arch Dermatol.* 1988;124(6):869-871.
3. Hamilton JB. Patterned loss of hair in men: types and incidence. *Ann N Y Acad Sci.* 1951;53(3):708-728.
4. Dedo DD. "How I do it"—plastic surgery: practical suggestions on facial plastic surgery: a preoperative classification of the neck for cervicofacial rhytidectomy. *Laryngoscope.* 1980;90(11, Pt 1):1894-1896.
5. Katz MI. Angle classification revisited 2: a modified Angle classification. *Am J Orthod Dentofacial Orthop.* 1992;102(3):277-284.
6. Gilbert S and McBurney E. Use of valacyclovir for herpes simplex virus-1 (HSV-1) prophylaxis after facial resurfacing: a randomized clinical trial of dosing regimens. *Dermatol Surg.* 2000;26(1):50-54.
7. Mass CS, Yu KC, Egan KK. Neuromodulators and injectable soft tissue substitutes. In: Papel ID, Frodel JL, Holt GR, et al., eds. *Facial Plastic and Reconstructive Surgery.* 3rd ed. New York, NY: Thieme; 2009:337-353.
8. Isse NG. Endoscopic facial rejuvenation: endoforehead, the functional lift. Case reports. *Aesthetic Plast Surg.* 1994;18(1):21-29.
9. Mitz V, Peyronie M. The superficial musculo-aponeurotic system (SMAS) in the parotid and cheek area. *Plast Reconstr Surg.* 1976;58(1):80-88.
10. Hamra ST. The deep-plane rhytidectomy. *Plast Reconstr Surg.* 1990;86(1):53-61.
11. Sheen JH. Spreader graft: a method of reconstructing the roof of the middle nasal vault following rhinoplasty. *Plast Reconstr Surg.* 1984;73(2):230-239.
12. Tebbetts JB. *Primary Rhinoplasty.* 2nd ed. Philadelphia, PA: Mosby; 2008.
13. Romo T, Al Moutran H, Paul BC, et al. Septal perforation—surgical aspects. Emedicine website. http://emedicine.medscape.com/article/878817-overview. Updated October 27, 2014. Accessed February 26, 2015.
14. Mustardé JC. The correction of prominent ears using simple mattress sutures. *Br J Plast Surg.* 1963;16:170-178.
15. Furnas DW. Correction of prominent ears by conchamastoid sutures. *Plast Reconstr Surg.* 1968;42(3):189-193.
16. Brent B. Auricular repair with autogenous rib cartilage grafts: two decades of experience with 600 cases. *Plast Reconstr Surg.* 1992;90(3):355-374, discussion 375-376.
17. Nagata S. A new method of total reconstruction of the auricle for microtia. *Plast Reconstr Surg.* 1993;92(2):187-201.
18. Millard Jr DR. In: *Cleft Craft.* Vols. 1-3. Boston, MA: Little Brown; 1976.
19. Qi Z, Liang W, Wang Y, et al. "X"-shaped incision and keloid skin-flap resurfacing: a new surgical method for auricle keloid excision and reconstruction. *Dermatol Surg.* 2012;38(8):1378-1382.
20. Hohman MH. Wound healing and optimization, including skin grafting, tissue expansion, and soft tissue techniques. In: Cheney ML, Hadlock TA, eds. *Facial Surgery: Plastic and Reconstructive.* 2nd ed. Boca Raton, FL: CRC Press; 2015:65-92.
21. Shan R. *Baker: Local Flaps in Facial Reconstruction.* 3rd ed. Philadelphia, PA: Saunders Elsevier; 2014.
22. Larrabee WF. A finite element model of skin deformation. *Laryngoscope.* 1986;96:399-405.
23. Zitelli JA. The bilobed flap for nasal reconstruction. *Arch Dermatol.* 1989;125(7):957-959.
24. Karapandzic M. Reconstruction of lip defects by local arterial flaps. *Br J Plast Surg.* 1974;27(1):93-97.
25. Urken ML, Cheney ML, Blackwell KE, et al. *Regional and Free Flaps for Head and Neck Reconstruction.* 2nd ed. Philadelphia, PA: Lippincott Williams & Wilkins; 2012.
26. Lengelé BG. Current concepts and future challenges in facial transplantation. *Clin Plast Surg.* 2009;36(3):507-521.
27. Hohman MH, Hadlock TA. Etiology, diagnosis, and management of facial paralysis: 2000 patients at a facial nerve center. *Laryngoscope.* 2014;124(7):E283-E293.
28. House JW, Brackmann DE. Facial nerve grading system. *Otolaryngol Head Neck Surg.* 1985;93(2):146-147.
29. Sunderland S. *Nerves and Nerve Injuries.* 2nd ed. New York, NY: Churchill Livingstone; 1978.
30. Seddon H. *Surgical Disorders of the Peripheral Nerves.* Baltimore, MD: Williams and Wilkins; 1972.

31. Pitanguy I, Ramos AS. The frontal branch of the facial nerve: the importance of its variations in face lifting. *Plast Reconstr Surg.* 1966;38(4):352-356.

32. Gantz BJ, Rubinstein JT, Gidley P, Woodworth GG. Surgical management of Bell's palsy. *Laryngoscope.* 1999;109(8):1177-1188.

33. Markowitz BL, Manson PN, Sargent L, et al. Management of the medial canthal tendon in nasoethmoid orbital fractures: the importance of the central fragment in classification and treatment. *Plast Reconstruct Surg.* 1991;87(5):843-853.

34. Champy M, Lodde JP, Muster D, et al. Osteosynthesis using miniaturized screw-on plates in facial and cranial surgery. Indications and results in 400 cases. *Ann Chir Plast.* 1977;22(4):261-264.

35. Zide MF, Kent JN. Indications for open reduction of mandibular condyle fractures. *J Oral Maxillofac Surg.* 1983;41(2):89-98.

4 Rhinology and Endoscopic Sinus Surgery

HISTORY, PHYSICAL EXAMINATION, AND ANCILLARY TESTS IN THE RHINOLOGIC PATIENT

HISTORY

- Nasal congestion/obstruction
  - Alternating cyclic engorgement of nasal turbinates is part of normal physiology, usually every 2-4 hours.
  - Increased obstruction when lying down or on dependent side with lateral recumbent position is normal.
- Purulent drainage
- Facial pain/pressure
- Loss of smell and taste
- History of environmental allergies (itchy, water eyes and nose and sneezing)
- Fever
- History of sinusitis
- History of sinonasal surgery
- Exposure to chemicals or metals
- Asthma
- Aspirin sensitivity
- Current medications
- Previous courses of antibiotics

ANCILLARY TESTS

1. Nasal endoscopy
2. Culture
3. Biopsy
4. Outcome measure
5. Radiologic studies
6. Allergy evaluation
7. Beta-2-transferrin for cerebrospinal fluid (CSF) leak suspicion
8. Pulmonary function test for coexisting reactive airway disease
9. Evaluation of smell
10. Measures of mucociliary function
11. Measures of nasal resistance and airflow

NASAL ENDOSCOPY

- Three passes
  1. Inferior pass: floor of nose, inferior turbinate, septum, Eustachian tube orifice, and nasopharynx
  2. Superior pass: nasal valve, septum, middle turbinate (MT), olfactory cleft, sphenoethmoid recess, and superior turbinate
  3. Middle pass: middle meatus, basal lamella attachment, ostiomeatal complex, and uncinate process
- Culture using endoscopic-directed middle meatal swabs if presence of bacterial sinusitis is suspected

- Biopsy (be aware not to biopsy encephaloceles or juvenile nasopharyngeal angiofibroma)

OUTCOME MEASURES

- Nasal Obstruction Symptom Evaluation (NOSE) scale for obstructive nasal symptoms
- Rhinosinusitis Disability Index (RSDI) and Chronic Sinusitis Survey (CSS)
- Sinonasal Outcomes Test (SNOT-22) for chronic rhinosinusitis (CRS) symptoms

RADIOLOGIC WORKUP

- Computed tomography (CT) of the paranasal sinuses (>4 weeks after treatment in most cases)
- Magnetic resonance imaging (MRI) for workup of tumors/masses, intracranial pathology and assessment of soft tissue

SMELL TESTS FOR EVALUATION OF ANOSMIA/HYPOSMIA

- University of Pennsylvania Smell Identification Test (UPSIT)
- Sniffing sticks
- Alcohol pad

OBJECTIVE MEASURES OF MUCOCILIARY TRANSPORT FUNCTION

- Saccharine ± color test in vivo (normal ~10 minutes; abnormal >30 minutes)
- Radioisotope transport testing in vivo
- Measuring ciliary activity in vitro
- Ciliary biopsy and electron microscopy for ciliary defect
- Nasal nitric oxide was found to be tenfold lower in primary ciliary dyskinesia (PCD) patients, but it cannot be used to exclude or to prove PCD

OBJECTIVE MEASURES OF NASAL RESISTANCE AND AIRFLOW

- Rhinomanometry and the nasal peak flowmeter both measure transnasal flow.
- Rhinomanometry (usually anterior because of the ease of testing) also simultaneously measures transnasal pressure, which allows calculation of nasal resistance (pressure/flow).
- No population threshold has been established for the resistance at which symptomatic obstruction occurs, but individual changes in measures after surgery and medical therapy are used.
- Intranasal dimensions of the nose can be assessed by acoustic rhinometry, CT, and computational fluid dynamics, MRI, fiberoptic videoendoscopy, and rhinostereometry.

ANATOMY OF THE PARANASAL SINUSES

COMPONENTS OF MUCOCILIARY CLEARANCE

- Pseudostratified ciliated columnar epithelium: anterior border begins at the limen nasi
- Ciliary activity causes the transport of mucus, an essential defense mechanism, at a frequency of 10-15 beats/min, and mucous blanket streams at a rate of 2.5-7.5 mL/min
- Double-layered mucous blanket: deep, less viscous, serous periciliary fluid (sol phase) and superficial, more viscous, mucous fluid (gel phase)
- Mucus-producing glands: goblet cells, seromucinous glands, and intraepithelial glands
- Inborn disorders of mucociliary transport (MCT) because of:
  - Ciliary dysfunction, as in PCD
  - Increased viscosity of the respiratory secretions, as in cystic fibrosis (CF)
- MCT is frequently impaired because of inflammation, infection, and exposure to ciliotoxic agents

EMBRYOLOGIC DERIVATIONS OF THE ETHMOTURBINALS

1. First ethmoturbinal: ascending portion is the agger nasi, and descending portion is the uncinate process
2. Second ethmoturbinal: ethmoid bulla
3. Third ethmoturbinal: basal lamella and attachment of MT to the lateral nasal wall
4. Fourth ethmoturbinal: attachment of the superior turbinate to the lateral nasal wall
5. Fifth and sixth: usually degenerate but can form a supreme turbinate

FIVE ANTERIOR-TO-POSTERIOR BONY LAMINA ENCOUNTERED IN ENDOSCOPIC SINUS SURGERY

1. Uncinate process
2. Ethmoid bulla
3. Vertical portion of the basal lamella
4. Vertical portion of the lamella of the superior turbinate
5. Anterior wall of the sphenoid sinus

OSTIOMEATAL COMPLEX

- Functional concept: final common pathway for drainage of anterior sinuses
- Structures within ostiomeatal complex (Fig. 4.1)
  - Uncinate process: sickle-shaped bone running anterosuperior to posteroinferior, with attachments along the lateral nasal wall. First structure encountered when MT is medialized
  - Ethmoid bulla
  - Hiatus semilunaris: two-dimensional slit that lies between the free edge of the uncinate process and the ethmoid bulla; connects the middle meatus into the infundibulum laterally

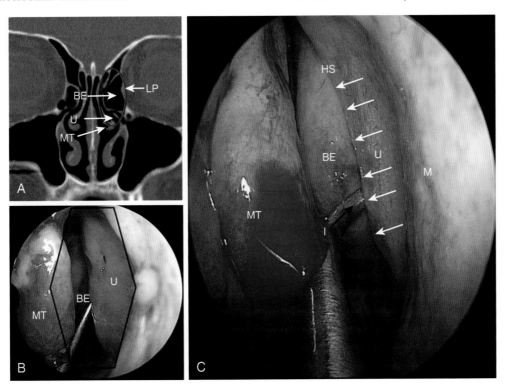

FIGURE 4.1 Left ostiomeatal complex (enclosed by *blue line*) is bound laterally by the medial orbital wall or lamina papyracea (*LP*) and medially by the MT. (**A**) Coronal CT section outlining ostiomeatal complex boundaries. (**B**) Endoscopic view of the left nasal cavity with the MT being medialized. (**C**) Closer view of the left middle meatus. The uncinate process extends anteriorly to the anterior maxillary line (*M*). Its posterior free margin parallels the ethmoid bulla. The hiatus semilunaris (*HS, white arrows*) is a two-dimensional cleft between the posterior free edge of the uncinate and the ethmoid bulla. It is the gap through which the nasal cavity communicates with the ethmoid infundibulum (*I*). The infundibulum (*black arrow*) is a three-dimensional space between the uncinate process and lamina papyracea. This endoscopic figure shows the maxillary ball probe being passed through the linear hiatus semilunaris into the infundibulum. *BE,* bulla ethmoidalis; *U,* uncinate process. (From Flint PW, Haughey BH, Lund VJ, et al. *Cummings Otolaryngology—Head and Neck Surgery.* 6th ed. Philadelphia, PA: Saunders; 2015, fig. 49-1.)

- Infundibulum: funnel-shaped three-dimensional space between the uncinate process medially and the lamina papyracea laterally
- MT
- Maxillary sinus ostium

SUPERIOR ATTACHMENT OF THE UNCINATE PROCESS (Fig. 4. 2)

Variable site of attachment:
- Laterally to lamina papyracea: most commonly resulting in a recessus terminalis; frontal recess drains medially to the uncinate and directly into the middle meatus
- Superiorly onto the skull base: frontal recess drains laterally into the infundibulum
- Medially to the MT: frontal recess drains laterally into the infundibulum

MIDDLE TURBINATE

- Boomerang-shaped structure
- Basal lamella is the entire MT attachment to the lateral nasal wall and skull base
- Basal lamella can be conveniently thought of in three parts from the anterior-to-posterior aspects (Fig. 4.3)
  - Anterior part: oriented in the sagittal plane (vertical) and attaches to the agger nasi region anteriorly and the cribriform plate superiorly
  - Middle: oriented in the coronal plane obliquely and attached to the lamina papyracea
  - Posterior: oriented in the axial place (horizontal) and attached to the lateral nasal wall at the lamina papyracea, maxilla, and perpendicular process of the palatine bone

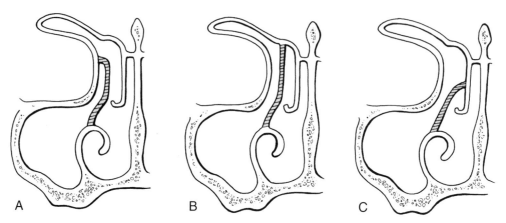

FIGURE 4.2 Coronal schematic view of the ostiomeatal complex showing the superior attachments of the uncinate process to the LP (**A**), the roof of the ethmoid (**B**), or the MT (**C**). If the uncinate process attaches to the roof of the ethmoid or to the MT, the frontal sinus drains into the infundibulum. If the uncinate attaches to the lamina papyracea, the frontal sinus drains medially, next to the MT. (From Flint PW, Haughey BH, Lund VJ, et al. *Cummings Otolaryngology—Head and Neck Surgery*. 6th ed. Philadelphia, PA: Saunders; 2015, fig. 49-2.)

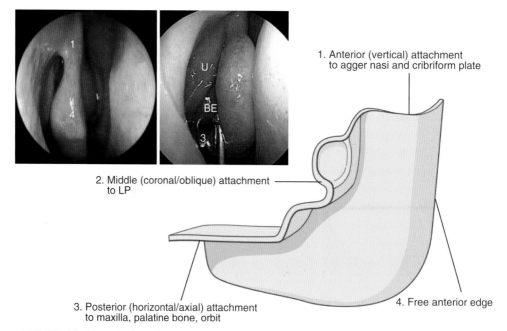

1. Anterior (vertical) attachment to agger nasi and cribriform plate

2. Middle (coronal/oblique) attachment to LP

3. Posterior (horizontal/axial) attachment to maxilla, palatine bone, orbit

4. Free anterior edge

FIGURE 4.3 Schematic view of the right MT viewed from the lateral aspect illustrates the anterior vertical (*1*), middle oblique (*2*), and posterior horizontal (*3*) attachments. Inset, endoscopic views of the right MT show the free anterior edge (*4*) and the anterior (*1*) and posterior (*3*) attachments. *BE*, bulla ethmoidalis; *U*, uncinate. (From Flint PW, Haughey BH, Lund VJ, et al. *Cummings Otolaryngology—Head and Neck Surgery*. 6th ed. Philadelphia, PA: Saunders; 2015, fig. 49-3.)

- Middle oblique part of the basal lamella is the only part of the MT that can be sacrificed without compromising the integrity of the turbinate: if the vertical or horizontal attachment is injured, MT will lateralize the obstructing middle meatus and posterior ethmoid complex

ETHMOID SINUSES

- The ethmoid complex is divided by the basal lamella into the anterior and posterior ethmoid cells (Fig. 4.4)
- Anterior ethmoid cells
  - Drain into the middle meatus
  - Ethmoid bulla: the largest and most prominent cell; it attaches laterally to the orbit
  - May have a cleft behind the bulla (retrobullar recess) or above the bulla (suprabullar recess)
  - Agger nasi at the attachment of the MT to the lateral wall is often pneumatized
    - Agger nasi cell is the most anterior of all ethmoid cells; it is present in >98% of CT scans
    - Key landmark in frontal sinus surgery
  - Posterior ethmoid cells drain into the superior (or supreme) meatus
    - 1-5 cells
  - Ethmoid cells may pneumatize into the adjacent sinuses and affect their drainage
    - Infraorbital or Haller cell into the maxillary sinus
    - Frontal, suprabullar, and supraorbital cells around the frontal sinus
    - Sphenoethmoid or Onodi cell over the sphenoid sinus, potentially placing the optic nerve and internal carotid artery (ICA) at risk if not recognized by surgeon

MAXILLARY SINUS

- Natural ostium
  - Drains into the inferior aspect (usually of the infundibulum) at a 45-degree angle
  - Elliptically shaped; accessory ostia are round and are present in the fontanelles in at least 10% of patients
  - Halfway between the anterior and posterior walls of the sinus
- Lateral nasal wall has two areas where bone is absent between the mucosa, called fontanelles
  - Anterior fontanelle is anterior to the uncinate bone
  - Posterior fontanelle

SPHENOID SINUS

- Natural os opens into the sphenoethmoidal recess
- Sphenoid os halfway to two-thirds up the anterior wall of the sinus
- Medial to the posterior end of the superior turbinate in the majority (83%) of cases
- Os is average of 7 cm from the nasal spine, at an angle of 30 degrees from the floor
- Walls of the sphenoid sinus contain several critical structures such as the ICA, optic nerve, and skull base
- Septations in the sphenoid frequently attach to the ICA

FRONTAL SINUS

- Originates embryologically from an anterior ethmoid cell
- Outflow tract has an hourglass shape, and the narrowest part is the internal frontal ostium
- Mucocilary flow is up the intersinus septum across the frontal sinus roof laterally and then medially along the floor of the frontal sinus down to the frontal recess
- Drains through the frontal recess into the middle meatus (commonly) or into the superior aspect of the infundibulum (less commonly), depending on the uncinated attachment
- Boundaries of the frontal recess
  - Medial: MT
  - Lateral: lamina papyracea
  - Anterior: posterior wall of the agger nasi
  - Posterior: ethmoid bulla

CELLS RELATED TO THE FRONTAL SINUS

- Frontal recess may contain anterior ethmoid cells (called frontal recess cells), which consequently narrow the frontal sinus drainage pathway (Fig. 4.5)
- Anterior to the frontal recess
  - Frontal cells
    - Type I: a single cell superior to the agger nasi cell
    - Type II: a tier of two or more cells above the agger nasi cell
    - Type III: a single cell that extends from the agger nasi cell into the frontal sinus, above the floor of the frontal sinus floor but <50% of the frontal sinus height
    - Type IV: an isolated cell within the frontal sinus (Kuhn) or a single cell that extends into the frontal sinus for >50% of the frontal sinus height (Wormald)

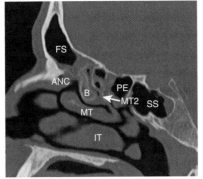
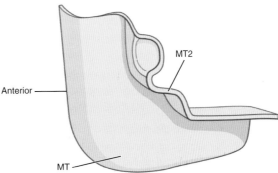

FIGURE 4.4 The oblique, second part of the MT2 attaches to the lamina papyracea via the basal lamella, separating the anterior ethmoid (*B*) from the posterior ethmoid (*PE*) cells. This part lies in a coronal/frontal plane and is best viewed on a sagittal view CT scan. *ANC,* Agger nasi cell; *FS,* frontal sinus; *IT,* inferior turbinate; *SS,* sphenoid sinus. (From Flint PW, Haughey BH, Lund VJ, et al. *Cummings Otolaryngology—Head and Neck Surgery.* 6th ed. Philadelphia, PA: Saunders; 2015, fig. 49-4.)

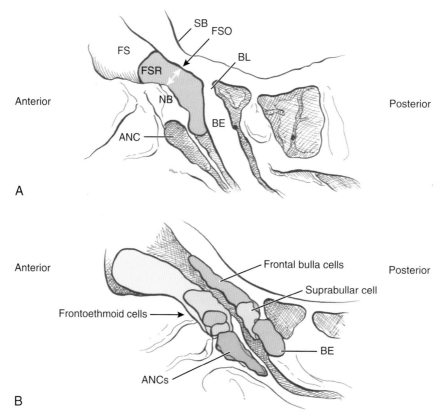

FIGURE 4.5 (A) The frontal sinus recess (*FSR*) is an hourglass-shaped space (*shaded area*) with the waist at the frontal sinus ostium (*FSO*), which is its narrowest part. In the simplest configuration, the boundaries of the frontal recess are limited by the ANC and nasal beak (*NB*) anteriorly, the bulla ethmoidalis (*BE*) and the bulla lamella (*BL*) posteriorly, the anterior skull base (*SB*) posterosuperiorly, the cribriform plate and MT medially, and the lamina papyracea laterally. **(B)** Frontoethmoid cells pneumatize around the frontal recess. Frontal cells lie anterior to the frontal recess; suprabullar, supraorbital ethmoid, and frontobullar cells lie posterior to the frontal recess. (From Flint PW, Haughey BH, Lund VJ, et al. *Cummings Otolaryngology—Head and Neck Surgery*. 6th ed. Philadelphia, PA: Saunders; 2015, fig. 49-9.)

- Posterior to the frontal recess
  - Supraorbital ethmoid cell: cells posterior to the frontal sinus, pneumatizing superiorly to the orbital roof
  - Interfrontal sinus cell: pneumatizes intersinus septum and drains into one frontal sinus, medially to the frontal ostium
  - Suprabullar cell: cell superior to the ethmoid bulla
  - Frontal bulla cell: cell superior to the ethmoid bulla pneumatizing into the posterior frontal table (anterior skull base)

BENT AND KUHN CLASSIFICATION OF FRONTAL CELLS

1. Type I: a single frontal recess cell above the agger nasi
2. Type II: a tier of cells above the agger nasi projecting into the frontal recess
3. Type III: single massive cell arising above the agger nasi, pneumatizing cephalad into the frontal sinus
4. Type IV: single isolated cell within the frontal sinus

ANATOMICAL VARIANTS (Fig. 4.6)

- Concha bullosa: defined as aeration of the MT; cavity lines with the same epithelium as the rest of the nasal cavity
- Paradoxic MT: curvature projecting laterally; may narrow or obstruct the nasal cavity, middle meatus, and infundibulum

- Atelectatic uncinate process: free edge of the uncinate adheres to the orbital wall; associated with an occluded infundibulum and hypoplastic opacified ipsilateral maxillary sinus, possibly with a more inferior location of the orbit and increased risk of orbital complications during surgery
- Haller cell: an infraorbital ethmoid cell; pneumatizes into the maxilla
- Onodi cell: a sphenoethmoidal cell, a posterior ethmoid air cell pneumatizing over the sphenoid

AIRSPACES WITHIN THE PARANASAL SINUSES

- Suprabullar recess: air cell space left between the ethmoid bulla and the fovea ethmoidalis when the bulla does not extend up to the fovea
- Sinus lateralis/retrobullar recess: air cell space found between the posterior surface of the ethmoid bulla and the vertical portion of the basal lamella
- Sinus terminalis: uncinate process terminates in the lamina papyracea; frontal recess drains medially to the uncinate process; this sinus is essentially a superior ending of the infundibulum (blind pocket)
- Agger nasi cell: remnant of the first ethmoturbinal, found superior, lateral, and anterior to the attachment of the MT; can also refer to ethmoid cells anterior to the frontal duct

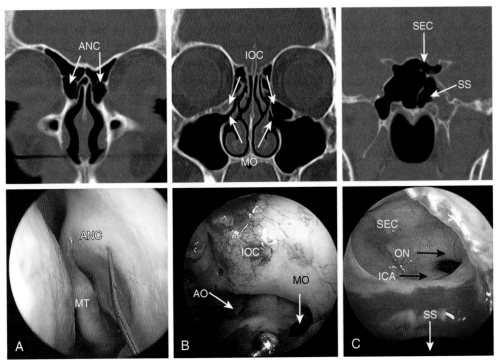

FIGURE 4.6 Ethmoid Cells. Top row shows a CT scan with corresponding endoscopic view below. (**A**) The ANC is the most anterior cell seen on a coronal CT scan, anterior to the MT. Endoscopically, it is seen as a bulge on the MT attachment and may narrow the superior ethmoid infundibulum. (**B**) Coronal CT section shows bilateral infraorbital ethmoid cells (*IOC*, Haller cells) narrowing the inferior ethmoid infundibulum and attaching laterally to the infraorbital canal. The maxillary sinus opens into the inferior part of the infundibulum at a 45-degree angle. Endoscopic view of the left infundibulum after uncinectomy shows the IOC narrowing the inferior infundibulum and potentially obstructing drainage of the natural maxillary ostium (*MO*). The natural MO is elliptically shaped and opens into the floor of the infundibulum at a 45-degree angle, not directly into the lateral wall. Accessory ostia (*AO*) are usually circular and are present here in the posterior fontanelle. (**C**) The sphenoethmoid cell (*SEC*), or Onodi cell, is a posterior ethmoid cell that is lateral and superior to the SS, which is usually smaller, pushed medially and inferiorly. The figures show arrows pointing to a left SEC on coronal and sagittal CT cuts. The endoscopic image demonstrates the relationship of the SEC to the SS and shows the optic nerve (*ON*) and ICA lying in relation to the SEC lateral wall. (From Flint PW, Haughey BH, Lund VJ, et al. *Cummings Otolaryngology—Head and Neck Surgery*. 6th ed. Philadelphia, PA: Saunders; 2015, fig. 49-5.)

ANTERIOR SKULL BASE

- Formed by the cribriform medially and the fovea ethmodalis laterally
- Slopes downward posteriorly
- Skull base is thinner medially (0.1 mm) along the lateral lamella of the cribriform plate
- Inverse relationship between maxillary sinus height and the height of the ethmoid cavity (ie, large maxillary sinus is related to lower-lying skull base)

KEROS CLASSIFICATION OF LATERAL LAMELLA OF CRIBRIFORM HEIGHT

1. Type 1: cribriform plate 1-3 mm below the fovea
2. Type 2: cribriform plate 4-7 mm below the fovea
3. Type 3: cribriform plate 8-16 mm below the fovea (highest risk of skull-base penetration)

RHINITIS

HISTORY AND PHYSICAL

- Single most important factor in attaining a proper diagnosis is a complete history
- Symptoms: nasal discharge, congestion/blockage, change in olfaction, postnasal drainage, episodes of sneezing, nasal itching, itchy eyes, and epiphora

- Symptom frequency: intermittent or persistent?
- Medication history
- History of asthma and sensitivity to aspirin or nonsteroidal antiinflammatory drugs (NSAIDs)
- History of head trauma
- History of prior nasal/sinus surgery
- History of hay fever/allergy testing
- Other systemic disorders
- Inciting factors including weather changes, certain odors or food, time of year, occupational history, chemical exposure at work, and improvement of symptoms on weekends/holidays (away from work)
- Examination should include nasal endoscopy

WORKUP

- Skin testing and/or serum testing for serum-specific immunoglobulin E (IgE) antibodies to relevant allergens
- Nasal cytology; scrapings from the inferior turbinate mucosa; high-power field of 5-25 eosinophils is compatible with a diagnosis of nonallergic rhinitis with eosinophilia syndrome (NARES) with negative allergy testing

TREATMENT PRINCIPLES

1. Avoidance of triggers
2. Topical corticosteroids for allergic and nonallergic rhinitis

3. Consider topical nasal (and oral) antihistamines and anticholinergic sprays, depending on etiology
4. Normal saline rinses as adjunct
5. In recalcitrant cases, may consider surgery, including turbinate reduction and potentially vidian neurectomy

CAUSES OF RHINITIS/RHINORRHEA

- Allergic rhinitis
- Churg-Strauss syndrome
- Infectious
- NARES
- Rhinitis sicca anterior
- Atrophic rhinitis
- Rhinitis medicamentosa
- Vasomotor rhinitis
- Hormonal rhinitis
- Medication-induced rhinitis
- CSF rhinorrhea

ALLERGIC RHINITIS

- Treat with avoidance of allergens, saline irrigations, oral and nasal antihistamines, nasal steroid sprays, oral decongestants, oral antileukotrienes, and nasal mast cell stabilizers
- Consider immunotherapy

CHURG-STRAUSS SYNDROME

- Asthma, eosinophilia (>10%), allergic rhinosinusitis, pulmonary infiltrates, vasculitis, and neuritis
- Treat with oral steroids, cyclophosphamide, and management of sinonasal symptoms

INFECTIOUS RHINITIS

- Viral (supportive Rx)
- Bacterial (commonly *Streptococcus pneumoniae*, *Haemophilus influenzae*, and *Moraxella catarrhalis*, treat with antibiotics)
- Rhinoscleroma (Mikulicz cells, Russell bodies on histopathology; treat with long-term ciprofloxacin or tertracycline)
- Rhinosporidiosis (*Rhinosporidium seeberi* is endemic in Africa and India): painless, friable, "strawberry" lesion; pseudoepitheliomatous hyperplasia on histopathology; treat with excision, antifungals, and dapsone

NONALLERGIC RHINITIS WITH EOSINOPHILIA SYNDROME

- Nasal eosinophilia (10-20% on smear) with negative allergy testing
- Symptoms and treatment are similar to allergic rhinitis

RHINITIS SICCA ANTERIOR

- Dry, raw nasal mucosa caused by changes in temperature/humidity, nose picking, and dust
- Symptoms include dryness, crusting, and epistaxis
- Treat with saline irrigation, topical antibiotics, and oil-based nasal ointments

ATROPHIC RHINITIS

- Transition from functional, ciliated respiratory epithelium to a nonfunctional lining of nonciliated squamous metaplasia, with a loss of mucociliary clearance and squamous metaplasia
- Destroyed MCT and loss of mucosal glands
- Crusting, fetor, mucosal atrophy, and widely patent nasal cavities are seen in patients who complain of nasal congestion
- Causes include aggressive turbinectomy, excessive nasal surgery, nutritional deficiencies (iron or vitamin A or D deficiency), chronic bacterial infection (eg, *Klebsiella ozaenae*, less common in antibiotic era), trauma, manifestations of granulomatous diseases, chronic cocaine abuse, and radiation therapy
- Symptoms include paradoxical nasal congestion/obstruction despite wide nasal cavity, nasal crusting, and odor
- Treatment options are limited: may include irrigations, humidification to provide moisture, and experimental surgical procedures

RHINITIS MEDICAMENTOSA

- Rebound congestion from decreased vasomotor tone, or increased parasympathetic activity, due of topical nasal decongestants or cocaine use
- Treat by discontinuing topical decongestants; consider short-term oral corticosteroids (for weaning)

VASOMOTOR RHINITIS

- Results from changes in vascular tone and permeability: stimulation of afferent sensory nerves is the most likely pathophysiologic mechanism, and it activates the parasympathetic nerves that supply the nasal mucosal glands
- Symptoms include clear watery rhinorrhea and occasionally sweating/epiphora
- More common in older adults
- Multiple triggers, including temperature change, eating (gustatory rhinitis often with hot/spicy food), and anxiety
- Treat with anticholinergic nasal sprays (ipratropium bromide); consider vidian neurectomy if refractory (risk of dry eye)

HORMONAL RHINITIS

- Fluctuating hormones with menstruation and puberty
- Rhinitis of pregnancy seen in >20%
- Increased in hypothyroidism and acromegaly

MEDICATION-INDUCED RHINITIS (Box 4.1)

- Aspirin and NSAIDs in patients with aspirin-exacerbated respiratory disease (AERD)
- Multiple psychotropic agents (eg, amitriptyline)
- Antihypertensives (eg, β-blockers and angiotensin-converting enzyme inhibitors)
- Hormonal replacement and oral contraceptives

INHALANT-INDUCED RHINITIS

- Proposed mechanism is the stimulation of chemical irritant receptors on sensory nerves (ie, C fibers) to induce neuropeptide release, which produces the vasodilation and edema associated with inflammation independent of immune-mediated responses
- Chemical exposures classifications:
  - Immunologic (high molecular-weight agents, eg, wheat, latex, compounds in insecticides, adhesives, and auto-body spray paint)
  - Annoyant (perfumes, exhaust fumes, cleaning agents, room deodorizers, floral fragrances, and cosmetics)
  - Irritant (air pollution, smoke, tobacco smoke, paint fumes, formaldehyde, and volatile organic compounds)

Box 4.1 MEDICATIONS THAT CONTRIBUTE TO RHINITIS

Intranasal Preparations
Cocaine
Topical nasal decongestants

Antihypertensives
α- and β-adrenoceptor antagonists
Reserpine
Hydralazine
Felodipine
Angiotensin-converting enzyme inhibitors
β-blockers
Methyldopa
Guanethidine
Phentolamine

Agents for Prostatic Hypertrophy
Doxazosin
Tamsulosin

Hormones
Oral contraceptives

Antiinflammatory Agents
Nonsteroidal antiinflammatory medications
Aspirin

Antiplatelet Agents
Clopidogrel

Antidepressants
Selective serotonin reuptake inhibitors

Nonbenzodiazepine Hypnotics
Zolpidem

Phosphodiesterase Type-5 Inhibitors
Sildenafil
Tadalafil
Vardenafil

Psychotropic Agents
Thioridazine
Chlordiazepoxide
Chlorpromazine
Amitriptyline
Perphenazine
Alprazolam

From Flint PW, Haughey BH, Lund VJ, et al. *Cummings Otolaryngology—Head and Neck Surgery*. 6th ed. Philadelphia, PA: Saunders; 2015, box 43-2.

can lead to the synthesis of proinflammatory mediators and neuromediators
  • Corrosive (ammonium chloride, hydrochloric acid, vinyl chloride, organophosphates, and acrylamide exposures causing mucosal burns and ulcerations)

CEREBROSPINAL FLUID RHINORRHEA

• Clear watery often unilateral rhinorrhea; worse with lowering head
• Patients will often report that the watery drainage occurs when they bend over to tie their shoes
• Treated with conservative or surgical therapy

NASAL OBSTRUCTION

DIFFERENTIAL DIAGNOSIS OF NASAL OBSTRUCTION

• Rhinitis (inflammatory)
• Chronic sinusitis (with or without nasal polyps)
• Rhinitis medicamentosa (chronic use of nasal decongestants)

• Deviated nasal septum
• Inferior turbinate hypertrophy
• Nasal valve collapse
• Adenoid hypertrophy (children)
• Choanal atresia (infants, congenital)
• Empty-nose syndrome (prior resection of inferior turbinates is the most likely cause)

EVALUATION OF NASAL OBSTRUCTION

• History and physical
    • Seasonal and/or daily variation of symptoms
    • History of nasal trauma
    • History of past nasal surgery
    • History and signs of allergic or nonallergic inflammation
    • Examine external and internal nasal valves (modified Cottle maneuver to assess nasal valves)
• Nasal endoscopy
• Sinus CT
• Allergy testing

TREATMENT OPTIONS FOR NASAL OBSTRUCTION

• Trial of nasal steroids and antihistamines
• Oral steroids for chronic sinusitis
• Trial of Breathe Right® nasal strips if nasal valve collapse is suspected
• Inferior turbinoplasty (submucosal resection and outfracture)
    • Radiofrequency coblation
    • Submucosal debridement
• Septoplasty
• Functional rhinoplasty (closed or open)
    • Extracorporeal septoplasty (caudal deviations)
    • Nasal valve repair

NASAL SEPTAL PERFORATION

CAUSES OF NASAL SEPTAL PERFORATION

• Iatrogenic (septoplasty)
• Trauma and septal hematoma
• Drug use (cocaine, inhaled narcotics)
• Malignancy
• Granulomatous disease (granulomatosis with polyangiitis [GPA], sarcoidosis)
• Corticosteroid nasal spray (overuse)
• Infection (tertiary syphilis)

TREATMENT OF NASAL SEPTAL PERFORATION

• Nasal hygiene: increase moisture (bactroban ointment); avoid digital manipulation
• Silastic buttons
• Surgical repair
• Extending perforation posteriorly

EPISTAXIS

WORKUP OF EPISTAXIS

• Unilateral versus bilateral
• Duration
• Frequency
• Severity (trickle vs. high flow)
• Time of day (morning vs. nighttime)
• Anterior (tends to be unilateral, flows from nostril)

- Posterior (may be bilateral, with significant bleeding from the oropharynx/oral cavity as it runs posteriorly)
- Source (Keisselbach's plexus, anterior ethmoid artery, posterior ethmoid artery, sphenopalatine artery, mucosal lesion, or neoplasm)
- Exacerbating factors (trauma, digital trauma, and temperature)
- Medical history (hypertension or coagulopathy)
- Family history
- Medications (aspirin, NSAIDs, and anticoagulants)

CAUSES OF EPISTAXIS

- Bleeding from blood vessels in Keisselbach's plexus is the most common cause in 90% cases (plexus in the anterior caudal septum is supplied by the anterior ethmoid artery, sphenopalatine artery, greater palatine artery, and superior labial artery)
- Mucosal trauma (digital manipulation)
- Toxic (inhaled drugs, including cocaine and heroin)
- Drugs (chemotherapy, anticoagulants, and alcoholism)
- Mucosal lesion (capillary hemangioma and telangiectasia)
- Neoplasm (juvenile nasopharyngeal angiofibroma [JNA] and malignant neoplasm)
- Congenital (hereditary hemorrhagic telangiectasias [HHT], hemophilia, and von Willebrand)
- Systemic (hypertension and coagulopathy)

TREATMENT OPTIONS FOR EPISTAXIS

- Nondissolvable packing (anterior pack: Kennedy Merocel vs. posterior pack)
- Dissolvable packing (hemostatic agents: surgicel Gelfoam, and Floseal)
- In-office cauterization (silver nitrate or laser)
- Cauterization under anesthesia (coblation, bipolar cautery, monopolar cautery, or laser)
- Manage underlying condition or cause (neoplasm, hypertension, and coagulopathy)

HEREDITARY HEMORRHAGIC TELANGIECTASIAS (FORMERLY OSLER WEBER RENDU)

- Diagnosis
  - Autosomal dominant (at least five genes identified)
  - Curacao criteria (definite if 3; suspected if 2; unlikely if <2)
    - Epistaxis
    - Mucosal telangiectasias (oral and sinonasal)
    - Visceral lesions (pulmonary arteriovenous malformation [AVM], cerebral AVM, hepatic AVM, and spinal AVM)
    - Family history (first-degree relative)
  - Medical management
    - Topical moisturizers (mupirocin and saline gel)
    - Topical rose geranium oil
    - Topical or oral estrogen agents (hormone replacement therapy and antiestrogen agents)
    - Topical timolol
    - Oral tranexamic acid
    - Topical or intravenous (IV) bevacizumab (Avastin)
    - In-office injected sclerotherapy
  - Surgical management
    - Cauterization (laser, bipolar, and radiofrequency)
    - Injected bevacizumab (Avastin)
    - Septodermoplasty
    - Young's procedure

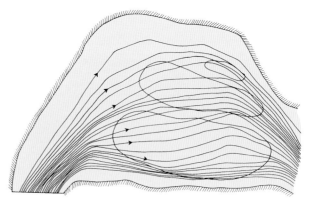

FIGURE 4.7 Streamline patterns for resting inspiratory flow (250 mL/sec) through an expanded (20 × normal size) scale model of a healthy human adult-male nasal cavity (sagittal view). Lines show the paths taken by small dust particles entering at the external nares. (From Scherer PW, Scherer PW, Hahn II, Mozell MM. The biophysics of nasal airflow. *Otolaryngol Clin North Am.* 1989;22:265 and Flint PW, Haughey BH, Lund VJ, et al. *Cummings Otolaryngology—Head and Neck Surgery.* 6th ed. Philadelphia, PA: Saunders; 2015, fig. 39-1.)

OLFACTORY PHYSIOLOGY AND DISORDERS

AIRFLOW THROUGH THE NASAL CAVITY (Fig. 4.7)

- Middle meatus (50%)
- Inferior meatus (35%)
- Olfactory cleft (15%)

OLFACTORY EPITHELIUM BASICS

- Much thicker than normal respiratory mucosa and is intermixed with respiratory epithelium (which increases with age)
- Mucus of epithelium traps odorant molecules
- Club-shaped bipolar neurons extend into the olfactory epithelium and are exposed via dendrites and cilia
  - Traverses toward the cribriform plate and becomes encased by Schwann cells
  - Travels through 1 of 20 foramen in the cribriform and enters the central nervous system (CNS) and synapse to the olfactory bulbs at the base of the brain
  - Humans have about 6 million olfactory neurons bilaterally
  - Uniquely capable of regeneration
- There are also basal cells, sustenacular (supporting) cells, and microvilli cells, which may be specialized sensory cells

OLFACTORY BULB BASICS (Fig. 4.8)

- Lies at the base of the frontal cortex in the anterior fossa
- Serves as the first relay station in the olfactory pathway, where the primary olfactory neurons synapse with secondary neurons
- These synapses and their postsynaptic partners form dense aggregates of neuropil called glomeruli

CENTRAL OLFACTORY CONNECTIONS

- Olfactory tubercule
- Prepiriform cortex
- Amygdaloid nuclei
- Nucleus of the terminal stria with further projections to a number of structures, including the hypothalamus

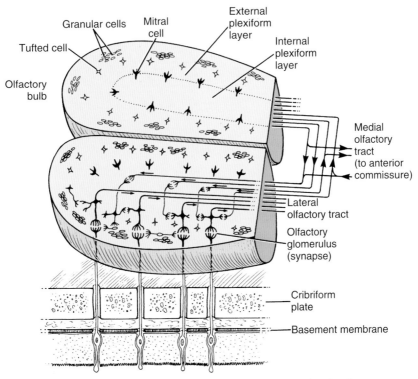

FIGURE 4.8 Structure of olfactory bulbs and their neural connections to one another, the olfactory mucosa, and the brain. (From Flint PW, Haughey BH, Lund VJ, et al. *Cummings Otolaryngology—Head and Neck Surgery*. 6th ed. Philadelphia, PA: Saunders; 2015, fig. 39-8.)

COMMON CHEMICAL SENSE BASICS

- Added chemoreceptivity in the mucosa of the respiratory tract is provided by free nerve endings of three cranial nerves
  1. Trigeminal (most important)
  2. Glossopharyngeal
  3. Vagus
- The trigeminal nerves sense the burn of ammonia and the bite of hot pepper
- In the nose, virtually all odorants stimulate olfactory and trigeminal nerves, even when no apparent pungency can be perceived

SMELL DETERMINANT BASICS

- Theories range from odor binding proteins (OBPs) and olfactory receptors to tonotopic organization and receptor specialization
- Agreed-upon factors on what a molecule must have to illicit smell
  1. Water solubility
  2. Sufficient vapor pressure
  3. Low polarity
  4. Some ability to dissolve in fat (lipophilicity): this may be aided by OBP
  5. Size: no known odorants possess a molecular weight of >294 kDa

OLFACTORY TESTS

1. UPSIT: most specific test
2. Gross perception
   - Odor sticks (eg, marker-type pen)
   - 12-inch alcohol smell test
3. Threshold: determine the threshold with serial dilutions of phenylethyl alcohol

TYPES OF OLFACTORY DISORDERS

1. Transport or conductive
2. Sensory
3. Neural olfactory loss

CAUSES OF TRANSPORT (CONDUCTIVE) OLFACTORY DISORDERS

1. Nasal inflammation resulting from rhinitis, sinusitis, or upper-respiratory infection (URI)
2. Polyps
3. Neoplasm
4. Mass effect
5. Septal deviation or nasal obstruction

CAUSES OF SENSORY OLFACTORY DISORDER

- From damage to the neuroepithelium caused by:
  1. Drugs
  2. Neoplasms
  3. External beam radiation therapy (XRT)
  4. Toxic-chemical exposure
  5. Viral URI:
     - Some patients never recover smell following URI
     - Overwhelming predominance of females in this group (80%)
     - Prognosis is poor, and etiology is not understood
     - Biopsy shows decreased or absence of receptors

CAUSES OF NEURAL OLFACTORY LOSS

1. Alcohol
2. Tobacco
3. Human immunodeficiency virus (HIV)
4. Age: olfaction decreases in the sixth to seventh decade from olfactory neuron loss

5. Neurologic: Parkinson's, Huntington's, and Alzheimer's diseases
   - Very high incidence of olfactory disorders in these dementia-related diseases
   - May preferentially involve the olfactory system
6. Kallmann syndrome: X-linked disorder characterized by hypogonadism and anosmia
7. Korsakoff psychosis
8. Metabolic
   - B_{12} or zinc deficiency
   - Hypothyroidism
   - Diabetes mellitus
   - Malnutrition
9. Trauma
   - 5-10% incidence of anosmia following head trauma
   - Shearing of olfactory neurons is the predominating theory

CEREBROSPINAL FLUID RHINORRHEA

CAUSES OF CEREBROSPINAL FLUID RHINORRHEA (Box 4.2)

- Traumatic
  - Accidental (eg, head trauma)
  - Iatrogenic (eg, endoscopic sinus surgery [ESS])
- Spontaneous
  - Typically involves meningoencephalocele
  - Likely secondary to increased intracranial pressure (associated with obstructive sleep apnea [OSA], obesity, or pseudotumor cerebri)
  - 15-50% of CSF leak repairs
  - Highest repair-failure rate

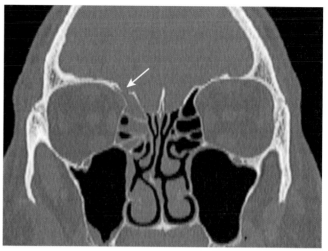

FIGURE 4.9 High-resolution sinus CT may be used to visualize even small bony defects of the SB. This coronal CT image was reconstructed from 1-mm direct axial CT image data using a robust image-processing software system. It should be noted that not all reformatted coronal images are of sufficient quality to permit this precise examination of the SB. A bony dehiscence (*arrow*) together with a positive β-2 transferrin study represents a likely site for an active CSF leak; however, in the absence of a positive β-2 transferrin study, the presence of a CSF leak should not be assumed from the presence of such a finding. (From Flint PW, Haughey BH, Lund VJ, et al. *Cummings Otolaryngology—Head and Neck Surgery*. 6th ed. Philadelphia, PA: Saunders; 2015, fig. 52-6.)

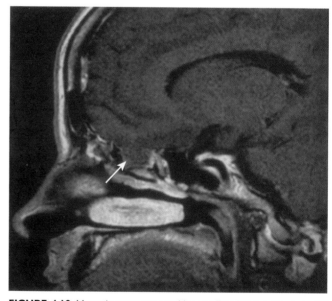

FIGURE 4.10 Magnetic resonance provides excellent imaging of anterior SB meningoencephaloceles. The arrow shows their characteristic appearance on this sagittal image. (From Flint PW, Haughey BH, Lund VJ, et al. *Cummings Otolaryngology—Head and Neck Surgery*. 6th ed. Philadelphia, PA: Saunders; 2015, fig. 52-7.)

- Neoplasm
- Congenital
- Infection

OPTIONS FOR CEREBROSPINAL FLUID RHINORRHEA EVALUATION

- High-resolution CT scan (0.5 mm) (Fig. 4.9) to evaluate bony skull base
- High-resolution MRI (Fig. 4.10) to evaluate for meningoencephalocele

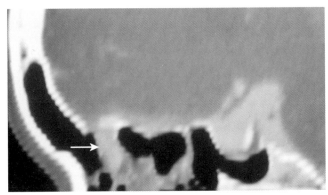

FIGURE 4.11 A CSF leak on CT cisternography is characterized by the presence of contrast material within the pneumatized paranasal sinuses. The contrast should be in direct continuity so that a precise site of communication can be reliably demonstrated, as shown in this sagittal CT image reconstruction from a positive CT cisternogram. The arrow points to the area of the contrast within the ethmoid sinuses. (From Flint PW, Haughey BH, Lund VJ, et al. *Cummings Otolaryngology—Head and Neck Surgery.* 6th ed. Philadelphia, PA: Saunders; 2015, fig. 52-3.)

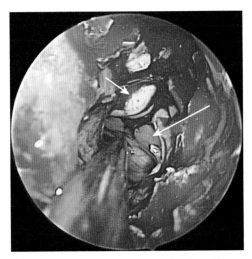

FIGURE 4.12 Intraoperative nasal endoscopy after the administration of intrathecal fluorescein provides a way to confirm a CSF leak and precisely localize the corresponding skull-base defect. In this endoscopic image obtained after ethmoidectomy and sphenoidotomy, a meningocele arises from the superior (*short arrow*) and superolateral (*long arrow*) aspects of the left SS. The meningocele has a greenish hue because the fluorescein colors the CSF within it. (From Flint PW, Haughey BH, Lund VJ, et al. *Cummings Otolaryngology—Head and Neck Surgery.* 6th ed. Philadelphia, PA: Saunders; 2015, fig. 52-5.)

- Presence of B-2 transferrin in nasal secretions is the gold standard (must collect 0.5 mL)
- CT cisternography (Fig. 4.11): thin section axial CT imaging in prone and supine positions before and after intrathecal contrast
- Radionuclide cisternography (technetium 99m or indium 111-labeled diethylenetriaminepentaacetic acid): identifies presence and side of leak
- Endoscopic and/or intraoperative evaluation with fluorescein (Fig. 4.12)

TREATMENT OPTIONS FOR CEREBROSPINAL FLUID RHINORRHEA

- Conservative management (particularly for traumatic leaks)
  - Bed rest with head of bed elevated
  - Stool softeners
  - Avoid Valsalva and nose blowing
  - Lumbar drain

Table 4.1 **Rhinosinusitis Symptoms**

Major	Minor
Facial pain/pressure	Headache
Facial congestion/fullness	Fever (nonacute)
Nasal obstruction/blockage	Halitosis
Nasal discharge/purulence with discolored posterior drainage	Fatigue
	Dental pain
Hyposmia/anosmia	Cough
Purulence on nasal exam	Ear pain, pressure, and/or fullness
Fever (acute rhinosinusitis only)	

Diagnosis of rhinosinusitis requires two major or one major and two minor symptoms.
From Flint PW, Haughey BH, Lund VJ, et al. *Cummings Otolaryngology—Head and Neck Surgery.* 6th ed. Philadelphia, PA: Saunders; 2015, table 46-1.

- Craniotomy and repair
- Endoscopic repair is the gold standard for amendable lesions
  - Grafts
    1. Bone: mastoid cortex, septal, and turbinate
    2. Cartilage: septal and pinna concha
    3. Fascia: fascia lata and temporalis
    4. Mucosa free grafts: septal, MT, and nasal floor
    5. Synthetic: dural substitutes (DuraMatrix, DuraGen, and AlloDerm)
  - Pedicled flaps (overlay)
    1. Nasoseptal
    2. Turbinate
  - Spontaneous leaks: must consider and treat increased intracranial pressure (eg, acetazolamide and CSF shunt)

RHINOSINUSITIS

DEFINITIONS OF RHINOSINUSITIS

- Rhinosinusitis: any inflammation of the nose and sinus mucosa
- Acute rhinosinusitis (ARS): rhinosinusitis lasting 4 weeks or less
- Recurrent ARS: four or more annual episodes of rhinosinusitis, without persistent symptoms in between
- CRS: rhinosinusitis lasting longer than 12 weeks

ETIOLOGIES OF ACUTE RHINOSINUSITIS

- Viral (most common): rhinovirus, parainfluenza virus, respiratory syncytial virus, influenza virus, and coronavirus
- Bacterial (acute bacterial sinusitis): *S. pneumoniae, H. influenzae, Moraxella catarrhalis, Staph. aureus,* and *Streptococcus pyogenes*
- Fulminant fungal: *Aspergillus, Mucor,* and *Rhizopus*

HALLMARK SYMPTOMS OF ACUTE RHINOSINUSITIS

1. Purulent rhinorrhea
2. Nasal obstruction
3. Facial pain and/or pressure

WORKUP AND DIAGNOSIS OF ACUTE BACTERIAL RHINOSINUSITIS (Table 4.1)

- Acute bacterial rhinosinusitis (ABRS) must be distinguished from viral URIs and noninfectious etiologies such as allergic rhinitis.

- Can be differentiated from these entities when:
  1. Symptoms or signs of ARS (hallmark symptoms) persist without evidence of improvement for at least 10 days or
  2. Symptoms of rhinosinusitis worsen within 10 days after an initial period of improvement ("double worsening").[1]
- Only 0.5-2% of viral rhinosinusitis is complicated by ABRS.[1]
- Diagnosis is made on clinical grounds: radiographic imaging should not be obtained for the diagnosis of ABRS unless complications are suspected.[1]

TREATMENT OF ACUTE BACTERIAL RHINOSINUSITIS

- Observation (reliable patients with adequate follow-up)
- First-line antibiotic: Augmentin (amoxicillin 875 mg with clavulanate)
- First-line antibiotic in penicillin allergic patients: fluoroquinolone (levofloxacin and moxifloxacin) or doxycycline
- Symptomatic treatment: saline irrigations, nasal steroids, and short-term decongestants for <3 consecutive days

COMPLICATIONS OF ACUTE BACTERIAL RHINOSINUSITIS (Table 4.2)

- Chandler classification of orbital complications
  1. Preseptal cellulitis
  2. Orbital cellulitis
  3. Subperiosteal abscess
  4. Orbital abscess
  5. Cavernous sinus thrombosis
- Intracranial complications
  1. Meningitis
  2. Epidural abscess
  3. Subdural abscess
  4. Intracranial abscess

CHRONIC RHINOSINUSITIS

PATHOPHYSIOLOGIC CONTRIBUTORS TO THE CHRONIC RHINOSINUSITIS

- Predominance of T helper 2 (Th2) cytokines
- Predominance of eosinophils
- Staphylococcal super-antigen
- Deficiency in innate immunity
- Impaired mucociliary clearance
- Biofilms
- Alterations in microbiome

SYMPTOMS OF CHRONIC RHINOSINUSITIS

- Nasal obstruction/congestion
- Hyposmia/anosmia
- Nasal discharge/postnasal drip
- Facial pressure
- Cough
- Wheeze (asthma)

WORKUP FOR CHRONIC RHINOSINUSITIS

- Examination: nasal endoscopy reveals inflammation, with polyps in some cases
- Lab testing
  - Endoscopic guided middle meatus cultures for concurrent bacterial infection (>80% accuracy)
  - Endoscopic biopsy for unilateral nasal mass/polyp or to differentiate from chronic granulomatous disease
  - Sweat chloride test/genetic test if CF is suspected

Table 4.2 Signs and Symptoms of the Complications of Acute Rhinosinusitis

Complication	Clinical Findings
Preseptal cellulitis	Eyelid edema, erythema, and tenderness Unrestricted extraocular movement Normal visual acuity
Subperiosteal abscess	Proptosis and impaired extraocular muscle movement
Orbital cellulitis	Eyelid edema and erythema, proptosis, and chemosis; no limited impairment of extraocular movements; normal visual acuity
Orbital abscess	Significant exophthalmos, chemosis, ophthalmoplegia, and visual impairment
Cavernous sinus thrombosis	Bilateral orbital pain, chemosis, proptosis, and ophthalmoplegia
Meningitis	Headache, neck stiffness, and high fever
Epidural abscess	Headache, fever, altered mental status, and local tenderness Unenhanced CT reveals a hypodense or isodense crescent-shaped collection in the epidural space
Subdural abscess	Headache, fever, meningismus, focal neurologic deficits, and lethargy with rapid deterioration; CT reveals a hypodense collection along a hemisphere or along the falx; MRI demonstrates low signal on T1 and high signal on T2 images with peripheral contrast enhancement
Intracerebral abscess	Fever, headache, vomiting, lethargy, seizures, and focal neurologic deficits; frontal deficits can include changes in mood and behavior; MRI demonstrates a cystic lesion with a distinct hypointense, strongly enhancing capsule on T2 images
Frontal bone osteomyelitis (Pott's puffy tumor)	Fluctuant forehead swelling

CT, Computed tomography; *MRI*, magnetic resonance imaging.
From Flint PW, Haughey BH, Lund VJ, et al. *Cummings Otolaryngology—Head and Neck Surgery.* 6th ed. Philadelphia, PA: Saunders; 2015, table 46-2.

- Allergy testing if concurrent allergic rhinitis is suspected
- Imaging studies
  - CT scan of paranasal sinuses without contrast is standard (conventional vs. in-office cone beam)
  - MRI if malignancy or other neoplasm is suspected

TREATMENT FOR CHRONIC RHINOSINUSITIS (Table 4.3)

- Medical treatment[6]
  - Oral steroids (level-1a evidence)
  - Topical steroids (level-1a evidence): steroid sprays, or budesonide or other steroid irrigations
  - Saline irrigations (level-1b evidence for symptomatic relief)
  - Short-term (<4 weeks) oral antibiotics (level-1b evidence)
  - Long-term (>4 weeks) oral antibiotics (level-III evidence)
  - Proton pump inhibitors (level-II evidence)

Table 4.3 Summary of Recommendations for Medical Therapy in Chronic Rhinosinusitis

Medical Therapy	EPOS12[a]	EBRR[b]
Oral antibacterial • Nonmacrolide • <3 to 4 weeks	CRSsNP: B+ CRSwNP: C+	CRS: option
Oral antibacterial • Macrolide • ≥12 weeks	CRSsNP: C+ CRSwNP: C+	CRS: option
Intravenous antibacterial	CRSsNP: did not review CRSwNP: did not review	CRS: recommend against
Topical antibacterial	CRSsNP: A− CRSwNP: no data	CRS: recommend against
Oral antifungal	CRSsNP: A− CRSwNP: A−	CRS: recommend against
Intravenous antifungal	CRSsNP: no data CRSwNP: no data	CRS: recommend against
Topical antifungal	CRSsNP: A− CRSwNP: A−	CRS: recommend against
Topical corticosteroid	CRSsNP: A+ CRSwNP: A+	CRSsNP: recommend CRSwNP: recommend
Systemic (oral) corticosteroid	CRSsNP: C+ CRSwNP: A+	CRSsNP: option CRSwNP: recommend
Saline irrigations	CRSsNP: A+ CRSwNP: D+	CRS: recommend
Antihistamines (in allergic patients)	CRSsNP: no data CRSwNP: D+	—
Leukotriene antagonists	CRSsNP: no data CRSwNP: A−	—
Anti-IgE monoclonal antibodies	CRSwNP: A−	—
Anti-IL-5 monoclonal antibodies	CRSwNP: D+	—

+, recommended; −, recommended against; A, directly based on category-I evidence; B, directly based on category-II evidence or extrapolated from category-I evidence; C, directly based on category-III evidence or extrapolated from category-I or category-II evidence; D, directly based on category-IV evidence or extrapolated from category-I, category-II, or category-III evidence.
CRSsNP, chronic rhinosinusitis without nasal polyps; CRSwNP, chronic rhinosinusitis with nasal polyps; IgE, immunoglobulin E; IL-5, interleukin 5.
[a]As reported in the European Position Paper on Rhinosinusitis and Nasal Polyps 2012.[2]
[b]Published evidenced-based reviews with recommendations.[3-5]
From Flint PW, Haughey BH, Lund VJ, et al. *Cummings Otolaryngology—Head and Neck Surgery.* 6th ed. Philadelphia, PA: Saunders; 2015, Table 44.3.

- Aspirin desensitization (level-II evidence for AERD)
- Antileukotrienes (level-Ib evidence; treats concurrent asthma symptoms)
- Antihistamines (topical or oral for concurrent allergic rhinitis)
- Anti-IgE (omalizumab monoclonal antibody; injection)
- Low-dose macrolides (antiinflammatory effect; 250 mg clarithromycin daily)
- Antifungals (oral vs. topical, effective in some patients but not shown to have a significant effect on CRS patients in randomized controlled trials)
- Surgical treatment of CRS
  - Functional endoscopic sinus surgery (FESS) is standard: OR (operating room) under general anesthesia versus in-office procedures

ETIOLOGIES OF CHRONIC RHINOSINUSITIS

1. Eosinophilic chronic sinusitis
2. Allergic fungal sinusitis
3. AERD (Aspirin exacerbated respiratory disease or Samter's triad)
4. Cystic fibrosis CF
5. Chronic granulomatous disease (Granulomatosis with polyangiitis [GPA], Sarcoidosis)
6. Churg-Strauss

EOSINOPHILIC CHRONIC SINUSITIS BASICS

- Chronic sinusitis with or without polyps
- Presence of thick mucin and eosinophils in tissue
- Concurrent asthma present in 50-70% of patients

ALLERGIC FUNGAL SINUSITIS BASICS

- Bent Kuhn criteria
  - Major criteria
    1. Type-1 hypersensitivity
    2. Nasal polyposis
    3. Characteristic CT scan signs: expansion of sinuses, asymmetry, and heterogeneously dense material in sinuses
    4. Positive fungal smear
    5. Eosinophilic mucin without tissue invasion
  - Minor criteria
    1. Asthma
    2. Unilateral predominance
    3. Serum eosinophilia
    4. Radiographic bone erosion
    5. Fungal culture
    6. Charcot-Leyden crystals
- Treatment
  - FESS to open sinuses and remove all fungal debris
  - Oral and topical steroids
  - Immunotherapy

ASPIRIN-EXACERBATED RESPIRATORY DISEASE (SAMTER'S TRIAD) BASICS

- Presence of polyps, asthma, and asthma exacerbated by Cox-1 inhibitors (aspirin, NSAIDs)
- Caused by abnormality of arachidonic acid cascade that leads to increased production of proinflammatory leukotrienes
- Cox-1 inhibitors will exacerbate increased production of leukotrienes, leading to severe worsening of asthma symptoms and/or allergy-like symptoms
- Treatment
  - Similar to treatment for CRS
  - Aspirin desensitization (requires daily aspirin maintenance after desensitization)

CYSTIC FIBROSIS BASICS[6]

- Pathophysiology: autosomal recessive defect in chloride ion channel
- Etiology: multiple mutations in CF conductance transmembrane conductance regulator (CFTR); F508 deletion is most common
- Clinical sinonasal manifestations
  - Severe chronic inflammation and polyposis
  - Chronic and recurrent bacterial infections (*Pseudomonas aeruginosa, Staph. aureus, Escherichia coli, Burkholderia cepacia, Acinetobacter* species, *Stenotrophomonas maltophilia, H. influenzae,* Streptococci, and anaerobes)
  - CT scans reveal underdeveloped paranasal sinuses
  - Viscous mucus secretions
- Medical treatment
  - Saline irrigations
  - Topical and oral steroids
  - Oral antibiotics
  - Topical antibiotics
  - Mucolytics (Dornase alfa)
  - Novel therapies
    - Ivacaftor (potentiates mutant CFTR on cell surface)
    - Lumacaftor (improves delivery of CFTR to cell surface)
    - Ataluren (induces translational reading of nonsense CFTR mutations)
- Surgical treatment
  - FESS allows improved debridement and irrigations
    - Modified endoscopic medial maxillectomy to promote gravity drainage of maxillary sinuses and allow for improved irrigations and debridement
  - Endoscopic debridements (in-office or under anesthesia)

GRANULOMATOSIS WITH POLYANGIITIS (FORMERLY WEGENER'S DISEASE) BASICS

- Small, medium vessel vasculitis; etiology unknown
- C-ANCA antibodies often present
- Clinical sinonasal manifestations
  - Severe chronic inflammation
  - Presence of granulation tissue
  - Concurrent infection (*Staph. aureus*)
  - Chronic mucosal crusting
  - Septal perforation and erosion of sinonasal structures (turbinates)
  - Saddle nose deformity
- Treatment
  - Oral corticosteroids
  - Immunosuppressive agents (cyclophosphamide and methotrexate)

- Sulfamethoxazole and trimethoprim (Bactrim) for disease in remission
- Topical saline rinses and steroids for symptomatic relief
- FESS in quiescent disease (disease in remission)

SARCOIDOSIS BASICS

- Noncaseating granulomatous disease
- Systemic clinical manifestations
  - Bihilar lymphadenopathy on chest x-ray
  - Fatigue, night sweats, and weight loss
  - Erythema nodosum
  - Uveitis
  - Peripheral lymphadenopathy
  - Heerfordt's syndrome (enlarged parotid glands, facial nerve palsy, uveitis, and fever)
- Clinical sinonasal manifestations
  - Severe chronic inflammation and polyps
  - Presence of mucosal nodules and/or cobble stoning of mucosa
  - Mucosal crusting
- Treatment
  - Oral corticosteroids
  - Immunosuppressive agents (cyclophosphamide and methotrexate)
  - Topical saline rinses and steroids for symptomatic relief
  - FESS in controlled inflammatory disease

CHURG-STRAUSS BASICS

- Small-to-medium vessel vasculitis, with etiology unknown
- P-ANCA antibodies often present
- American College of Rheumatology criteria for diagnosis
  1. Asthma
  2. Eosinophilia of more than 10% in peripheral blood
  3. Paranasal sinusitis
  4. Pulmonary infiltrates
  5. Histologic proof of vasculitis with extravascular eosinophils
  6. Mononeuritis multiplex or polyneuropathy
- Three clinical phases
  1. Prodromal phase (asthma and upper-respiratory involvement)
  2. Peripheral eosinophilia (pulmonary or gastrointestinal [GI] involvement)
  3. Disseminated (lung, CNS, kidney, GI, and skin)
- Treatment
  - Oral corticosteroids
  - Immunosuppressive agents (cyclophosphamide and methotrexate)
  - FESS

SINONASAL NEOPLASMS

DIFFERENTIAL DIAGNOSIS OF BENIGN SINONASAL NEOPLASMS

1. Osteoma
2. Fibrous dysplasia
3. Ossifying fibroma
4. Chordoma
5. Cementoma
6. Hemangioma
7. Inverted papilloma (Figs. 4.13-4.16)
8. JNA (Figs. 4.17-4.19)
9. Pleomorphic adenoma
10. Schwannoma
11. Neurofibroma

DIFFERENTIAL DIAGNOSIS OF MALIGNANT SINONASAL NEOPLASMS

1. Esthesioneuroblastoma
2. Lymphoma
3. Ewing sarcoma
4. Chondrosarcoma
5. Rhabdomyosarcoma
6. Nasopharyngeal carcinoma
7. Small cell carcinoma
8. Squamous cell carcinoma
9. Sinonasal undifferentiated carcinoma (SNUC)

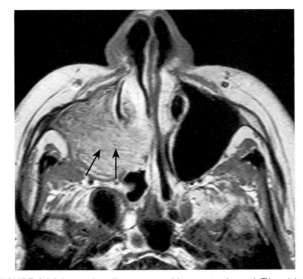

FIGURE 4.13 Typical endoscopic appearance of an inverted papilloma. A polypoid lesion with a pale, papillary surface protrudes from the middle meatus and extensively fills the left nasal cavity. (From Flint PW, Haughey BH, Lund VJ, et al. *Cummings Otolaryngology—Head and Neck Surgery*. 6th ed. Philadelphia, PA: Saunders; 2015, fig. 48-1.)

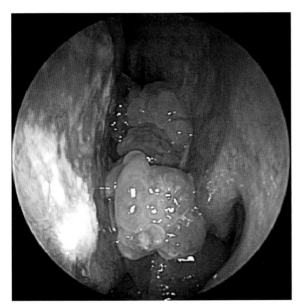

FIGURE 4.14 Inverted papilloma on an axial contrast-enhanced, T1-weighted, spin-echo MRI. The maxillary sinus is occupied by a solid mass that protrudes into the nasal fossa through an accessory ostium. The lesion exhibits a cerebriform-columnar pattern, which is typically seen in inverted papilloma (*arrows*). (From Flint PW, Haughey BH, Lund VJ, et al. *Cummings Otolaryngology—Head and Neck Surgery*. 6th ed. Philadelphia, PA: Saunders; 2015, fig. 48-2.)

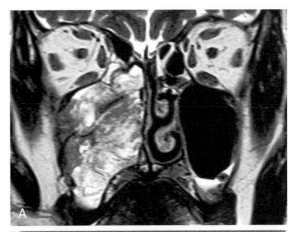

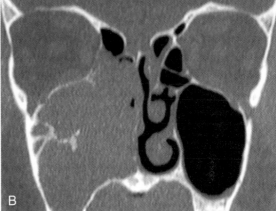

FIGURE 4.15 Inverted papilloma on an MRI and a CT scan, both in the coronal plane. The maxillary sinus is completely occupied by an expansile lesion that destroyed the medial wall and invaded the right nasal fossa. (**A**) The T2-weighted spin-echo MRI demonstrates the cerebriform-columnar pattern of the lesion and permits visualization of the bony spur along the lateral maxillary sinus wall, where the lesion originates. (**B**) The CT scan does not provide a good characterization of soft tissue–density opacification but gives a superior view of the sclerotic bony spur. (From Flint PW, Haughey BH, Lund VJ, et al. *Cummings Otolaryngology—Head and Neck Surgery*. 6th ed. Philadelphia, PA: Saunders; 2015, fig. 48-3.)

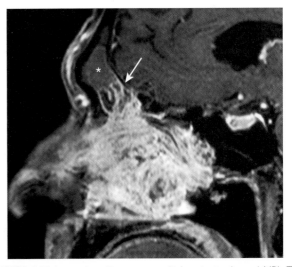

FIGURE 4.16 Inverted papilloma on a sagittal contrast-enhanced MRI. The advantage of this acquisition plane is the excellent assessment of tumor growth into the most caudal part of the frontal sinus. The upper part of the sinus is filled with inflammatory secretions (*asterisk*). The sagittal plane also permits accurate evaluation of the relationships between the tumor and the floor of the anterior cranial fossa, which is not invaded (*arrow*). (From Flint PW, Haughey BH, Lund VJ, et al. *Cummings Otolaryngology—Head and Neck Surgery*. 6th ed. Philadelphia, PA: Saunders; 2015, fig. 48-5.)

10. Adenocarcinoma
11. Adenocystic carcinoma
12. Mucoepidermoid carcinoma
13. Hemangiopericytoma (both benign and malignant types)
14. Melanoma
15. Peripheral nerve sheath tumor

DIFFERENTIAL DIAGNOSIS OF CONGENITAL SINONASAL NEOPLASMS

1. Dermoid
2. Teratoma
3. Glioma
4. Encephalocele

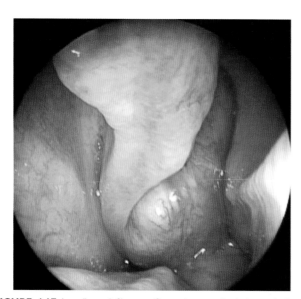

FIGURE 4.17 Juvenile angiofibroma. On endoscopy, the lesion typically appears as a polypoid hypervascularized mass that bulges from the lateral wall behind the MT, which is laterally compressed. The choana is completely obstructed. (From Flint PW, Haughey BH, Lund VJ, et al. *Cummings Otolaryngology—Head and Neck Surgery.* 6th ed. Philadelphia, PA: Saunders; 2015, fig. 48-7.)

DIFFERENTIAL DIAGNOSIS OF INFLAMMATORY SINONASAL NEOPLASMS

1. Nasal polyp
2. Antrochoanal polyp
3. Inverting papilloma

DIFFERENTIAL DIAGNOSIS OF VASCULAR SINONASAL NEOPLASMS

1. Hemangioma
2. Lobular capillary hemangioma (pyogenic granuloma)
3. Hamartoma

DIFFERENTIAL DIAGNOSIS OF TRAUMATIC SINONASAL NEOPLASMS

1. Encephalocele
2. Septal hematoma
3. Pyogenic granuloma

DIFFERENTIAL FOR SINONASAL "BLUE CELL" TUMORS

1. Rhabdomyosarcoma
2. Esthesioneuroblastoma
3. Lymphoma
4. Melanoma
5. Poorly differentiated carcinoma (SNUC)
6. Hemangiopericytoma
7. Immature teratoma
8. Carcinoid
9. Peripheral nerve sheath tumor

STAGING SYSTEMS FOR JUVENILE NASOPHARYNGEAL ANGIOFIBROMA

- Radkowski (most universally accepted system)
  - Stage 1A: limited to nose or nasopharynx
  - Stage IB: extension into at least one paranasal sinus

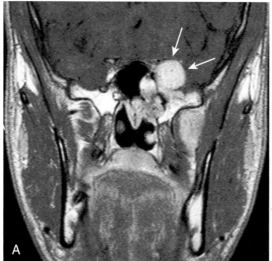
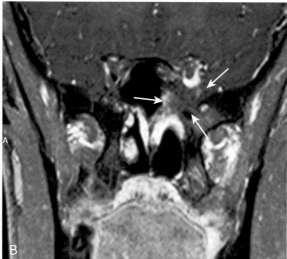

FIGURE 4.18 Juvenile angiofibroma on coronal contrast-enhanced MRIs obtained before and after endoscopic resection. (**A**) Pretreatment image shows encroachment of both the floor and lateral wall of the left SS and infratemporal fossa. Intracranial extension is demonstrated in close proximity to the superior orbital fissure (*arrows*). (**B**) MRI obtained after surgical resection shows solid tissue (*arrows*) along the lateral SS wall; the lack of contrast enhancement suggests residual scar tissue. (From Flint PW, Haughey BH, Lund VJ, et al. *Cummings Otolaryngology—Head and Neck Surgery.* 6th ed. Philadelphia, PA: Saunders; 2015, fig. 48-8.)

- Stage IIA: minimal extension through the sphenopalatine foramen; includes a minimal part of the medial pterygomaxillary fossa
- Stage IIB: full occupation of pterygomaxillary fossa with Holman-Miller sign (bowing of the posterior wall of the maxillary sinus on CT); lateral or anterior displacement of maxillary artery branches; may have superior extension with orbital bone erosion
- Stage IIC: extension through the pterygomaxillary fossa into the cheek, temporal fossa, or posterior to the pterygoids
- Stage IIIA: skull-base erosion with minimal intracranial extension
- Stage IIIB: skull-base erosion with extensive intracranial extension ± cavernous sinus
- Modified Sessions
- Fisch

STAGING SYSTEMS FOR ESTHESIONEUROBLASTOMA

- Kadish
  - Stage A: tumor limited to the nasal cavity
  - Stage B: extension to the paranasal sinuses
  - Stage C: extension beyond the nasal cavity/paranasal sinuses
  - Stage D: metastatic disease
- Dulgerov
  - Stage T1: tumor of the nasal cavity and/or paranasal sinuses, sparing the most superior ethmoid cells
  - Stage T2: tumor involving the nasal cavity and/or paranasal sinuses (including sphenoid) with extension to or erosion of the cribriform plate
  - Stage T3: tumor extending to the orbit or protruding into the anterior fossa
  - Stage T4: tumor involving the brain
- Biller
  - Stage T1: tumor of the nasal cavity/paranasal sinuses (excluding sphenoid) with or without erosion of the anterior fossa bone

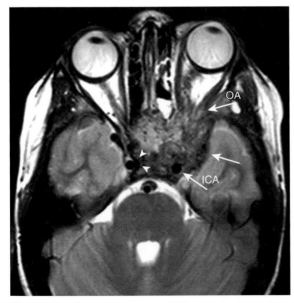

FIGURE 4.19 Juvenile angiofibroma on axial T2-weighted, spin-echo MRI. The lesion invades the left orbital apex (*OA*); the lateral wall of the left SS (*arrows*) is completely destroyed, and the ICA is encased. On the right side, a bony barrier (*arrowheads*) still separates the lesion from the ICA. (From Flint PW, Haughey BH, Lund VJ, et al. *Cummings Otolaryngology—Head and Neck Surgery*. 6th ed. Philadelphia, PA: Saunders; 2015, fig. 48-9.)

- Stage T2: extension into the orbit or protrusion into the anterior fossa
- Stage T3: involvement of the brain that is resectable with margins
- Stage T4: unresectable
- Hyams (histologic grade)
  - Grade I: prominent neurofibrillary matrix, tumor cells with uniform nuclei, some rosettes, and absence of nuclear pleomorphism, mitotic activity, or necrosis
  - Grade II: some neurofibrillary matrix, nuclear pleomorphism, and mitotic activity; absence of mitoses and necrosis
  - Grade III: minimal neurofibrillary matrix and rosettes; more prominent mitotic activity and nuclear pleomorphism; some necrosis may be seen
  - Grade IV: no neurofibrillary matrix or rosettes seen; marked nuclear pleomorphism and necrosis, and increased mitotic activity

STAGING SYSTEMS FOR INVERTED PAPILLOMA

- Krouse[7]
  - Stage T1: limited to one area of the nasal cavity
  - Stage T2: involvement of the medial wall of the maxillary or ethmoid sinuses and/or the osteomeatal unit
  - Stage T3: involvement of the superior, inferior, posterior, anterior, or lateral walls of the maxillary sinus
  - Stage T4: tumors with extrasinonasal spread or malignancy
- Cannaday[8]
  - Group A: confined to the nasal cavity, medial maxillary sinus, and ethmoid sinus (recurrence rate = 3%)
  - Group B: involving the lateral maxillary sinus, sphenoid sinus, or frontal sinus (recurrence rate = 19.8%)
  - Group C: extrasinus extension (recurrence rate = 35.5%)

SURGICAL APPROACHES

1. Open craniofacial
2. Endoscopic assisted (combined open and endoscopic)
3. Endoscopic and expanded endoscopic approaches

SURGERY OF THE PARANASAL SINUSES

INDICATIONS FOR ENDOSCOPIC SINUS SURGERY

- Chronic sinusitis with or without polyps refractory to medical treatment: most common indication, to relieve obstruction and allow for delivery of medication
- Recurrent sinusitis (≥4 episodes a year): should be confirmed endoscopically or on CT scan, while the patient is symptomatic, to rule out disorders that mimic sinusitis such as migraines
- Acute complications of rhinosinusitis, (ie; intracranial or orbital)
- Antrochoanal polyps
- Sinus mucoceles: marsupialized to avoid continued expansion and risk of intracranial and orbital complications
- Excision of sinonasal tumors
- Excision of skull-base tumors
- CSF leak repair
- Orbital decompression (eg, Graves ophthalmopathy)

- Optic nerve decompression
- Dacryocystorhinostomy (DCR)
- Choanal atresia repair
- Foreign body removal
- Intractable epistaxis control
- Noninvasive fungal sinusitis
- Invasive fungal sinusitis
- Headache and facial pain—controversial—contact points on CT and/or endoscopy with clear reduction in headache in response to intranasal decongestants after both thorough neurologic and radiographic evaluation and failure of medical therapy

INDICATIONS FOR SURGICAL INTERVENTION IN ACUTE BACTERIAL SINUSITIS

- Impending complications of sinusitis
- Nonresponse to medical therapy
- Immunosuppressed patient

FUNCTIONAL ENDOSCOPIC SINUS SURGERY PRINCIPLES

- Restore mucociliary function by reestablishing physiologic sinus ventilation and drainage
- Remove irreversibly diseased mucosa and bone and preserve normal tissue
- Allow for delivery of topical therapies
- Ostiomeatal complex is the primary target of ESS because minimal inflammation in this area can lead to disease in the maxillary, anterior ethmoid, and frontal sinuses

EXTERNAL APPROACHES TO THE PARANASAL SINUSES

- Maxillary sinus: Caldwell-Luc procedure and canine fossa trephination
- Ethmoid sinuses: external ethmoidectomy (results in external scar; loss of bone lateral to the frontal recess and loss of mucosa often result in scar tissue and stenosis of the frontal recess)
- Frontal sinus: frontal sinus trephination, osteroplastic flap with or without obliteration (has significant rate of long-term failure and mucocele formation)

MAJOR COMPLICATIONS OF ENDOSCOPIC SINUS SURGERY

- CSF leak
- Blindness
- Diplopia
- ICA injury
- Major bleeding
- Orbital hematoma

OTHER COMPLICATIONS OF ENDOSCOPIC SINUS SURGERY

- Nasolacrimal duct injury
- Hyposmia
- Minor epistaxis
- Adhesions
- Periorbital ecchymosis
- Facial pain

Box 4.3 BASIC STEPS IN ENDOSCOPIC SINUS SURGERY

1. Patient positioning
2. Diagnostic nasal endoscopy
3. Topical anesthetic injections
4. Medialization of the MT to expose the ostiomeatal complex (basal lamella–relaxing incision is optional)
5. Uncinectomy with a zero-degree endoscope
6. Maxillary antrostomy: use a 30- or 45-degree endoscope to identify the maxillary sinus ostium and floor of the orbit, and then follow it up to the medial orbital wall (lamina papyracea)
7. Removal of the ethmoid bulla; identification of the lamina papyracea in its medial wall
8. Identification of the basal lamella of the MT in the horizontal and oblique segments
9. Removal of the inferomedial part of the vertical MT basal lamella to penetrate into the posterior ethmoid sinus
10. Ethmoidectomy; stay low, between the superior turbinate medially and the lamina papyracea laterally
11. Identification of the sphenoid face
12. Identification of the posterior skull base, in either the posterior ethmoid (possible in the absence of polyps or in a single tier of cells) or following the sphenoid face up to the skull base
13. Clearance of the skull base in a posterior to anterior direction, removing the ethmoid partitions
14. Sphenoid sinusotomy (if needed) through the medial inferior triangle of the posterior ethmoid box or by identifying it in the sphenoethmoidal recess
15. Optional: identification of the frontal recesses, frontal sinusotomy
16. Optional: medialization of the medial MT by creating adhesion between the medial surface and septum (suture or pack)
17. Optional: placement of a middle meatal spacer

From Flint PW, Haughey BH, Lund VJ, et al. *Cummings Otolaryngology—Head and Neck Surgery*. 6th ed. Philadelphia, PA: Saunders; 2015, box 49-3.

MANAGEMENT OF POSTOPERATIVE ORBITAL HEMATOMA

- Surgical emergency
- Immediate decompression of the orbit via a lateral canthotomy with cantholysis and/or formal external or endoscopic orbital decompression
- Surgical hemostasis of bleeding vessels
- Ophthalmology consultation
- IV mannitol
- IV acetazolamide
- IV steroids

FACTORS INCREASING RISK OF ORBITAL OR SKULL-BASE INJURIES (Box 4.3)

- Lamina papyracea lies medial to maxillary ostium
- Dehiscence of the lamina
- Maxillary sinus hypoplasia
- Low or sloping fovea ethmoidalis
- Sphenoid sinus septations are attached to the carotid canal
- Carotid canal or optic nerve dehiscence
- Presence of sphenoethmoid (also known as Onodi) cell

COMMON CAUSES OF FAILURE OF ENDOSCOPIC SINUS SURGERY

- Lateralized MT
- Missed middle meatal antrostomy (recirculation)
- Maxillary ostium stenosis
- Frontal recess scarring
- Residual ethmoidal air cells
- Adhesions

INDICATIONS FOR USE OF IMAGE GUIDANCE

- Revision sinus surgery
- Distorted sinus anatomy of development, postoperative, or traumatic origin
- Extensive sinonasal polyposis
- Pathology involving the frontal, posterior ethmoid, and sphenoid sinuses
- Disease abutting the skull base, orbit, optic nerve, or carotid artery
- CSF rhinorrhea or conditions where there is a skull-base defect

REVISION SINUS SURGERY

- Initial surgery represents the greatest chance for long-term success
- Comprehensive postsurgical care with directed debridement, sinonasal irrigations, and appropriate medical therapy is critical to achieving high success rates in primary surgery
- Causes of failure
  - Misattribution of symptoms: initial surgery performed for misattributed symptoms (eg, headache, facial pain, odontogenic disease, temporomandibular joint [TMJ] dysfunction, and reflux)
  - Medical factors
    - Persistent microbial disease
    - Biofilm formation
    - Persistent inflammatory disease (eg, chronic sinusitis with nasal polyposis, presence of asthma, and AERD)
    - Systemic comorbidities (eg, granulomatous diseases, allergy, CF, immunoglobulin deficiencies, and HIV)
  - Environmental factor: smoking
  - Iatrogenic factors
    - Submaximal dissection of the instrumented sinuses (eg, retained ethmoid cells and residual agger nasi remnants)
    - Incomplete uncinate dissection and posteriorly placed maxillary antrostomy not incorporating natural os resulting in possible recirculation phenomenon
    - MT lateralization and middle meatal obstruction, common in setting of partial middle turbinectomy
    - Failure to recognize and address anatomic variants such as infraorbital ethmoid (Haller) and sphenoethmoid (Onodi) cells

FRONTAL SINUS SURGERY

- Use an instrument in the frontal recess only with good reason. Remove all cells obstructing the frontal recess including Agger Nasi, frontal, subrabullar and supraorbital cells.
- Functional drainage of the frontal sinus relies on preservation of the mucosa of the frontal recess
- If the mucosa of the frontal recess cannot be preserved, a Draf III procedure is the remaining endoscopic option
- Maintain bony support around the frontal recess whenever possible

ENDOSCOPIC FRONTAL SINUS APPROACHES

- Balloon dilation
- Draf I: complete ethmoidectomy with removal of the bulla and suprabullar cells
- Draf IIa: enlargement of the frontal outflow tract with removal of all occupying cells (frontal sinusotomy)
- Draf IIb (unilateral frontal sinus drill out): removal of the floor of the frontal sinus, from the lamina papyracea to the septum, to produce the largest possible unilateral outflow tract
- Draf III (endoscopic modified Lothrop): complete drill out of the floor of the frontal sinuses, frontal beak, and intersinus septum and an adjacent part of the nasal septum

EXTERNAL FRONTAL SINUS APPROACHES

- Frontal trephine
- External ethmoidectomy
- Osteoplastic flap with or without obliteration
  - If obliteration of the sinus is required, remove all mucosa and drill the cavity
  - Obliteration is associated with a high rate of long-term failure

APPROACHES TO BENIGN OR MALIGNANT NASAL MASSES

- Endoscopic excision
- Midface degloving
- Lateral rhinotomy ± lip-split and subciliary incisions
- Combined craniofacial (facial incisions with bicoronal incisions)
- Transpalatal
- Infratemporal fossa
- Facial translocation

ENDOSCOPIC SKULL-BASE RECONSTRUCTION OPTIONS

- Septal mucosal flap: septal branch of sphenopalatine artery
- MT flap: MT branch of sphenopalatine artery
- Inferior turbinate flap: inferior turbinate branch of sphenopalatine artery
- Pericranial flap: supraorbital and supratrochlear arteries
- Temporoparietal fascia flap: anterior branch of the superficial temporal artery
- Palatal flap: descending palatine artery

ENDOSCOPIC DACRYOCYSTORHINOSTOMY

CLASSIFICATION OF LACRIMAL OBSTRUCTION

- Anatomic
  - 70% of cases have complete blockage; better outcome with DCR
    - Children with nasolacrimal duct obstruction often have imperforate Hasner valve amenable to probing
    - Young adults tend to have pathology of the canaliculi
    - Middle-aged patients tend to have dacryoliths, which are amenable to DCR
    - Elderly patients tend to have lacrimal duct obstruction, which is amenable to DCR
  - Functional failure in 30% of cases: of proximal pump mechanism or critical narrowings

PHYSICAL EXAMINATION

- Exclude lid laxity, malposition, punctal anomalies, and blepharitis.
- Palpate over lacrimal sac to search for reflux of mucopurulence.

- Dye disappearance test: drop of 2% fluorescein into both conjunctival fornices—normal test is symmetric and with complete disappearance of dye within 5 minutes.
- A cotton swab is used in the inferior meatus to confirm the flow of fluorescein (positive Jones I test).
- For abnormal results, perform Jones II test.
  - Bowman lacrimal probe places an inferior or a superior canaliculus to palpate the common internal punctum.
    - Soft stop: impeded progress of the lacrimal probe before entering the lacrimal sac requires further assessment.
    - Hard-stop: probe impacts the medial bony wall of the lacrimal sac, which implies no stenosis of the canalicular system.
  - Finally, a 25-G blunt lacrimal needle is placed into the inferior punctum to irrigate the lacrimal system with clear (nonflourescein dyed) saline.
    - If the patient tastes saline, this rules out a complete obstruction but not a functional problem.
    - If the patient does not taste saline, anatomic obstruction is likely.

INTERPRETATION OF JONES II TEST RESULTS

1. Reflux of clear saline fluid from the same punctum being irrigated indicates obstruction proximal to the common canaliculus because fluorescein did not fill the lacrimal sac during Jones I and is not present in sufficient quantity to stain refluxing saline.
2. Reflux of clear fluid from the opposite punctum indicates obstruction of the common canaliculus or common internal punctum.
3. Reflux of fluorescein-stained fluid through the opposite punctum indicates nasolacrimal duct obstruction (fluorescein present in lacrimal sac stains refluxing saline).

RADIOLOGIC EVALUATION

- Scintillogram: nuclear medicine equivalent of the dye disappearance test; assesses functional and anatomic obstructions
- Dacryocystogram (DCG) requires syringing the lacrimal puncta with radiopaque dye; gives results similar to Jones II test results

SURGICAL TECHNIQUE

- Advantages over external DCR
  - Lack of an incision
  - No disruption of the lacrimal pump mechanism
- Key elements
  - Creation of the widest possible marsupialization of the medial wall of the lacrimal sac
  - Identification of the common internal punctum (most proximal portion of the lacrimal system that can be successfully managed by DCR)

- Endoscopic anatomical landmarks
  - Axilla of the MT: upper one-third of the sac just superior to the anterior insertion of the MT
  - Maxillary line: corresponds intranasally to the junction of the uncinate and maxilla, extranasally to the suture line between the lacrimal bone and maxilla within the lacrimal fossa; inferior two-thirds of the sac is oriented vertically, just under the maxillary line
- Steps of surgery
  - Flap elevation or removal of mucosa around maxillary line
  - Frontal process of the maxilla covering the anterior portion of the lacrimal sac is now removed with punch or drill; frontal process of the maxilla and the lacrimal bone are the two bone segments on either side of the lacrimomaxillary suture that need to be removed
  - Superior and inferior lacrimal puncta dilated and cannulated with Bowman probes
  - Once the probe is evident in the lacrimal sac, the sac is incised from top to bottom
  - May consider stenting (eg, with silicone Crawford tubes) for a period of several weeks to months

OUTCOMES OF DACRYOCYSTORHINOSTOMY

- Anatomic obstruction >95% success rate (free flow of fluorescein; asymptomatic patient)
- Functional obstruction approximately 80% success rate
- 5% rate of complications, including hemorrhage, orbital fat exposure, orbital hematoma, and synechiae/granulation tissue obstruction of the ostium

REFERENCES

1. American Academy of Otolaryngology—Head and Neck Surgery (AAO-HNS). Clinical practice guideline (update): adult sinusitis. *Otolaryngol Head Neck Surg.* 2015;152(suppl 2):S1-S39.
2. Fokkens WJ, Lund VJ, Mullol J, et al. EPOS 2012: European position paper on rhinosinusitis and nasal polyps 2012. A summary for otorhinolaryngologists. *Rhinology.* 2012;50:1-12.
3. Soler ZM, Oyer SL, Kern RC, et al. Antimicrobials and chronic rhinosinusitis with or without polyposis in adults: an evidenced-based review with recommendations. *Int Forum Allergy Rhinol.* 2013;3:31-47.
4. Rudmik L, Hoy M, Schlosser RJ, et al. Topical therapies in the management of chronic rhinosinusitis: an evidence-based review with recommendations. *Int Forum Allergy Rhinol.* 2013;3(4):281-298.
5. Poetker DM, Jakubowski LA, Lal D, et al. Oral corticosteroids in the management of adult chronic rhinosinusitis with and without nasal polyps: an evidence-based review with recommendations. *Int Forum Allergy Rhinol.* 2013;3:104-120.
6. Reh DD, Woodworth BA, Poetker D, eds. Rhinology maintenance of certification review. *Am J Rhinol Allergy.* May-Jun. 2014;28(suppl 1): S18.
7. Krouse JH. Development of a staging system for inverted papilloma. *Laryngoscope.* 2000;110:965-968.
8. Cannaday SB, Batra PS, Sautter NB, et al. New staging system for sinonasal inverted papilloma in the endoscopic era. *Laryngoscope.* 2007;117:1283-1287.

Head and Neck Surgery

PRINCIPLES OF RADIATION THERAPY

TYPES OF RADIATION

- Photon: most common form
- Electron: superficial penetration ideal for skin
- Neutron: high-energy particle and highly toxic
  - Selectively used for salivary gland malignancies
- Proton: low-energy particle with a sharp falloff of dose beyond the target (Bragg peak)
  - Increasingly used for skull base where dose to critical adjacent structures must be minimized
- Carbon ion: high-energy particle with a sharp Bragg peak

UNITS OF RADIATION ENERGY

- Gray (Gy): 1 Gy equals 1 J of energy deposited per kilogram material
- Radiation-absorbed dose (rad): 100 rad = 1 Gy
- Doses range from 30 to 70 Gy

RADIATION SOURCES

- Cobalt (Co-60), iridium (Ir-192), and cesium (Cs-137)
- Linear accelerator
- X-rays and electron energy of 4-25 MeV
- Accelerated electrons strike tungsten to produce x-rays

RADIATION DELIVERY

- Conventional radiation
- Intensity modulated radiation therapy (IMRT)
- Brachytherapy
- Stereotactic body radiation therapy (SBRT)

CONVENTIONAL RADIATION

- Manual blocks are cut to shape the beam.
- Multileaf collimators are introduced to shape the radiation field.

INTENSITY MODULATED RADIATION THERAPY

- Inverse planning
  - Ideal radiation dose distribution is based on imaging
  - Computer algorithm is applied to achieve the ideal distribution
- Precise control
  - Multiple small "beamlets" converge on targets
  - Multiple beamlet conformations contour the dose
  - Minimization of the dose to critical structures

- Salivary glands
- Pharyngeal constrictors
- Temporal lobe
- Optic nerve
- Cochlea
- Spinal cord

BRACHYTHERAPY

- Radioisotopes applied to tumor bed
- Permanent implants (beads) or interstitial catheters
- Rapid dose falloff of radiation
- Lip cancer
- Nasopharyngeal recurrence
- Base of tongue recurrence

INDICATIONS FOR POSTOPERATIVE RADIOTHERAPY

- Advanced-stage disease: pT3, pT4
- Multiple positive nodes
  - Without extracapsular extension (radiation alone)
  - With extracapsular extension (concurrent chemoradiation)
- Positive surgical margins
  - Reresection preferable if possible
  - Concurrent chemoradiation if reresection is not possible
- Perineural invasion

TIMING OF RADIATION THERAPY

- Adjuvant: 4-6 weeks after surgery
  - Delays in initiation and completion of postoperative adjuvant radiation are associated decreased locoregional control and overall survival
- Primary: 2 weeks after any necessary dental extractions

PRETREATMENT CONSIDERATIONS

- Dental evaluation
- Nutritional status
  - Avoid prophylactic gastrostomy tube unless patient has preexisting dysphagia, aspiration, or severe weight loss
    - Longer duration of tube use compared with as needed tube placement or temporary nasogastric tube use
    - Higher likelihood of long-term dysphagia
- Swallowing evaluation
- Airway safety: determination of the potential need for a tracheotomy
- Treatment planning and simulation
  - Thermoplastic mask immobilization

> **Box 5.1   SALIENT FEATURES OF ALTERED FRACTIONATION SCHEMES**
>
> **Hyperfractionation**
> - Smaller fraction size (115-120 cGy) compared with conventional fractionation (180-200 cGy)
> - BID to TID fractionation
> - Larger total dosage (7440-8460 cGy) than conventional fractionation (7000 cGy)
> - Similar overall treatment duration as conventional fractionation
>
> **Accelerated Fractionation**
> - Similar fraction size as conventional fractionation (180-200 cGy)
> - BID to TID fractionation
> - Similar total dosage as conventional fractionation
> - Shortened overall treatment duration compared with conventional fractionation
>
> **Hypofractionation**
> - Larger fraction size (600-800 cGy) compared with conventional fractionation (180-200 cGy)
> - Fractions delivered several days apart
> - Lower total dosage (2100-3200 cGy) than conventional fractionation (7000 cGy)
> - Shortened overall treatment duration compared with conventional fractionation

BID, Twice a day; *TID*, three times a day.
Adapted from Shah JP, Patel SG, Singh B. *Jatin Shah's Head and Neck Surgery and Oncology*. 4th ed. Philadelphia, PA: Mosby; 2012, fig. 19-4.

FRACTIONATION (Box 5.1)

- Conventional fractionation
  - Daily treatment, 5 days/wk, 7 weeks
  - Example: 2 Gy/fraction, 1 fraction/day, 5 days/wk, 7 weeks (60-70 Gy total)
- Hyperfractionation
  - Decrease dose per fraction; increase in the number of fractions
  - Larger total dose
  - Example: 1.15 Gy/fraction, 2 fractions/day, 5 days/wk, 7 weeks (81.5 Gy total)
  - Possible therapeutic advantage over conventional radiation, but greater burden on patients leads to poorer compliance
  - Theoretical improvement in locoregional control
- Accelerated fractionation
  - Conventional dose per fraction with an increased number of fractions
  - Similar total dose and decreased treatment duration
  - Example: 1.6 Gy/fraction, 3 fractions/day, 5 days/wk, for 5 weeks
  - Reduce tumor repopulation as a cause of radiotherapy (RT) failure
  - Increased toxicity
- Hypofractionation
  - Larger doses per fraction with decreased number of fractions
  - Smaller total dose and decreased treatment duration
  - Decreased side effects
  - Examples: 6 Gy/fraction, 1 fraction q3day (every 3 days) for 15 days (30 Gy total)
  - Used in melanoma or in palliative regimens

COMPLICATIONS OF RADIATION THERAPY

- Mucositis (World Health Organization scale)
  - Grade 1: soreness with erythema
  - Grade 2: erythema, ulcers, and can eat solids
  - Grade 3: ulcers and liquid diet only
  - Grade 4: alimentation is not possible
- Xerostomia
  - Prevention
    - IMRT to spare salivary glands
    - Submandibular gland transfer
  - Treatment
    - Saliva substitutes and mucosal lubricants
    - Stimulation of saliva
      - Sugar-free hard candy or gum
      - Pilocarpine: parasympathomimetic agent that is often limited by side effects of sweating, headaches, flushing, and increased bowel and bladder function
- Dental caries
- Osteoradionecrosis (ORN)
  - Mandible
    - Risk factors
      - Radiation dose >60 Gy
      - Poor oral hygiene or poor dentition
      - Location of primary tumor: the posterior mandible is most commonly affected
      - Extent of mandible in radiation field
      - Poor nutritional status
      - Concurrent chemoradiation
    - IMRT is less likely to cause ORN than conformal radiation fields are
    - Marx classification system[1]
      - Staging based upon response to hyperbaric oxygen (HBO)
      - Stage I: exposed bone treated with HBO alone
      - Stage II: diagnosed if there was no response to HBO at stage I and debridement is undertaken followed by further HBO
      - Stage III: diagnosed if there was no response to stage II treatment and resection and reconstruction are undertaken
    - Temporal bone
    - Maxilla
  - Chondroradionecrosis of the larynx
  - Soft-tissue fibrosis
  - Dysphagia: potential percutaneous endoscopic gastrostomy (PEG) dependence
  - Cranial neuropathy
  - Atherosclerosis and long-term risk of stroke
  - Long term risk of secondary malignancies such as sarcomas

PREVENTION OF RADIATION COMPLICATIONS

- Pretreatment dental examination
  - Extraction of diseased teeth (at least 2 weeks before starting radiation treatments)
  - Fabrication of custom molded fluoride trays for use during radiation
- Posttreatment dental care
  - Routine dental follow-up and daily fluoride application
  - HBO before dental extractions[1]: 20 dives at 2.4 atmospheres for 90 minutes before extraction and 10 dives after extraction

PRINCIPLES OF CHEMOTHERAPY

ROLE OF CHEMOTHERAPY

- Sensitizes radiation
- Palliation
- Not curative as a single agent

DRUGS USED

- Platinum agents
  - Cisplatin
    - Leads to DNA crosslink formation
    - Crosslinks activate multiple cellular pathways including apoptosis
    - Most common chemotherapy used
    - High-dose q3 weeks cisplatin protocol: delivered every 3 weeks (100 mg/m^2 on days 1, 22, and 43)
      - Category-1 evidence
      - More toxic
    - Low-dose weekly cisplatin protocol: weekly (40 mg/m^2)
      - Category-2b evidence
      - Better tolerated
    - Side effects
      - Nephrotoxicity
      - Ototoxicity
      - Alopecia
      - Nausea and vomiting
      - Neutropenia
  - Carboplatin
    - Similar mechanism of action as cisplatin
    - More myelosuppressive
    - Better tolerated than cisplatin (less ototoxic)
    - Mixed results in studies comparing its efficacy to cisplatin
- 5-Fluorouracil (5-FU)
  - Causes derangements in DNA synthesis and repair
  - Causes severe mucositis
  - Less commonly used now in favor of platinum agents
- Taxanes
  - Stabilize microtubules and arrest cells in G2/M phase
  - In induction chemotherapy regimens, addition of taxanes to cisplatin and 5-FU (TPF) leads to better outcomes compared with cisplatin and 5-FU alone
- Targeted agents
  - Cetuximab
    - Epidermal growth factor highly overexpressed in head and neck squamous cell carcinoma (HNSCC)
    - Cetuximab is a monoclonal antibody that binds epidermal growth factor receptor (EGFR)
    - Improved survival when given concurrently with radiation compared with radiation alone[2]

RATIONALE FOR CONCURRENT CHEMOTHERAPY AND RADIATION

- Improves the therapeutic ratio of radiation
  - Chemotherapeutic drug affects tumor and normal tissues differently
- Postoperative addition of chemotherapy to radiation
  - RTOG 95-01[3]
    - High-risk patients (+ margins, extracapsular extension or 2 or more positive nodes) received 60-66 Gy with concurrent cisplatin
    - Improved locoregional control and disease-free survival, with no significant difference in overall survival compared with RT alone
  - EORTC 22931[4]
    - High-risk patients (+ margins, extracapsular extension, perineural invasion, vascular tumor embolism, oral cavity, or oropharynx primary with level IV or V lymph nodes) received 66 Gy with concurrent cisplatin
    - Improved locoregional control, disease-free survival, and overall survival compared with RT alone

- Meta-analysis[5] of these two trials determined that the addition of cisplatin to adjuvant postoperative radiation was only helpful when extracapsular extension or positive margins were noted
- MACH-NC meta-analysis: patient age—decrease in the efficacy of concurrent chemotherapy with increasing age; no benefits noted in patients over age 70[6,7]

INDUCTION CHEMOTHERAPY

- Chemotherapy given before definitive surgery or radiation
- With few exceptions, this has not resulted in better outcomes
- TPF (taxane, platinum, and fluorouracil) induction has been demonstrated to be superior to a two-drug induction regimen, but not superior to concurrent chemoRT
- Two randomized control trials failed to show a benefit with induction chemotherapy (PARADIGM and DeCIDE trials)[8,9]

MANAGEMENT OF THE NECK

- Management of regional lymphatics determined by the extent of disease at initial staging
- Types of neck dissections
  - Radical: resection of levels I-V with sacrifice of internal jugular vein, sternocleidomastoid muscle, and spinal accessory nerve
  - Modified radical: resection of levels I-V with sparing of at least one of the nonlymphatic structures taken in a radical neck dissection
  - Selective neck dissection
    - Supraomohyoid neck dissection: levels I-III
    - Lateral neck dissection: levels II-IV
    - Posterolateral neck dissection: levels II-V, suboccipital lymph nodes
      - Most often employed for cutaneous melanoma or Merkel cell carcinoma of the posterior scalp
    - Central neck dissection level VI nodal contents
    - Extended: removal of an additional lymphatic group or nonlymphatic structure (eg, retropharyngeal node dissection, supraclavicular node dissection, external carotid artery, or the vagus nerve)
  - Anatomic landmarks of neck levels (Fig. 5.1)
    - Level Ia: bounded by the anterior bellies of the digastric muscle laterally, the mandible superiorly, the hyoid inferiorly, and the mylohyoid deeply
    - Level Ib: bounded anteriorly by the anterior belly of the digastric, superiorly by the body of the mandible, and posteriorly by the posterior belly of the digastric
    - Level II: upper jugular group that extends from the skull base superiorly to the hyoid bone inferiorly
      - Level IIa: inferior to the spinal accessory nerve
      - Level IIb: superior to the spinal accessory nerve
    - Level III: midjugular group that extends from the carotid bifurcation (surgical landmark) or the hyoid (radiographic landmark) to the junction of the omohyoid muscle and the internal jugular vein (surgical landmark) or the inferior border of the cricoid cartilage (radiographic landmark)
    - Level IV: lower jugular group that extends from the junction of the omohyoid with the internal jugular vein (surgical landmark) or the inferior border of the cricoid cartilage (radiographic landmark) to the clavicle
    - Level V: posterior triangle nodes that are bordered by the trapezius muscle posteriorly and the posterior border of the sternocleidomastoid muscle anteriorly; the inferior border is the clavicle

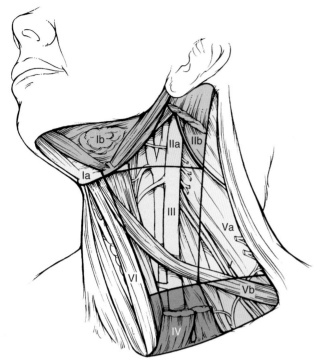

FIGURE 5.1 Neck Dissection Levels. The six sublevels of the neck used to describe the location of lymph nodes within levels I, II, and V. Level Ia, submental group; level Ib, submandibular group; level IIa, upper jugular nodes along the carotid sheath, including the subdigastric group; level IIb, upper jugular nodes in the submuscular recess; level Va, spinal accessory nodes; and level Vb, the supraclavicular and transverse cervical nodes. (From Flint PW, Haughey BH, Lund VJ, et al. *Cummings Otolaryngology—Head and Neck Surgery.* 6th ed. Philadelphia, PA: Saunders; 2015, fig. 119-2.)

- Va: nodes located above a horizontal plane at the inferior border of the cricoid cartilage
- Vb: nodes located below a horizontal plane at the inferior border of the cricoid cartilage
- Level VI: central compartment nodes bounded by the hyoid bone superiorly, the common carotid arteries laterally, and the innominate artery inferiorly; includes the paraesophageal, paratracheal, precricoid (Delphian), and perithyroidal nodes
- Level VII: superior mediastinal nodes bounded by the superior border of the manubrium superiorly, the left common carotid artery and the innominate artery on the left, and the arch of the aorta inferiorly

NECK DISSECTION IN THE N0 NECK

- Elective neck dissection for detection of occult disease
  - Diagnostic: additional pathologic information for risk stratification and determination of adjuvant needs
  - Therapeutic: occult N1 disease without adverse features may not require postoperative radiation
  - Management of the neck (surgery or radiation) indicated when the risk of nodal involvement reaches 20%
- Oral cavity primary with >4-mm invasion, where RT is not already planned
  - Supraomohyoid neck dissection (levels I-III)
  - Consider bilateral dissection for midline lesions (floor of mouth and tongue)
- Oropharynx: T1 or T2 treated surgically where RT is not already planned
  - Ipsilateral dissection for tonsil primary (at least levels II-IV)
  - Bilateral dissection for the base of tongue
- Supraglottis: T1 or T2 treated surgically where RT is not already planned (bilateral level II-IV dissection)

- Hypopharynx: T1 or T2 treated surgically where RT is not already planned (ipsilateral vs. bilateral level II-IV dissection)
- T3 or T4 primary disease with N0 neck
  - Surgical management of primary should include neck dissection
  - Ipsilateral: lateral tongue not crossing the midline, retromolar trigone, buccal mucosa, lateral alveolar ridge, and tonsil
  - Bilateral: oral tongue crossing the midline, anterior floor of the mouth, soft palate, base of the tongue, supraglottis, glottis, and hypopharynx

NECK DISSECTION FOR N+ DISEASE

- Neck dissection is indicated when the primary site is managed surgically
  - Modified radical neck dissection is indicated for positive disease
  - Selective neck dissections should be considered in small-volume neck disease
- Salvage neck dissection
  - Removal of metastatic disease of the neck that was previously treated
  - Common practice is to perform a positron emission tomography (PET) scan at 3 months after completion of the non-surgical treatment, and neck dissections for fluorodeoxyglucose (FDG)-avid residual disease
  - Perform surgery if needed within 3-6-month window after chemoradiation to avoid radiation-induced fibrosis
- Incisions for radical neck dissection (Fig. 5.2)
- Complications of neck dissection
  - Nerve injury
    - Spinal accessory nerve: more common with level IIb dissection
    - Vagus nerve
    - Recurrent laryngeal nerve (RLN) (level VI dissection)
    - Phrenic nerve
    - Sympathetic chain
    - Brachial plexus
    - Marginal mandibular branch of facial nerve
    - Hypoglossal nerve
  - Hematoma
  - Infection
  - Seroma
  - Chyle leak (left neck)
  - Lymphatic leak (right neck)
  - Skin-flap necrosis
  - Carotid rupture

LYMPHOMAS OF THE HEAD AND NECK

- Second most common primary malignancy of the head and neck
- 8% of supraclavicular masses are consistent with lymphoma
- Hodgkin lymphoma
  - Often presents with an enlarged node in the neck that may wax and wane
- Non-Hodgkin lymphoma
  - Oropharyngeal (OP) or nasopharyngeal mass
  - Waldeyer's ring
  - Epstein-Barr infection
- Extranodal natural killer (NK)/T-cell lymphoma
  - Midline lethal granuloma
  - Destruction of the nose, sinuses, or the face
- Thyroid lymphoma (more common than anaplastic thyroid carcinoma)
  - Hashimoto's disease is a risk factor

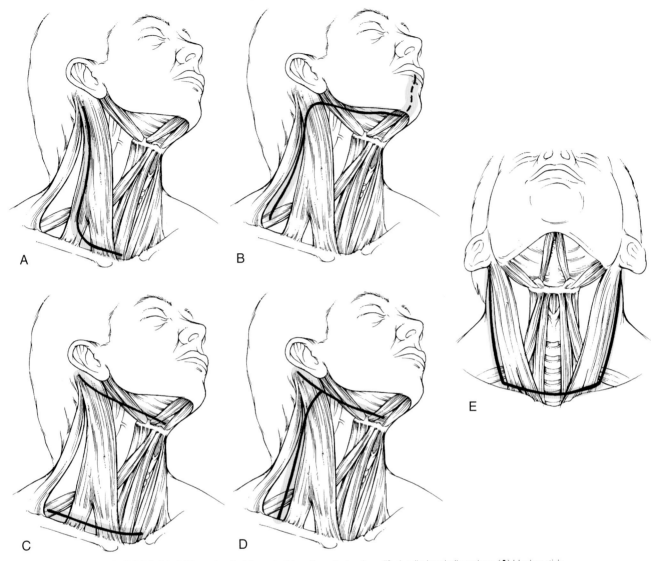

FIGURE 5.2 Neck Dissection Incisions. Incisions for radical and modified radical neck dissections. (**A**) Hockey stick. (**B**) Boomerang. (**C**) McFee. (**D**) Modified Schobinger. (**E**) Apron or bilateral hockey stick. (From Flint PW, Haughey BH, Lund VJ, et al. *Cummings Otolaryngology—Head and Neck Surgery*. 6th ed. Philadelphia, PA: Saunders; 2015, fig. 119-4.)

- Burkitt's lymphoma: endemic in Africa and may present as a jaw mass
- Salivary gland involvement
  - Mucosa-associated lymphoid tissue lymphoma
  - Sjögren syndrome
- B symptoms (temperatures >38°, drenching night sweats, and >10% weight loss)
- Persistent cough and mediastinal adenopathy
- Diagnosis requires fresh tissue (no formalin) which can be obtained by an excisional biopsy or occasionally a core needle biopsy

ORAL CAVITY MALIGNANCIES

SUBSITES OF THE ORAL CAVITY

- Lips (skin-vermilion junction to the gingiva)
- Buccal mucosa
- Oral tongue
- Floor of the mouth
- Hard palate
- Alveolar ridge
- Retromolar trigone

ORAL CAVITY STAGING (Table 5.1)

RISK FACTORS FOR ORAL CAVITY CANCER

- Tobacco (smoking imparts greater risk than chewing tobacco does)
- Alcohol (synergistic risk with tobacco)
- Betel nut (commonly used in Asia)
- Inflammatory disorders of the oral cavity
  - Submucosa fibrosis (often associated with Betel nut use)
  - Lichen planus (erosive and atrophic subtypes)
  - Poor oral hygiene
- Sun exposure (lip cancer)

CLINICAL PRESENTATION

- Irregularity of mucosal epithelium
  - Leukoplakia: white patch that does not rub off (no histopathologic correlate)
    - May represent mild, moderate or severe dysplasia
    - Most commonly hyperkeratosis secondary to irritant
  - Erythroplakia: red, velvet-textured lesion that cannot be classified as another entity; high likelihood of dysplasia or carcinoma on biopsy

Table 5.1	**American Joint Committee on Cancer Staging**
Primary Tumor	
TX	Unable to assess primary tumor
T0	No evidence of primary tumor
Tis	Carcinoma *in situ*
T1	Tumor <2 cm in greatest dimension
T2	Tumor >2 cm and <4 cm in greatest dimension
T3	Tumor >4 cm in greatest dimension
T4 (lip)	Primary tumor invades cortical bone, inferior alveolar nerve, floor of mouth, or skin of face (eg, nose and chin)
T4a (oral)	Tumor invades adjacent structures (eg, cortical bone, into deep tongue musculature, and maxillary sinus) or skin of face
T4b (oral)	Tumor invades masticator space, pterygoid plates, or skull base or encases the internal carotid artery
Regional Lymphadenopathy	
NX	Unable to assess regional lymph nodes
N0	No evidence of regional metastasis
N1	Metastasis in a single ipsilateral lymph node; <3 cm in greatest dimension
N2a	Metastasis in a single ipsilateral lymph node; >3 cm and <6 cm
N2b	Metastasis in multiple ipsilateral lymph nodes; all nodes <6 cm
N2c	Metastasis in bilateral or contralateral lymph nodes; all nodes <6 cm
N3	Metastasis in a lymph node >6 cm in greatest dimension
Distant Metastases	
MX	Unable to assess for distant metastases
M0	No distant metastases
M1	Distant metastases

Tumor, Node, and Metastasis Staging

Stage 0	Tis	N0	M0
Stage I	T1	N0	M0
Stage II	T2	N0	M0
Stage III	T3	N0	M0
	T1 to T3	N1	M0
Stage IVa	T4a	N0	M0
	T4a	N1	M0
	T1 to T4a	N2	M0
Stage IVb	Any T	N3	M0
	T4b	Any N	M0
Stage IVc	Any T	Any N	M1

From Flint PW, Haughey BH, Lund VJ, et al. *Cummings Otolaryngology—Head and Neck Surgery.* 6th ed. Philadelphia, PA: Saunders; 2015, table 93-1, and Edge SB. *The American Joint Committee on Cancer: American Joint Committee on Cancer Staging Manual.* 7th ed. New York, NY: Springer; 2010.

- Pain
  - Pain at the site of mucosal abnormality
  - Referred otalgia
  - Odynophagia
- Bleeding
- Neck mass
- Weight loss

HISTOLOGY OF ORAL CAVITY LESIONS

- Benign
  - Frictional keratosis
  - Mucocele
  - Hairy leukoplakia: Epstein-Barr mediated, more common in human immunodeficiency virus (HIV)/AIDS
  - Papilloma
  - Pyogenic granuloma
  - Fibroma (typically buccal and labial mucosa)
  - Pleomorphic adenoma (often on hard palate)
  - Granular cell tumor (dorsal surface of tongue)
- Malignant
  - SCC (90-95%)
    - Field cancerization
    - 4% annual risk of second primary neoplasms
  - Minor salivary gland tumors (mucoepidermoid carcinoma, adenoid cystic carcinoma, adenocarcinoma)
  - Mucosal melanoma
  - Lymphoma
  - Sarcoma

IMAGING OF ORAL CAVITY TUMORS

- Computed tomography (CT) scan: good for evaluation of bone involvement, fast, and inexpensive; dental artifacts can be limiting in the oral cavity
- Magnetic resonance imaging (MRI): excellent for evaluation of soft tissues, perineural invasion, and bone involvement; limitations include motion artifact, cost, and claustrophobic conditions
- PET/CT scan: may improve definition of the extent of primary disease and detection of pathologic nodes that do not meet size criteria on CT/MRI; limitations include cost and availability

EARLY-STAGE DISEASE MANAGEMENT

- Surgery is the preferred modality
  - Less morbidity than radiation therapy with equivalent efficacy
  - No randomized trials comparing surgery to radiation for early-stage disease
- Radiation considered in patients unable to tolerate surgery

LIP CANCER

- 25% of oral cavity cancers
- Lower lip > upper lip because of sun exposure
- Prognosis is better for lower lip than for upper lip or oral commissure
- Optimal resection margins are not well defined
  - Final margins >5 mm are generally recommended
  - Initial operative margin may shrink by 50%, so at least a 1-cm operative margin is generally recommended
- Brachytherapy has a high success rate in lip cancer
- Reconstruction depends on the extent of resection
  - A <50% defect of the lip can often be closed primarily
  - Larger lesions may require local flaps (ie, Abbe, Estlander, Karapandzik, or Gilles fan flap) or free tissue transfer (Fig. 5.3)

FLOOR OF MOUTH

- Locally invasive with a higher rate of occult metastasis; bilateral lymphatic drainage to central Floor of mouth (FOM)
- Surgery is the preferred modality
  - Careful attention to the lingual nerve and Wharton's duct
  - Be prepared to reroute the Wharton's duct

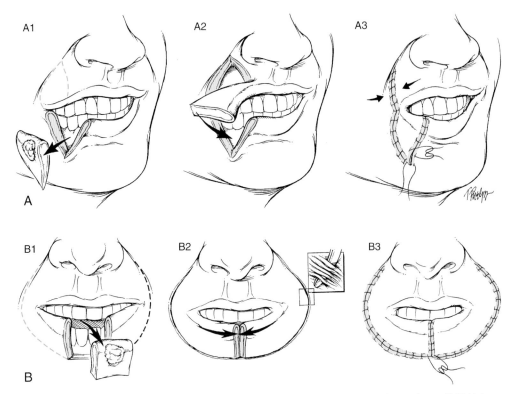

FIGURE 5.3 (**A**) Abbe-Estlander flap for a left lower-lip resection that extended to the oral commissure. (**A1**) Wedge resection of lateral lower-lip carcinoma. (**A2**) Initial mobilization of upper-lip tissue that preserves the commissure, consistent with Abbe-Estlander flap reconstruction. (**A3**) Final inset of flap; arrows mark the site of advancement and tension with closure. (**B**) Karapandzic fan flap for midline lower-lip defect. (**B1**) Rectangular-shaped full-thickness resection of lower-lip carcinoma. (**B2**) Initial mobilization of circumoral advancement flaps; the neurovascular pedicle (inset) is preserved bilaterally. (**B3**) Final inset of reconstruction. (From Flint PW, Haughey BH, Lund VJ, et al. *Cummings Otolaryngology—Head and Neck Surgery.* 6th ed. Philadelphia, PA: Saunders; 2015, figs. 93-13 and 93-14.)

- Reconstruct to prevent tongue tethering
- Consider tongue and mandible extension
- Defect closure
  - Primary closure for small lesions
  - Healing by secondary intention
  - Skin grafts
  - Local flaps (eg, platysmal flap and supraclavicular flap)
  - Free tissue transfer for larger defects

ORAL TONGUE

- Surgery is the first-line treatment
- Speech and swallowing considerations affect reconstructive considerations
- Depth of invasion directs decision on management of the N0 neck
  - Depth >4 mm imparts risk of occult disease >20%[10]
    - Supraomohyoid neck dissection
    - Consider sentinel lymph node biopsy (SLNB) at high-volume centers
- Deep margin assessment can be difficult
  - Skeletal muscle is often friable, leading to unreliable association with tumor
  - Muscle fibers contract with resection leading to a narrower pathologic margin
  - Low threshold to treat close margins (reresection or radiation)

RETROMOLAR TRIGONE

- Mucosal space between the third mandibular molar and the maxillary tuberosity

- Continuous with buccal mucosa, hard and soft palate, anterior tonsillar pillar, maxillary tuberosity, and the upper and lower alveolar ridges
- Early extension to the closely approximated mandible
- 5-Year survival of early-stage disease 70%
- Surgery is the first-line treatment
  - Difficult exposure
  - May require a lip split for access
  - Marginal mandibulectomy is often necessary for deep margin (Fig. 5.4)
  - Edentulous patients are more likely to have mandibular invasion
    - Porous bone
    - Lower threshold for segmental resection

HARD PALATE AND ALVEOLAR RIDGE

- Surgery is the first-line treatment
- Radiation achieves good oncologic control but increases the risk of ORN
- Hard palate: reverse smoking is a risk factor
- Mucosa lies directly on the bone
  - Bone resection is often necessary in early-stage disease
  - Marginal mandibulectomy for stages I and II
  - Segmental mandibulectomy
    - Mandible enveloped by tumor
    - Cortical bone involvement
    - Tumor invades into tooth roots
  - Infrastructural maxillectomy
    - Reconstruct with regional flaps or free flaps
    - Prosthetic rehabilitation

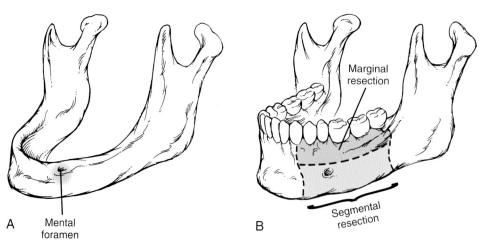

FIGURE 5.4 Mandible Variants and Surgical Approaches. (**A**) Edentulous mandible, which demonstrates why marginal mandibulectomy is difficult to perform without iatrogenic fracture in these patients. (**B**) Examples that compare marginal versus segmental mandibulectomy. (From Flint PW, Haughey BH, Lund VJ, et al. *Cummings Otolaryngology—Head and Neck Surgery.* 6th ed. Philadelphia, PA: Saunders; 2015, fig. 93-15.)

BUCCAL CARCINOMA

- Often misdiagnosed as trauma: T1 presentation unusual
- 5-Year survival 75-85% for stage I, 65% for stage II, 18-27% stage III/IV
- 5-10% of oral cancers in North America
- Common cancer in India and Southeast Asia
  - Oral submucous fibrosis: 19-fold increased risk of buccal cancer
  - Betel quid use
- Surgery is the first-line treatment
- Buccal space involvement common
- 40% of T2 tumors are node positive; 50% of T3 tumors are node positive
- Perifacial and submandibular nodes are typically first echelon
- Most common site of verrucous carcinoma
- Difficult exposure
- All defects must be reconstructed to prevent trismus
  - Skin graft for small tumors
  - Free tissue transfer for larger tumors
- Adjuvant radiation or chemoradiation is commonly indicated

NECK MANAGEMENT IN EARLY-STAGE DISEASE

- Risk of occult metastasis is dependent on the depth of invasion
- Selective neck dissection with thickness >2-4 mm
- Preoperative assessment of tumor depth is difficult
  - Imaging unreliable
  - Consider full-thickness punch biopsy
- Intermediate thickness lesions may be approached in two stages
  - Primary >2 mm thick: perform neck dissection
  - Primary <2 mm thick: observe the neck clinically
- Consideration of SLNB

EXTENT OF PROPHYLACTIC NECK DISSECTION

- Levels I-III (supraomohyoid)
- Oral tongue cancers may skip to level IV
- Level IIB lymph nodes controversial
  - May be unnecessary in absence of gross disease

- Level IIB dissection can cause spinal accessory nerve weakness and injury
- Midline lesions may drain bilaterally and require bilateral neck dissection

INDICATIONS FOR ADJUVANT TREATMENT

- Positive or close margins (if not reresected)
- Bone invasion
- Pathologically positive nodes: controversy regarding N1 disease
- Perineural invasion

OROPHARYNGEAL MALIGNANCIES

OROPHARYNX SUBSITES

- Palatine tonsils
  - Most common site of OP SCC (75%)
- Base of tongue/lingual tonsils (tissue posterior to the circumvallate papillae)
- Soft palate and uvula
- Anterior and posterior tonsillar pillars (palatoglossus and palatopharyngeus muscles)
- Posterior pharyngeal wall

CANCERS OF THE OROPHARYNX

- SCC
  - Traditional: negative for human papillomavirus (HPV) (p16 negative) and mediated by alcohol and tobacco
    - Spindle cell variant (sarcomatoid): highly aggressive
    - Verrucous: relatively radioresistant
    - Basaloid
    - Adenosquamous
    - Often larger primary site disease, and smaller nodal disease
  - HPV-mediated (p16 positive)
    - HPV-16 is most commonly involved
    - Oncogenic HPV types: 16, 18, 31, and 33
    - Younger patients
    - Better prognosis (less so in patients with a history of smoking)
    - Often larger and more cystic nodal disease and smaller primary site disease

- Lymphoma: two-thirds of Waldeyer's ring resides in the oropharynx
  - Palatine tonsil is the most common extranodal site of non-Hodgkin lymphoma
- Minor salivary gland neoplasms
  - Adenoid cystic carcinoma (most common minor salivary gland tumor of the oropharynx)
  - Mucoepidermoid carcinoma (second most common minor salivary gland tumor of the oropharynx)
- Sarcomas (rare)

PRESENTATION

- Early-stage disease is often asymptomatic
- Most common symptom is a neck mass
- Otalgia
- Odynophagia
- Dysphagia
  - Weight loss
  - Malnutrition
- Globus sensation
- Voice changes
- Hemoptysis
- Difficulty breathing

WORKUP

- Physical exam
  - Flexible fiberoptic laryngoscopy
  - Palpation
  - Neck exam for lymphadenopathy
  - Evaluate access to oropharynx
    - Trismus
    - Dentition
- Biopsy
  - Primary site and/or lymph node
    - Fine-needle aspiration (FNA) of lymph node
  - HPV testing (p16 testing as a surrogate for HPV)
- Cross-sectional imaging
  - CT scan with contrast
  - MRI with contrast
  - PET/CT scan

STAGING (Table 5.2)

TREATMENT

- Early stage (stage I or II)
  - Single modality therapy
  - Radiation
  - Surgery
- Advanced-stage disease
  - Concurrent chemoradiation: surgery reserved for salvage
  - Surgery with adjuvant radiation or chemoradiation

SURGICAL APPROACHES

- Transoral techniques
  - Transoral robotic surgery (TORS) (Fig. 5.5)
    - da Vinci robot: Food and Drug Administration approved for T1 and T2 OP cancers
    - Three-dimensional (3D), high-definition view
    - Assistant sits at the head of the bed and surgeon sits at the operating console
    - Close margins are acceptable because of proximity to the carotid artery
  - Transoral laser microsurgery (TLM)
    - Micrographic surgical technique

Table 5.2	**Tumor/Node/Metastasis Staging System for the Oropharynx**
Primary Tumor (T)	
TX	Primary tumor cannot be assessed
T0	No evidence of primary tumor
Tis	Carcinoma in situ
T1	Tumor ≤2 cm in greatest dimension
T2	Tumor >2 cm but ≤4 cm in greatest dimension
T3	Tumor >4 cm in greatest dimension
T4a	Moderately advanced local disease; tumor invades the larynx, deep or extrinsic muscle of the tongue, medial pterygoid, hard palate, or mandible (mucosal extension to lingual surface of the epiglottis does not constitute invasion of the larynx)
T4b	Very advanced local disease; tumor invades the lateral pterygoid muscle, pterygoid plates, lateral nasopharynx, or skull base or encases the carotid artery
Regional Lymph Nodes (N)	
NX	Regional lymph nodes cannot be assessed
N0	No regional lymph node metastasis
N1	Metastasis in a single ipsilateral lymph node ≤3 cm in greatest dimension
N2	Metastasis in a single ipsilateral lymph node >3 cm but ≤6 cm in greatest dimension or in multiple ipsilateral lymph nodes with none >6 cm in greatest dimension or in bilateral or contralateral lymph nodes with none >6 cm in greatest dimension
N2a	Metastasis in a single ipsilateral lymph node >3 cm but ≤6 cm in greatest dimension
N2b	Metastasis in multiple ipsilateral lymph nodes with none >6 cm in greatest dimension
N2c	Metastasis in bilateral or contralateral lymph nodes with none >6 cm in greatest dimension
N3	Metastasis in a lymph node >6 cm in greatest dimension
Distant Metastasis (M)	
MX	Distant metastasis cannot be assessed
M0	No distant metastasis
M1	Distant metastasis

From Flint PW, Haughey BH, Lund VJ, et al. *Cummings Otolaryngology—Head and Neck Surgery*. 6th ed. Philadelphia, PA: Saunders; 2015, table 97-4, and Edge SB. *The American Joint Committee on Cancer: Cancer Staging Manual*. 7th ed. New York, NY: Springer; 2009.

- Initial cuts are made through the tumor to define the normal tissue: tumor interface
- Careful communication with pathology and inking of margins are required
- Benefits of transoral techniques
  - No facial disassembly to access the tumor (eg, mandibulotomy and pharyngotomy)
  - Shorter hospital stay
  - Faster resumption of oral diet
  - Tracheostomy often unnecessary
- Open techniques
  - Transhyoid pharyngotomy (Fig. 5.6)
    - Dissection superior to the hyoid with pharyngotomy in the vallecular space
    - Pharyngotomy must be made away from the tumor: best for lateral lesions of the base of tongue or inferior tonsil
    - Advantage: preservation of pharyngeal plexus
    - Disadvantage: less exposure compared with other open approaches

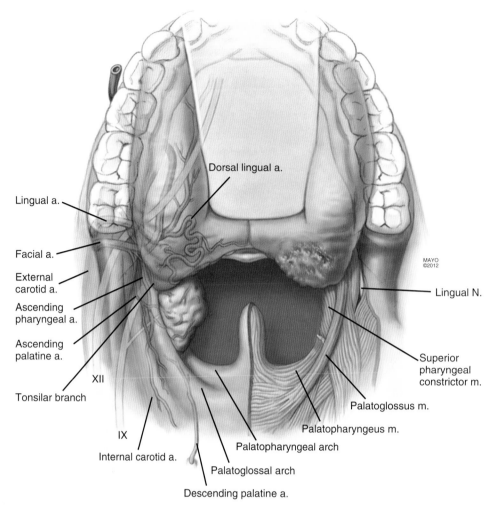

FIGURE 5.5 Anatomy of the Tongue Base in Transoral Robotic Surgery. Important adjacent structures include the lingual artery, facial artery, and lingual nerve. (From Van Abel KM, Moore EJ. Surgical management of the base of tongue. *Operat Techn Otolaryngol.* 2013;24:74-85, fig. 4.)

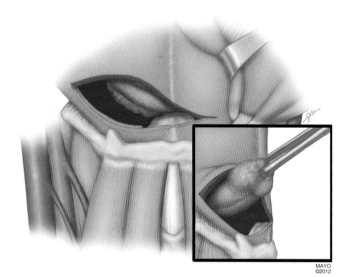

FIGURE 5.6 Transhyoid Pharyngotomy. A suprahyoid incision leads to the pharyngotomy, leaving a cuff of muscle along the hyoid bone for closure. The point of entry is at the hyoepiglottic ligament. (From Van Abel KM, Moore EJ. Surgical management of the base of tongue. *Operat Tech Otolaryngol.* 2013;24:74-85.)

- Lip split with mandibulotomy (Fig. 5.7)
  - Midline or parasymphyseal cut
  - Plating performed before mandibulotomy
  - Advantages: wide exposure and preservation of alveolar nerve and pharyngeal plexus
  - Disadvantage: facial scar and potential for mandible nonunion or malocclusion
- Visor flap (Fig. 5.8)
  - With or without lingual release/pull through
  - Cosmetically preferable
  - May require transection of bilateral mental nerves
  - By itself, it may limit posterior access
- Lingual release (Fig. 5.9)
  - Circumferential incision at the floor of the mouth: alveolar ridge junction
  - Used for total glossectomy
  - Advantage: wide exposure of the oral tongue in conjunction with the base of the tongue
  - Disadvantage: release of all lingual attachments to the mandible

SURVEILLANCE

- 3-Month posttreatment PET/CT
  - If negative findings, may follow clinically with no further imaging required[11]

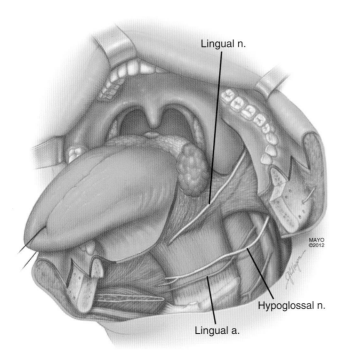

FIGURE 5.7 Lip Split with Mandibulotomy. Demonstration of the important neurovascular, bony, and muscular structures exposed through the mandibulotomy. The mandible bony cuts are performed in stair-step fashion. (From Van Abel KM, Moore EJ. Surgical management of the base of tongue. *Operat Tech Otolaryngol.* 2013;24:74-85.)

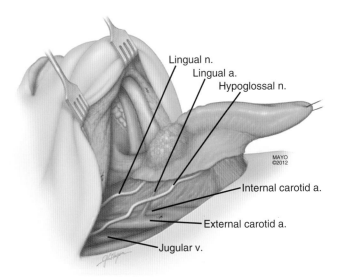

FIGURE 5.9 Lingual Release (Pull Through). Extension of cuts to the retromolar trigone and into the tonsillar fossa and pharynx allows for enough mobility of the tongue, so that it can be dropped beneath the mandible and visualized in the neck. (From Van Abel KM, Moore EJ. Surgical management of the base of tongue. *Operat Tech Otolaryngol.* 2013;24:74-85.)

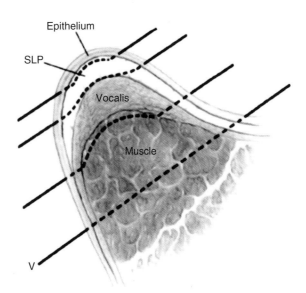

FIGURE 5.10 Vocal fold layers showing potential planes of dissection: epithelium, superficial lamina propria (*SLP*), vocalis ligament, and thyroarytenoid (*vocalis*) muscle (*V*). (From Myers EN, Carrau RL. *Operative Otolaryngology: Head and Neck Surgery.* 2nd ed. Philadelphia, PA: Saunders; 2008, fig. 46.2.)

- If equivocal, further imaging may be warranted
- Salvage surgery
  - Approximately 90% of recurrences occur within the first 2 years[12]
  - Salvage surgery has been shown to improve survival if resectable[13,14]
  - Confers importance of close and routine clinical follow-up

LARYNGEAL MALIGNANCIES

LAYERS OF TRUE VOCAL FOLD (Fig. 5.10)

- Squamous epithelium
- Superficial lamina propria (Reinke's space)

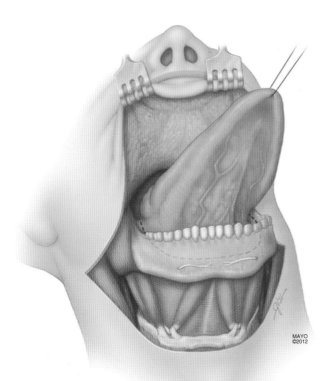

FIGURE 5.8 Visor Flap. The superior flap is raised in the subplatysmal plane up to the submandibular level. Intraoral mucosal cuts are then performed transorally along the lingual surface of the mandible (hatched line). (From Van Abel KM, Moore EJ. Surgical management of the base of tongue. *Operat Tech Otolaryngol.* 2013;24:74-85.)

- Intermediate lamina propria (vocalis ligament)
- Deep lamina propria (vocalis ligament)
- Vocalis muscle (vocal fold body)

SITES OF LARYNX

- Supraglottis
- Glottis
- Subglottis

SUBSITES OF SUPRAGLOTTIS

- Epiglottis
- Aryepiglottic (AE) folds
- Arytenoids
- False vocal cords

SUBSITES OF GLOTTIS

- True vocal cords
- Anterior commissure
- Posterior commissure
- Ventricle

SITES OF LARYNGEAL LYMPHATIC SPREAD

- Prelaryngeal
- Pretracheal
- Paralaryngeal
- Paratracheal
- Upper jugular
- Mid jugular
- Lower jugular
- Mediastinal (considered distant metastasis)

STRUCTURES DEFINING CLASSIFICATION OF T4B (SURGICALLY UNRESECTABLE)

- Carotid artery
- Mediastinum
- Prevertebral space

STAGING (Box 5.2)
LARYNGEAL CARCINOMA BARRIERS TO SPREAD

1. Quadrangular membrane (above false cords) for supraglottis
2. Conus elasticus (between true cords and cricoid) for glottis and subglottis
3. Cricothyroid membrane
4. Thyrohyoid membrane
5. Inner perichondrium

LARYNGEAL CARCINOMA PATHWAYS TO SPREAD

1. Broyle's tendon: vocalis tendon insertion into thyroid cartilage
2. Preepiglottic space
3. Paraglottic space

PARTIAL PROCEDURES FOR SUPRAGLOTTIC CARCINOMA

1. Supraglottic laryngectomy (T1, T2, and limited T3 supraglottis)
   a. Remove epiglottis, AE folds, false cords, preepiglottic space, and portions of the hyoid, and thyroid cartilage
   b. Spare arytenoids and true cords

Box 5.2 TUMOR/NODE/METASTASIS SYSTEM FOR THE LARYNX (EPITHELIAL MALIGNANCIES)

Primary Tumor (T)

T_x Primary tumor cannot be assessed
T_0 No evidence of primary tumor
T_{IS} Carcinoma in situ

Supraglottis

T1 Tumor limited to one subsite of the supraglottis with normal vocal cord mobility
T2 Tumor invades the mucosa of more than one adjacent subsite of the supraglottis or glottis or region outside the supraglottis (eg, mucosa of base of tongue, vallecula, or medial wall of piriform sinus) without fixation of the larynx
T3 Tumor limited to the larynx with vocal cord fixation and/or invasion of the postcricoid area, preepiglottic tissues, or paraglottic space with or without minor thyroid cartilage erosion (eg, inner cortex)
T4a Tumor invades through the thyroid cartilage and/or invades tissues beyond the larynx (eg, trachea; soft tissues of neck, including deep extrinsic muscles of the tongue; strap muscles; thyroid; or esophagus)
T4b Tumor invades the prevertebral space, encases the carotid artery, or invades mediastinal structures

Glottis

T1 Tumor limited to the vocal cords; may involve anterior or posterior commissure; normal vocal cord mobility
T1a Tumor limited to one vocal cord
T1b Tumor involves both vocal cords
T2 Tumor extends to the supraglottis and/or subglottis or impairs vocal cord mobility
T3 Tumor limited to the larynx with vocal cord fixation and/or invades paraglottic space and/or causes minor thyroid cartilage erosion (eg, inner cortex)
T4a Tumor invades through the thyroid cartilage and/or invades tissues beyond the larynx (eg, trachea; soft tissues of neck, including deep extrinsic muscles of the tongue, strap muscles, thyroid, or esophagus)

T4b Tumor invades the prevertebral space, encases the carotid artery, or invades mediastinal structures

Subglottis

T1 Tumor limited to the subglottis
T2 Tumor extends to the vocal cords with normal or impaired mobility
T3 Tumor limited to the larynx with vocal cord fixation
T4a Tumor invades the cricoid or thyroid cartilage and/or invades tissues beyond the larynx (eg, trachea; soft tissues of neck, including deep extrinsic muscles of the tongue, strap muscles, thyroid, or esophagus)
T4b Tumor invades the prevertebral space, encases the carotid artery, or invades mediastinal structures

Regional Lymph Nodes (N)

NX Regional lymph nodes cannot be assessed
N0 No regional lymph node metastasis
N1 Metastasis in a single ipsilateral lymph node, <3 cm in greatest dimension
N2 Metastasis in a single ipsilateral lymph node, >3 cm but not >6 cm in greatest dimension, or in multiple ipsilateral lymph nodes, none >6 cm in greatest dimension or in bilateral or contralateral lymph nodes, none >6 cm in greatest dimension
N2a Metastasis in a single ipsilateral lymph node, >3 cm but not >6 cm in greatest dimension
N2b Metastasis in multiple ipsilateral lymph nodes, none >6 cm in greatest dimension
N2c Metastasis in bilateral or contralateral lymph nodes, none >6 cm in greatest dimension
N3 Metastasis in a lymph node >6 cm in greatest dimension

Distant Metastasis (M)

MX Distant metastasis cannot be assessed
M0 No distant metastasis
M1 Distant metastasis

From Flint PW, Haughey BH, Lund VJ, et al. *Cummings Otolaryngology—Head and Neck Surgery.* 6th ed. Philadelphia, PA: Saunders; 2015, box 106-3, and Edge SB, Byrd DR, Compton CC, et al., eds. *AJCC Cancer Staging Manual.* 7th ed. New York, NY: Springer; 2010:57-62.

2. Supracricoid laryngectomy with cricohyoidopexy/cricoepiglottopexy (select T3-T4 glottic and supraglottic cancers without the following: arytenoid fixation, cricoid cartilage contact/ invasion, major preepiglottic space involvement, invasion of thyroid cartilage perichondrium, hyoid, and posterior arytenoid mucosa)
   a. Remove the entire thyroid cartilage, bilateral true and false cords, one arytenoid and the paraglottic space
   b. Spares cricoid, hyoid, and at least one arytenoid

PARTIAL PROCEDURES FOR GLOTTIC CARCINOMA

1. Endoscopic cordectomy (T1 glottic in the mid third)
2. Laryngofissure and cordectomy (T1 glottic in the mid third)
3. Vertical partial laryngectomy (T1-T2 glottic carcinomas: the tumor does not extend beyond one-third of the opposite cord; <10 mm anterior subglottic extension; <5 mm posterior subglottic extension; no posterior commissure, cricoarytenoid joint, AE fold, posterior surface of arytenoids, or paraglottic space involvement; FEV1 >50%)
   a. Remove one vocal fold from the arytenoid cartilage (AC) to vocal process, false cord, ventricle, paraglottic space, and overlying thyroid cartilage
4. Supracricoid laryngectomy with cricohyoidopexy/ cricoepiglottopexy

FOUR PRINCIPLES OF ORGAN PRESERVATION SURGERY

- Local control: organ preservation procedures should only be used when local control rates approximate that of total laryngectomy
- Accurate assessment of the 3D extent of the tumor: comprehensive appreciation of the extent of the tumor is necessary
- Cricoarytenoid unit is the basic functional unit of the larynx
  - Consists of an AC, cricoid cartilage, associated musculature, superior laryngeal nerve, and RLN
  - Preservation of the cricoarytenoid unit (not vocal folds) allows for physiologic speech/swallow without permanent need for tracheostomy
- Resection of normal tissue to achieve an expected functional outcome: resection of normal tissue in a standard approach is necessary to achieve consistent functional outcomes

VERTICAL PARTIAL LARYNGECTOMY

- Indications: transglottic or very extensive bilateral glottic carcinoma
  - Tumor involvement of the anterior commissure
  - Extension to vocal process of the AC
  - Selected superficial transglottic lesions
  - Carcinoma recurring after external beam radiation therapy (XRT)
- Contraindications
  - Fixed True vocal cord (TVC)
  - > 10 mm anterior subglottic extension or > 5 mm posterior subglottic extension
  - Involvement of the posterior commissure
  - Invasion of both arytenoids
  - Bulky transglottic lesions
  - Lesions invading thyroid cartilage

SUPRAGLOTTIC PARTIAL LARYNGECTOMY: STRUCTURES REMOVED (Fig. 5.11)

- Superior portion of thyroid cartilage
- Epiglottis

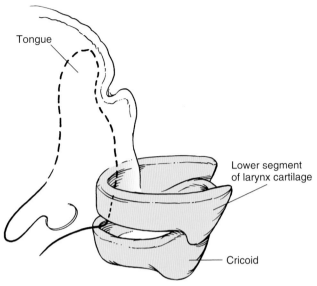

FIGURE 5.11 Supraglottic Laryngectomy. Laryngoplasty is performed with three closure stitches circumferentially around the inferior half of the thyroid cartilage, and submucosally into the tongue base, as is done in the supracricoid partial laryngectomy. (From Flint PW, Haughey BH, Lund VJ, et al. *Cummings Otolaryngology—Head and Neck Surgery.* 6th ed. Philadelphia, PA: Saunders; 2015, fig. 109-114.)

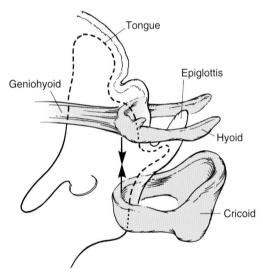

FIGURE 5.12 Supraglottic Laryngectomy with Cricohyoidoepiglottopexy. Laryngoplasty is performed using circumferential cricoid, hyoid, epiglottic, and tongue-base sutures. (From Flint PW, Haughey BH, Lund VJ, et al. *Cummings Otolaryngology—Head and Neck Surgery.* 6th ed. Philadelphia, PA: Saunders; 2015, fig. 109-112.)

- Preepiglottic space
- False vocal cords
- ± Hyoid bone

SUPRACRICOID PARTIAL LARYNGECTOMY: STRUCTURES REMOVED (Fig. 5.12)

- Entire thyroid cartilage
- Bilateral true vocal cords
- Bilateral false vocal cords
- ± single arytenoid

SUPRAGLOTTIC CANCER: ONCOLOGIC CONTRAINDICATIONS FOR SUPRAGLOTTIC PARTIAL LARYNGECTOMY

- Cricoid or thyroid cartilage invasion
- Arytenoid mucosa involvement
- Posterior or anterior commissure involvement
- Impaired TVC motion
- Impaired Base of tongue (BOT) motion
- BOT invasion <1 cm from circumvallate papillae
- Invasion of FOM via vallecular involvement

SUPRAGLOTTIC CANCER ONCOLOGIC CONTRAINDICATIONS FOR SUPRACRICOID PARTIAL LARYNGECTOMY-CRICOHYOIDOPEXY

- Arytenoid fixation
- >1.5 cm extension anteriorly (cricothyroid membrane) and >0.5 cm posterolaterally
- Cricoid involvement
- Extensive preepiglottic space invasion with bulging beneath the vallecula or extension to the thyrohyoid membrane
- Hyoid bone involvement
- External perichondrial thyroid cartilage involvement or extralaryngeal spread

CONTRAINDICATIONS FOR PARTIAL LARYNGECTOMY

1. Fixed cords
2. Cartilage invasion
3. Subglottic extension
4. Interarytenoid invasion
5. Subglottic invasion
6. Cervical metastasis (relative contraindication)

ADVANTAGES OF SURGERY FOR GLOTTIC CANCER

- Equivalent voice outcomes for T1 disease
- Faster than radiation
- Better salvage options for recurrence that are less morbid
- Avoid long-term speech/swallow dysfunction from radiation

ADVANTAGES OF RADIATION FOR GLOTTIC CANCER

- Better voice outcomes, especially in patients with T2-T4 disease
- Equivalent local control
- Avoid issues with unfavorable surgical access
- Avoid need for second-look OR procedures

TYPES OF CORDECTOMY (Table 5.3)

TOTAL LARYNGECTOMY

- Indications
  - T3/T4 tumors with thyroid cartilage destruction
  - Posterior commissure or bilateral arytenoid involvement (seen in advanced supraglottic tumors)
  - Circumferential submucosal disease
  - Subglottic extension with cricoid cartilage involvement
  - RT or chemoradiation failures

Table 5.3	**Types of Cordectomy**
Type	**Description**
Type I	Subepithelial
Type II	Subligamental
Type III	Transmuscular
Type IV	Total/complete
Type Va	Extended, including contralateral true vocal cord
Type Vb	Extended, including arytenoid
Type Vc	Extended, including ventricular fold
Type Vd	Extended, including subglottis

- Completion laryngectomy for failed conservation laryngeal surgery
- Hypopharyngeal tumors that spread to the postcricoid mucosa
- Thyroid tumors that invade both sides of the larynx
- Advanced tumors of unusual histology that are incurable by conservation surgery or chemoradiation (eg, adenocarcinoma and sarcomas)
- Extensive pharyngeal or tongue-base resections in patients at high risk for aspiration
- Radiation necrosis of the larynx
- Severe irreversible aspiration

VETERANS AFFAIRS LARYNX TRIAL (1991)[15]

- 332 randomized stage III-IV glottic or supraglottic SCC patients
- Arms
  - Cohort 1: total laryngectomy + postop radiation
  - Cohort 2: induction chemotherapy + radiation
    - Proceed to total laryngectomy + postop radiation if not at least a partial response
- No significant difference in 2-year overall survival (68% vs. 68%), but 64% of Cohort 2 had their larynx preserved
- Controversial as to whether the 64% of preserved larynx patients were functional
- Effect: supports that chemoradiation is as effective as laryngectomy with the potential to preserve function

RTOG 91-11 INTERGROUP TRIAL (2003, 2013)[16,17]

- 547 randomized patients with stage III-IV glottic or supraglottic SCC
- Excluded T1N+ or large-volume T4 disease
- Arms
  - Cohort 1: induction chemotherapy + radiation (or laryngectomy if no response)
  - Cohort 2: concurrent chemoradiation
  - Cohort 3: radiation alone
- Larynx preservation is superior with concurrent chemoRT (88%) versus induction (75%, $p = 0.005$) or versus RT alone (70%, $p < 0.001$)
- Locoregional control is superior with concurrent chemoRT (78%) versus induction (61%) or versus RT alone (56%)
- Decreased distant metastasis in chemo groups (Cohorts 1 and 2), but 2-year and 5-year overall survival no different among the 3 cohorts
- Use of induction chemotherapy + radiation (Cohort 1) not supported
- Effect: supports that concurrent chemoradiation protocols should become the standard of care

- 10-Year follow-up: still no significant difference in overall survival, with chemo groups (Cohorts 1 and 2) showing improved larynx preservation over RT alone

PREVENT LARYNGECTOMY STOMAL STENOSIS

- Bevel tracheal cuts
- Minimize tracheal tension
- Cut medial heads of sternocleidomastoid muscles
- Minimize suctioning
- Minimize laryngectomy tube use

COMPLICATIONS FROM TOTAL LARYNGECTOMY

- Early complications
  - Drain failure
  - Hematoma
  - Infection
  - Pharyngocutaneous fistula
  - Wound dehiscence
  - Hypoglossal nerve injury
- Late complications
  - Stomal stenosis
  - Pharyngoesophageal stenosis or stricture
  - Hypothyroidism

CONSIDERATIONS FOR TOTAL LARYNGECTOMY

- Neck dissections
  - Bilateral selective neck dissections recommended for supraglottic involvement
  - Unilateral neck dissection can be considered for T3 glottic carcinoma
  - Salvage neck dissection recommended for chemoradiation failures
- Thyroidectomy
  - Thyroid involvement in larynx cancer is rare
  - The thyroid is at higher risk when there is subglottic extent because of paratracheal and parapharyngeal lymphatic spread
  - The thyroid is at higher direct risk when there is transglottic spread, such as thyroid cartilage or cricoid invasion by tumor
  - Depending on extent of the cancer, hemithyroidectomy may be performed on the side of the cancer, or total thyroidectomy for advanced disease
- Pedicled flap closure in radiated tissue to prevent fistula
  - 30% risk of pharyngocutaneous fistula in laryngectomy patients who had prior RT
  - Pharyngeal mucosal closure options include primary closure, constrictor muscle overlay, pedicled flap buttress, and free-flap buttress
  - Controversial whether pedicled flap or free flap decreases incidence
- Primary versus secondary tracheoesophageal puncture (TEP)
  - Primary TEP means fewer procedures and can be done safely in a patient with prior RT: easier to perform at time of total laryngectomy
  - Secondary TEP is likely better for:
    - Patients who have received high RT doses and are at high risk for wound healing issues
    - Patients with subglottic cancer who will need high-dose postoperative RT
    - Patients who have poor understanding of the TEP process at time of total laryngectomy and need further counseling

VOCAL REHABILITATION AFTER TOTAL LARYNGECTOMY (Fig. 5.13)

1. Esophageal voice
2. Electrolarynx
3. TEP

TREATMENT OF PHARYNGOCUTANEOUS FISTULA

- Local wound care
- Nasogastric (NG) tube
- Nil per os (NPO)
- Total parenteral nutrition (TPN)
- Strict glycemic control
- Correct hypothyroidism
- Debridement
- Local closure
- Regional flaps

HYPOPHARYNGEAL MALIGNANCIES

ETIOLOGY OF HYPOPHARYNGEAL SQUAMOUS CELL CARCINOMA

- More likely to demonstrate submucosal spread
- More direct correlation with alcohol intake than other HNSCC
- Association with Plummer-Vinson syndrome
  - Dysphagia, iron deficiency anemia, hypopharyngeal webs
- More likely to present in advanced stages (>75% are stage III-IV at time of diagnosis)

SUBSITES OF HYPOPHARYNX

- Pyriform sinuses
- Postcricoid space
- Posterior pharyngeal wall

BORDERS OF PYRIFORM SINUS

- Medial border: AE fold
- Lateral border: thyroid cartilage
- Superior border: glossoepiglottic fold
- Inferior border: cricopharyngeus
- Posterior border: lateral pharyngeal wall

BORDERS OF POSTCRICOID SPACE

- Superior border: posterior ACs
- Inferior border: esophageal introitus
- Lateral border: tracheoesophageal groove

BORDERS OF PARAGLOTTIC SPACE

- Anterolateral: thyroid cartilage
- Inferomedial: conus elasticus
- Medial: ventricle and quadrangular membrane
- Posterior: pyriform sinus

INNERVATION

- Motor
  - Superior pharyngeal nerve
  - Pharyngeal branches of the CNIX and CNX
  - External branch of the superior laryngeal nerve
- Sensory
  - Internal branch of the superior laryngeal nerve
  - Glossopharyngeal nerve (CNIX)
  - Vagus nerve (CNX)

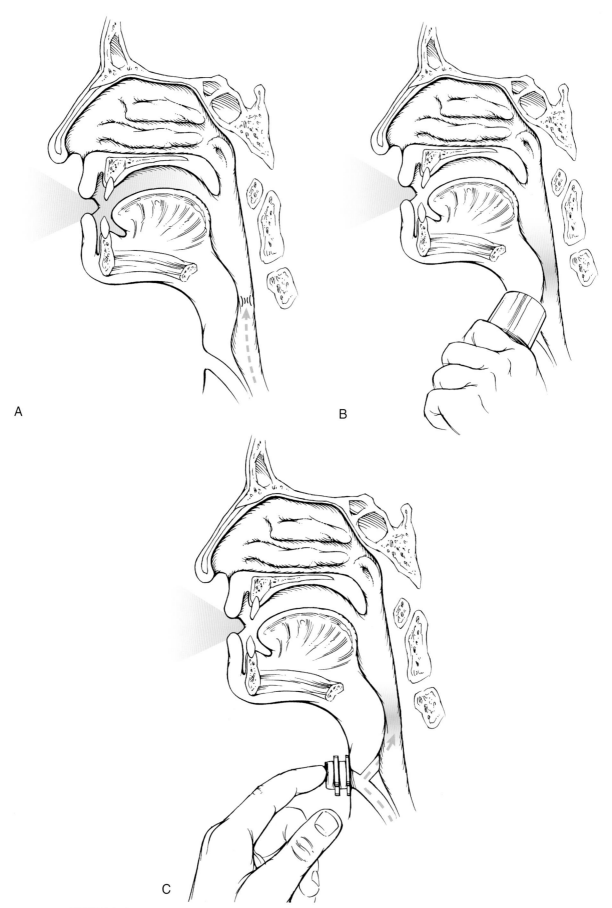

FIGURE 5.13 Forms of Speech after Total Laryngectomy (**A**) Electrolarynx speech. (**B**) Esophageal speech. (**C**) TEP speech. (From Flint PW, Haughey BH, Lund VJ, et al. *Cummings Otolaryngology—Head and Neck Surgery*. 6th ed. Philadelphia, PA: Saunders; 2015, figs. 112-4-112-6.)

- Chemoradiation (organ preservation)
- Surgery plus postoperative radiation
- Neck usually must be addressed (surgery or radiation) bilaterally given the rich lymphatic innervation
- Radiation is commonly employed in the treatment plan because retropharyngeal lymph nodes are common and are not typically addressed with surgery

SURGICAL OPTIONS

- Partial pharyngectomy
- Partial laryngopharyngectomy
- CO_2 laser excision
- Total laryngectomy with partial pharyngectomy
- Total laryngopharyngectomy
- Total laryngopharyngoesophagectomy

ADVANTAGES OF LASER EXCISION

- No tracheostomy is required
- Preservation of suprahyoid musculature facilitates more normal swallowing
- No reconstruction is needed
- Voice preservation
- Decreased hospital stay

COMPLICATIONS FROM OPEN SURGERY

- Pharyngocutaneous fistula
- Stricture
- PEG dependency
- Tracheostomy dependency

INDICATIONS FOR TOTAL LARYNGOPHARYNGECTOMY

- Cancer involves postcricoid mucosa
- Cancer extends beyond the midline
- Advanced cancer of the posterior hypopharyngeal wall

RECONSTRUCTION OPTIONS

- Primary closure
- Regional flap (pectoralis major, platysma)
- Secondary intention (CO_2 laser approach)
- Gastric pull-up (when resection extends below the cervicothoracic junction of the esophagus)
- Colonic interposition
- Radial forearm free flap
- Anterolateral thigh free flap
- Jejunal free flap

PRIMARY CLOSURE

- Essential to estimate the extent of resection before surgery
- Resection requires a minimum of 1.5-cm margins
- Primary closure requires a minimum of 3 cm of pharynx (side to side)
- Contraindications to primary closure
  - Cancer extends past the midline
  - Cancer extends to the postcricoid mucosa
  - Cancer extends to the cervical esophagus

JEJUNAL FREE FLAP

- Advantages
  - Large segment that can be used for anastomosis as high as the nasopharynx
  - Intrinsic mucous production may assist in swallowing
  - Tolerates postoperative RT

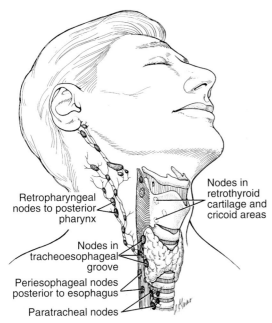

FIGURE 5.14 Hypopharynx Lymphatic Drainage. Hypopharyngeal carcinomas metastasize primarily to the superior jugular and midjugular nodes. However, metastasis to the retropharyngeal, paratracheal, paraesophageal, and parapharyngeal space nodes may be present. (From Flint PW, Haughey BH, Lund VJ, et al. *Cummings Otolaryngology—Head and Neck Surgery.* 6th ed. Philadelphia, PA: Saunders; 2015, fig. 102-2.)

LYMPHATIC DRAINAGE IN THE HYPOPHARYNX (Fig. 5.14)

- Jugulodigastric
- Midjugular
- Spinal accessory chain
- Paratracheal
- Paraesophageal
- Retropharyngeal

MOST COMMON PRESENTING SYMPTOMS

- Dysphagia
- Neck mass
- Sore throat
- Hoarseness
- Otalgia

DIFFERENTIAL DIAGNOSIS

- SCC (>95%)
- Lymphoma
- Adenocarcinoma
- Sarcoma

PLUMMER-VINSON SYNDROME

- Specifically associated with postcricoid SCC
- Primarily affects women (85%)
- Dysphagia, iron deficiency anemia, and hypopharyngeal/esophageal webs
- Chronic irritation from webs progress to carcinoma
- Syndrome etiology likely the result of nutritional deficiency

HYPOPHARYNX AND CERVICAL ESOPHAGUS STAGING (Table 5.4)

TREATMENT OPTIONS

- Radiation (for very early stage)

Table 5.4 Tumor and Lymph Node Staging

Primary Tumor (T)

Hypopharynx

TX	Primary tumor cannot be assessed
T0	No evidence of primary tumor
T1	Tumor limited to one subsite of the hypopharynx and ≤2 cm in greatest dimension
T2	Tumor invades more than one subsite of the hypopharynx or an adjacent site or measures >2 cm but >4 cm in greatest dimension without fixation of the hemilarynx
T3	Tumor >4 cm in greatest dimension or with fixation of the hemilarynx
T4a	Tumor invades the thyroid/cricoid cartilage, hyoid bone, thyroid gland, esophagus, or central compartment soft tissue (including prelaryngeal strap muscles and subcutaneous fat)
T4b	Tumor invades the prevertebral fascia, encases the carotid artery, or involves mediastinal structures

Cervical Esophagus

TX	Primary tumor cannot be assessed
T0	No evidence of primary tumor
Tis	Carcinoma in situ
T1	Tumor invades the lamina propria, muscularis mucosae, or submucosa
T1a	Tumor invades the lamina propria or muscularis mucosae
T1b	Tumor invades the submucosa
T2	Tumor invades the muscularis propria
T3	Tumor invades the adventitia
T4	Tumor invades the adjacent structures
T4a	Resectable tumor invades the pleura, pericardium, or diaphragm
T4b	Unresectable tumor invades other adjacent structures, such as the aorta, vertebral body, or trachea

Regional Lymph Nodes (N)

Hypopharynx

NX	Regional lymph nodes cannot be assessed
N0	No regional lymph node metastasis
N1	Metastasis in a single ipsilateral lymph node ≤3 cm in greatest dimension
N2a	Metastasis in a single ipsilateral lymph node >3 cm but not >6 cm in greatest dimension
N2b	Metastasis in multiple ipsilateral lymph nodes with none >6 cm in greatest dimension
N2c	Metastasis in bilateral or contralateral lymph nodes with none >6 cm in greatest dimension
N3	Metastasis in a lymph node >6 cm in greatest dimension

Cervical Esophagus

NX	Regional lymph nodes cannot be assessed
N0	No regional lymph node metastasis
N1	Metastasis in one to two regional lymph nodes
N2	Metastasis in three to six regional lymph nodes
N3	Metastasis in seven or more regional lymph nodes

Distant Metastasis (M)

MX	Distant metastasis cannot be assessed
M0	No distant metastasis
M1	Distant metastasis present

Grade (G)

GX	Grade cannot be assessed, stage as G1
G1	Well differentiated
G2	Moderately differentiated
G3	Poorly differentiated
G4	Undifferentiated, stage as G3

From Flint PW, Haughey BH, Lund VJ, et al. *Cummings Otolaryngology—Head and Neck Surgery.* 6th ed. Philadelphia, PA: Saunders; 2015, table 102-2.

- Lower mortality/morbidity rates compared with gastric pull-up
- Disadvantages
  - Short ischemia time
  - Dysphagia from jejunum peristalsis
  - Poor vocal rehabilitation from TEP prosthesis (wet "gurgly" voice) compared with Anterolateral thigh (ALT)
  - Morbidity from second incision in the abdomen
  - Need for two microvascular anastomotic sites

NECK DISSECTION CONSIDERATIONS

- Bilateral necks should be addressed for all but the earliest T1 lesions with surgery or radiation
- Significantly worse prognosis with N+ disease
- Occult lymphadenopathy is common enough that elective neck dissection is warranted for N0 disease
- Recommendation for level II-IV neck dissection for N0 disease
- Recommendation for level I-V neck dissection for N+ disease
- Contralateral neck disease more likely in unilateral N+ disease
- Postoperative radiation is typically administered for extracapsular spread or multiple involved lymph nodes

- Paratracheal and retropharyngeal lymph node spread is common and needs to be addressed

NASOPHARYNGEAL MALIGNANCIES

MAIN CAUSES OF NASOPHARYNGEAL CARCINOMA

- Genetic factors
  - Family clusters: 15% of nasopharyngeal carcinoma (NPC) patients have a first-degree family member with NPC
  - HLA-B, C, D haplotypes are associated with increased risk
- Environmental factors
  - High-nitrosamine (preservative) diet of salted fish, eggs, and vegetables
  - Risk associated with early exposure or during weaning period
- Epstein-Barr virus (EBV)
  - Viral capsid antigen (VCA) and early antigen (EA)
  - Majority of population: elevated immunoglobulin G (IgG) VCA and IgG EA

- NPC patients: elevated IgA VCA (highly sensitive) and IgA EA (highly specific)
- NPC patients: elevated Epstein-Barr nuclear antigens (EBNAs) and latent membrane proteins (LMPs)

DEMOGRAPHICS OF NASOPHARYNGEAL CARCINOMA

- 75% of NPC patients are male
- 20% of NPC patients will have a first-degree relative with NPC
- >50% of NPC patients are diagnosed between age 30 and 50 years
- Highest world incidence is in Guangzhou, China (30 per 100,000)
- 99% of NPC patients have symptoms at diagnosis

MAIN FACTORS IN DEVELOPMENT

- Genetic factors: risk of NPC in a first-degree family member is as high as 20-fold
- Environmental factors
  - Diets high in preservatives such as nitrosamines
  - Geographic centers such as Southern China
- EBV

MOST COMMON NASOPHARYNGEAL CARCINOMA SYMPTOMS

- Neck mass (usually high level V and level II)
- Otitis media with effusion/Eustachian tube dysfunction
- Unilateral hearing loss
- Blood in saliva
- Nasal obstruction
- Tinnitus
- Cranial nerve palsy

MOST COMMON CRANIAL NERVES AFFECTED

- CNV
- CNVI
- CNIX
- CNX
- CNXII

DIFFERENTIAL DIAGNOSIS OF NASOPHARYNGEAL MASSES

- NPC
- Adenoid cystic carcinoma
- Chordoma
- Craniopharyngioma
- Angiofibroma
- Lymphoma
- Thornwaldt cyst
- Adenoid hypertrophy

JUVENILE NASOPHARYNGEAL ANGIOFIBROMA STAGING (CHANDLER)

- Stage I: tumor confined to the nasopharynx
- Stage II: tumor extends to the nasal cavity or sphenoid
- Stage III: tumor involves the maxillary sinus, ethmoid sinus, infratemporal fossa, orbit, cheek, and cavernous sinus
- Stage IV: tumor is intracranial

NASOPHARYNGEAL CARCINOMA STAGING (Table 5.5)

Table 5.5	**The 2009 Union Internationale Contre Cancer Tumor/Node/Metastasis Staging of Nasopharyngeal Carcinoma**
Stage	**Description**
T Classification	
Tx	Primary tumor cannot be assessed
T0	No evidence of tumor
T1	Confined to the nasopharynx or extends to the oropharynx and/or nasal cavity
T2	Tumor extends to the parapharyngeal space
T3	Tumor involves sinuses and/or the skull base
T4	Intracranial, infratemporal/masticator space involvement, cranial nerve involvement, orbit, or hypopharynx
N Classification	
N0	No nodal involvement
N1	Unilateral cervical lymph nodes ≤6 cm, or unilateral or bilateral retropharyngeal nodes ≤6 cm, above the supraclavicular fossa
N2	Bilateral cervical lymph nodes ≤6 cm, above supraclavicular fossa
N3a	Lymph node >6 cm
N3b	Supraclavicular lymph node
M Classification	
M0	No distant metastasis
M1	Distant metastasis (includes mediastinal nodes)
Stage Classification	
Stage I	T1N0M0
Stage II	T1N1M0, T2N0M0, and T2N1M0
Stage III	T3N0M0, T3N1M0, and T1 to T3N2M0
Stage IVa	T4, any NM0
Stage IVb	Any TN3M0
Stage IVc	Any T; any N, M1

From Flint PW, Haughey BH, Lund VJ, et al. *Cummings Otolaryngology—Head and Neck Surgery.* 6th ed. Philadelphia, PA: Saunders; 2015, table 96-1.

WORLD HEALTH ORGANIZATION CLASSIFICATION OF NASOPHARYNGEAL CARCINOMA

- Type I: SCC (keratinizing)—5-year survival is 35%
- Type IIa: nonkeratinizing carcinoma (EBV+)
- Type IIb: undifferentiated carcinoma (EBV+)
  - 5-Year survival: 60%
  - Most common in endemic regions
- Basaloid SCC

WORKUP

- MRI for evaluation of tumor extent and skull-base involvement
- PET/CT for evaluation of distant metastasis
- Audiogram

- EBV serologies
  - IgA VCA: highly sensitive
  - IgA EA: highly specific
- Dental evaluation
- Speech and swallow evaluation

MAGNETIC RESONANCE IMAGING EVALUATION FOR EXTENSION

- Superior: cavernous sinus, meninges, foramina lacerum, foramen rotundum, and foramen ovale
- Inferior: oropharynx
- Posterior: clivus, sphenoid, and retropharyngeal lymph nodes
- Lateral: pterygopalatine fossa and infratemporal fossa

DIFFERENTIAL DIAGNOSIS

- Juvenile nasopharyngeal angiofibroma (JNA)
- Thornwaldt cyst
- Adenoid hypertrophy
- Squamous papilloma
- Craniopharyngioma
- Chordoma
- Adenoid cystic carcinoma

TREATMENT OPTIONS

- State I-II: radiation alone
- Stage III-IV: chemoRT
- Persistent disease: salvage surgery
- Recurrent disease: reirradiation or salvage surgery

EARLY SIDE EFFECTS OF RADIATION

- Mucositis
- Xerostomia
- Sinusitis
- Otitis media with effusion

LATE SIDE EFFECTS OF RADIATION

- CNVIII palsy (sensorineural hearing loss)
- CNXII palsy
- Trismus

COMPLICATIONS OF REIRRADIATION

- Transverse myelitis
- Temporal lobe necrosis
- Trismus
- Sensorineural hearing loss
- Choanal stenosis
- Palatal dysfunction
- Cranial nerve palsy

LOCOREGIONAL RECURRENCES

- 5-10% of NPC patients will ultimately develop local recurrences
- 50% will be salvageable by surgery
- 10% of patients will ultimately develop neck recurrence or residual neck disease
- Success of salvage surgery correlates with T-stage classification
- Close follow-up with low threshold for biopsy is therefore important to allow for early detection and treatment

CONTRAINDICATIONS TO SURGERY IN NASOPHARYNGEAL CARCINOMA

- Clival erosion
- Intracranial involvement
- Carotid artery encasement

SURGICAL APPROACHES

- Endoscopic
- Lateral rhinotomy with medial maxillectomy
- Maxillary swing

PROGNOSIS

- Patients with stage I-II disease treated with radiation alone have a 5-year OS of 80% or higher
- Patients with stage III-IV disease treated with chemoRT have a 5-year OS of 70%
- N3 disease is associated with poorer survival and higher rates of distant metastasis
- Distant metastasis remains the main cause of death

SINONASAL MALIGNANCIES

MOST COMMON SITES OF MALIGNANCY

- Maxillary sinus (#1)
- Nasal cavity
- Ethmoid sinus

MOST COMMON SYMPTOMS

- Nasal obstruction
- Localized facial pain
- Epistaxis
- Nasal discharge

SYMPTOMS OF ADVANCED DISEASE

- Epiphora
- Palatal numbness
- Diplopia
- Facial numbness
- Decreased vision
- Neck mass
- Proptosis
- Trismus

RISK FACTORS

- Wood-dust exposure (adenocarcinoma)
- Leather-related occupational exposure (adenocarcinoma)
- Smoking (SCC)

CLINICAL EXAM

- Ophthalmologic exam (proptosis, epiphora, visual acuity changes, and extraocular muscle impingement)
- Neurologic exam (numbness and paresthesias)
- Dental exam (trismus, palatal lesions, and loose dentition)
- Nasal endoscopy exam (outflow obstruction and CSF leakage)

MUCOSAL MELANOMA FEATURES

- Sinonasal cavity is the most common site of mucosal melanoma presentation
- Very aggressive and high grade (all lesions are at least T3 and stage III)
- Majority of patients develop distant metastases

COMPUTED TOMOGRAPHY IMAGING OF PARANASAL SINUSES

- Advantages
  - Complementary to MRI
  - Faster
  - Less expensive
  - Better tolerated
  - Evaluate bony expansion, remodeling, or destruction
  - Evaluate calcifications (associated with esthesioneuroblastomas, sarcomas)
  - Evaluate widening of bony fissures or foramina

MAGNETIC RESONANCE IMAGING OF PARANASAL SINUSES

- Advantages
  - Complementary to CT
  - Rule out encephalocele before biopsy
  - Evaluate perineural invasion
  - Differentiate postobstructive changes from true tumor
  - Better evaluate orbital invasion (differentiates periorbita from tumor)
  - Better evaluate intracranial invasion (differentiates dura from tumor)

POSITRON EMISSION TOMOGRAPHY/ COMPUTED TOMOGRAPHY IMAGING OF PARANASAL SINUSES

- Advantages
  - Evaluate distant metastases
  - Posttreatment surveillance

DIAGNOSIS OF PERINEURAL INVASION

- Asymmetric nerve enlargement or enhancement
- Obliteration of perineural fat planes
- Denervation changes in end organs (muscles of facial expression or mastication)
- Widening of nerve foramina

KADISH SYSTEM FOR ESTHESIONEUROBLASTOMA

- Kadish A: confined to the nasal cavity
- Kadish B: extends to the paranasal sinuses
- Kadish C: extends beyond the nasal cavity and paranasal sinuses
- Kadish D: lymph node or distant metastasis

INFRASTRUCTURAL LESION SPREAD

- Through the maxillary sinus floor into the oral cavity
- Through the maxillary sinus medial wall into the nasal cavity
- Through the maxillary sinus anterior wall into the soft tissues of the cheek

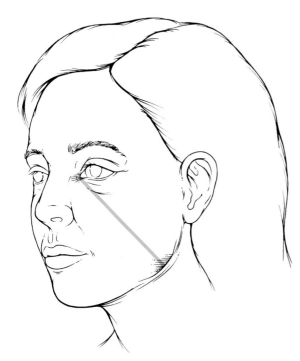

FIGURE 5.15 Ohngren's Line. An imaginary line is drawn from the medial canthus to the angle of the jaw, which gives a rough estimate of the dividing line between tumors that may be resected with a good prognosis (below the line) and those with a poor prognosis (above the line). (From Flint PW, Haughey BH, Lund VJ, et al. *Cummings Otolaryngology—Head and Neck Surgery*. 6th ed. Philadelphia, PA: Saunders; 2015, fig. 82-4.)

OHNGREN'S LINE (Fig. 5.15)

- Imaginary plane from the medial canthus of the eye to the angle of mandible
- Infrastructural lesions (anterior and inferior to line): present earlier and are more amenable to resection
- Suprastructural lesions (posterior and superior to line): present at more advanced stages, more likely to involve critical structures, and less amenable to resection

SINONASAL MASSES

1. Papilloma
   a. Fungiform
   b. Cylindric
   c. Keratotic
   d. Inverted
2. Osteoma/ossifying fibroma
3. Fibrous dysplasia
4. JNA
5. NPC
6. SCC
7. Adenocarcinoma
8. Adenoid cystic carcinoma
9. Sarcoma
   a. Rhabdomyosarcoma
   b. Leiomyosarcoma
   c. Chondrosarcoma
   d. Fibrosarcoma
10. Hemangiopericytoma
11. Lymphoma
12. Melanoma
13. Esthesioneuroblastoma
14. Plasmacytoma

- Through the maxillary sinus lateral wall into the masticator space

SUPRASTRUCTURAL LESION SPREAD

- Through the posterior wall of the maxillary sinus to the pterygopalatine fossa
- Through the maxillary sinus roof into the orbit
- Through the ethmoid cavities to the anterior cranial fossa

SINONASAL CARCINOMA SUBSITES

1. Paranasal sinuses
2. Nasal cavity
3. Anterior cranial fossa
4. Pterygopalatine fossa
5. Infratemporal fossa
6. Orbital cavity

MOST COMMON SITES OF SINONASAL MALIGNANCIES

- Maxillary sinus (50-70%)
- Nasal cavity (15-30%)
- Ethmoid sinus (10-20%)

MOST COMMON SINONASAL MALIGNANCIES

- Epithelial
  - SCC
  - Adenoid cystic carcinoma
  - Adenocarcinoma
- Nonepithelial
  - Lymphoma
  - Esthesioneuroblastoma
  - Sinonasal undifferentiated carcinoma
  - Mucosal melanoma

MAXILLARY SINUS CARCINOMA STAGING (Table 5.6)

Table 5.6	Maxillary Sinus Carcinoma Staging
Stage	Definition
T1	Tumor limited to maxillary sinus mucosa with no erosion or destruction of bone
T2	Tumor causing bone erosion or destruction including extension into the hard palate and/or the middle of the nasal meatus, except extension to the posterior wall of the maxillary sinus and pterygoid plates
T3	Tumor invades any of the following: bone of the posterior wall of the maxillary sinus, subcutaneous tissues, floor or medial wall of the orbit, pterygoid fossa, or ethmoid sinuses
T4a	Tumor invades the anterior orbital contents, skin of cheek, pterygoid plates, infratemporal fossa, cribriform plate, or sphenoid or frontal sinuses
T4b	Tumor invades any of the following: orbital apex, dura, brain, middle cranial fossa, cranial nerves other than maxillary division of trigeminal nerve (V2), nasopharynx, or clivus

NASAL CAVITY AND ETHMOID SINUS STAGING (Table 5.7)

Table 5.7	Nasal Cavity and Ethmoid Sinus Staging.
Stage	Definition
T1	Tumor restricted to any one subsite, with or without bony invasion
T2	Tumor invading two subsites in a single region or extending to involve an adjacent region within the nasoethmoidal complex, with or without bony invasion
T3	Tumor extends to invade the medial wall or floor of the orbit, maxillary sinus, palate, or cribriform plate
T4a	Tumor invades any of the following: anterior orbital contents, skin of the nose or cheek, minimal extension to the anterior cranial fossa, pterygoid plates, or sphenoid or frontal sinuses
T4b	Tumor invades any of the following: orbital apex, dura, brain, middle cranial fossa, cranial nerves other than (V2), nasopharynx, or clivus

MUCOSAL MELANOMA STAGING (Table 5.8)

Table 5.8	Mucosal Melanoma Staging
Stage	Definition
Primary Tumor	
T3	Mucosal disease
T4a	Moderately advanced disease; tumor involves deep soft tissue, cartilage, bone, or overlying skin
T4b	Very advanced disease; tumor involves brain, dura, skull base, lower cranial nerves (IX, X, XI, and XII), masticator space, carotid artery, prevertebral space, or mediastinal structures
Lymph Nodes	
NX	Regional lymph nodes cannot be assessed
N0	No regional lymph node metastases
N1	Regional lymph node metastases present
Distant Metastasis	
M0	No distant metastasis
M1	Distant metastasis present

From Flint PW, Haughey BH, Lund VJ, et al. *Cummings Otolaryngology—Head and Neck Surgery*. 6th ed. Philadelphia, PA: Saunders; 2015, table 82-2.

SURGICAL APPROACHES

1. Endoscopic approach
2. Transoral approach
3. Midface degloving approach (Fig. 5.16)
4. Lateral rhinotomy approach (Fig. 5.17)
   a. Lynch incision: extend superiorly to the medial eyebrow (access the medial canthal ligament and lacrimal duct)
   b. Subciliary incision: extend across the lower-eyelid crease (access the orbital floor)

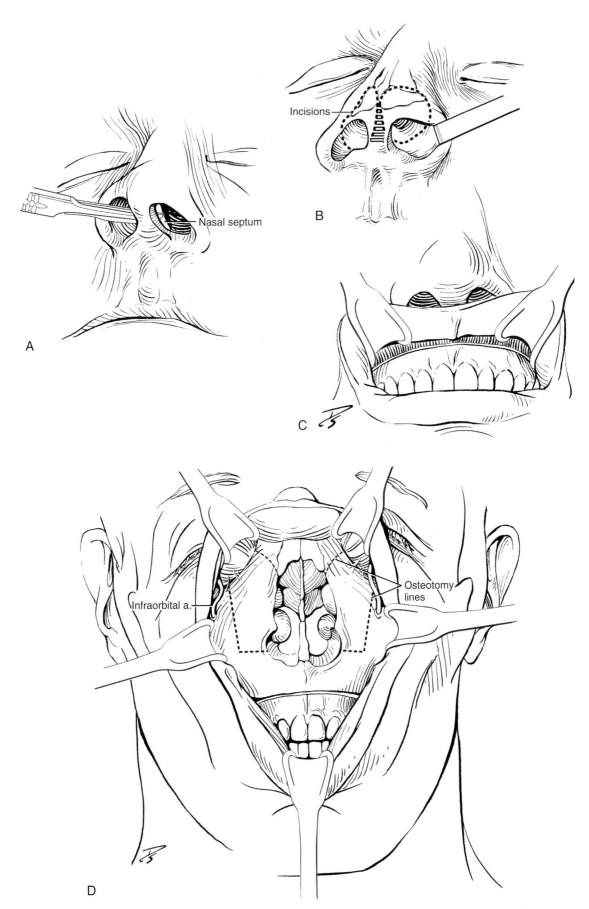

FIGURE 5.16 Midface Degloving. (**A**) Release of the nasal septum. (**B**) Further incisions are extended over the alar cartilages to the pyriform aperture. (**C**) Mucosal incisions are made into the soft tissues of the gingivolabial sulcus. (**D**) The upper-lip and midface tissues are retracted superiorly to expose the tumor. (From Cohen JI, Clayman GL. *Atlas of Head & Neck Surgery.* 1st ed. Philadelphia, PA: Saunders; 2011.)

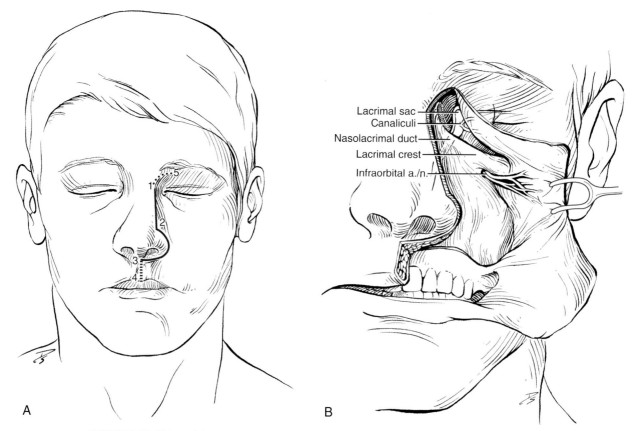

FIGURE 5.17 (**A**) Lateral rhinotomy incision. (**B**) Soft-tissue dissection, exposing critical structures including the lacrimal sac, nasolacrimal duct, and infraorbital nerve. (From Cohen JI, Clayman GL. *Atlas of Head & Neck Surgery.* 1st ed. Philadelphia, PA: Saunders; 2011.)

5. Weber-Ferguson incision: extend inferiorly as the upper-lip split (access to the palate) (Fig. 5.18)
6. Craniofacial resection (Fig. 5.19)
7. Robotic approach

TYPES OF RESECTION

1. Medial maxillectomy (middle turbinate, inferior turbinate, ethmoid sinus, and maxillary sinus)
2. Infrastructural maxillectomy (adds the upper alveolar ridge with the adjoining hard palate)
3. Subtotal maxillectomy (entire maxilla)
4. Total maxillectomy (adds the orbital floor)
5. Radical maxillectomy (total maxillectomy plus orbital exenteration)
6. Craniofacial resection (anterior cranial-base removal including the cribriform plate, ethmoid sinuses, and dura)

RECONSTRUCTION

- Obturator coverage with facial and dental prostheses
  - Faster with shorter hospitalization
  - Easier to survey for recurrence
  - Requires prosthodontics team with specialized expertise
  - Radiation and healing cause contraction that requires numerous obturator adjustments
- Microvascular free-flap reconstruction
  - May better restore facial contour and profile
  - May better support orbital floor
  - Can accept dental implants
  - May better withstand effects of postoperative radiation
  - May have better mastication and speech intelligibility and less oronasal reflux

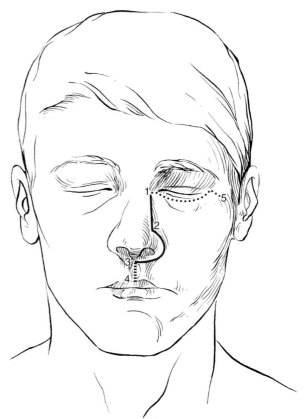

FIGURE 5.18 Weber-Fergusson Incision. The lateral rhinotomy incision is extended laterally along the infraorbital crease. (From Cohen JI, Clayman GL. *Atlas of Head & Neck Surgery.* 1st ed. Philadelphia, PA: Saunders; 2011.)

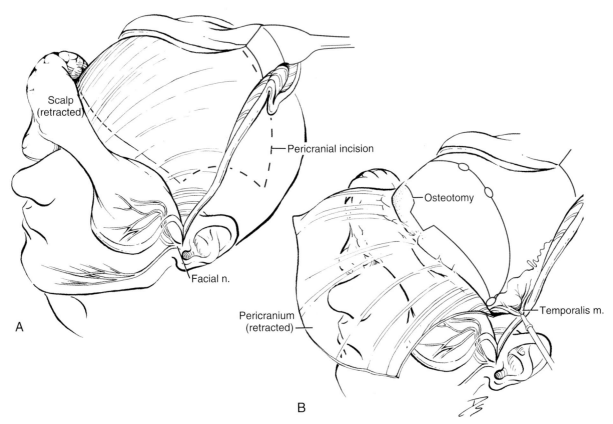

FIGURE 5.19 Bifrontal Approach. (**A**) The incision begins in a preauricular crease anterior to the tragus, and then is elevated in a subgaleal plane superficial to the pericranium between the superior temporal lines. An incision is made through the temporalis fascia (superficial and deep layers) 1.5 cm posterior to the superior orbital rim, extending parallel to the zygomatic arch. Dissection proceeds deep to the deep layer of the temporalis fascia to preserve the frontal branch of the facial nerve, which is superficial to the fascia. (**B**) The scalp flap is elevated anteriorly to expose the superior orbital rims and supraorbital nerves. (From Cohen JI, Clayman GL. *Atlas of Head & Neck Surgery.* 1st ed. Philadelphia, PA: Saunders; 2011.)

CONTRAINDICATIONS TO ENDOSCOPIC SURGERY

- Facial soft-tissue extension
- Anterolateral frontal sinus involvement
- Palate involvement
- Dural involvement beyond the midpupillary line
- Mandible involvement
- Orbital extension

CONTRAINDICATIONS TO OPEN SURGERY

- Trismus (pterygoid muscle involvement)
- Skull-base invasion (optic chiasm or cavernous sinus involvement)
- Significant brain parenchymal invasion
- Carotid artery encasement

NONSURGICAL MANAGEMENT

- Very advanced or nonresectable cases
- Unlikely to improve survival but may slow tumor growth into critical structures
- Options
  - Induction chemotherapy followed by surgery if there is a response
  - Surgical debulking followed by topical 5-FU
  - Proton beam or carbon ion radiation

SALIVARY NEOPLASMS

DISTRIBUTION OF SALIVARY NEOPLASMS

- Parotid: 70% (75% benign and 25% malignant)
- Submandibular: 22% (57% benign and 43% malignant)
- Minor salivary: 8% (18% benign and 85% malignant)

HISTOLOGY

- Benign
  - Pleomorphic adenoma (45%)
  - Warthin tumor (6%)
  - Benign cyst (1.0%)
- Malignant
  - Mucoepidermoid carcinoma (15.7%)
  - Adenoid cystic carcinoma (10.0%)
  - Adenocarcinoma (8.0%)
  - Malignant mixed tumor (5.7%)
  - Acinic cell carcinoma (3.0%)

NONTUMOR DIFFERENTIAL DIAGNOSIS FOR PAROTID SWELLING

- Viral parotitis
- Bacterial parotitis: often in elderly, malnourished, dehydrated, or immunocompromised patients
- Sialolithiasis
- Sjögren syndrome
- Inflammatory/reactive lymph node

SYMPTOMS SUGGESTIVE OF MALIGNANCY

- Most malignant salivary tumors present only with a painless mass
- Pain
- Facial nerve paresis or paralysis
- Tongue weakness or numbness (submandibular malignancies)
- Fixation of mass to overlying skin or underlying structures
- Cervical lymphadenopathy

SYMPTOMS OF DEEP LOBE OR PARAPHARYNGEAL SPACE INVOLVEMENT

- Decreased gag reflex (CNIX and CNX)
- Aspiration (CNIX and CNX0)
- Asymmetric palate elevation (CNX)
- Hoarseness (CNX)
- Dysphagia (CNX)
- Shoulder weakness (CNXI)
- Tongue atrophy/paresis (CNXII)
- Ptosis (sympathetic chain)

FINE-NEEDLE ASPIRATION

- High sensitivity, specificity, and predictive value
- Higher diagnostic accuracy for benign compared with malignant salivary tumors
- Diagnostic difficulties
  - Variation in expected cytology of pleomorphic adenoma
  - Benign-malignant look-alike lesions that are confused on FNA
    - Basal cell adenoma versus adenoid cystic carcinoma
    - Salivary duct obstruction versus mucoepidermoid carcinoma
    - Oncocytic lesion versus acinic cell carcinoma
- Utility or necessity of FNA
  - Avoid unnecessary surgical resection for lymphomas and inflammatory masses
  - Enables better preoperative counseling of patients
  - Enables better surgical planning
    - Extent of resection
    - Management of facial nerve
    - Likelihood of neck dissection
  - No evidence of seeding or needle tracking of tumors

IMAGING

- Routine use for small masses not warranted because it would not change the treatment plan
- Useful for lesions that may be malignant
  - Provide accurate delineation of location and extent of tumor
  - Provide relationship to major neurovascular structures
  - Provide information on perineural spread, skull-base invasion, and intracranial extension
- MRI characteristics in salivary tumors
  - Bilateral high T2 signal that does not enhance: more likely Warthin's tumor
  - Unilateral high T2 signal that enhances: more likely pleomorphic adenoma
  - Intermediate to low T2 signal: more likely to be malignant
- Parapharyngeal space
  - Prestyloid compartment: deep lobe parotid tumors and minor salivary gland tumors
  - Poststyloid compartment: neurogenic and glomus tumors
    - Neurogenic tumors: enhance with gadolinium
    - Glomus tumors: serpiginous flow voids (salt-pepper)

STAGING (Table 5-9)

Table 5.9	2010 American Joint Committee on Cancer Tumor/Node/Metastasis Staging for Major Salivary Gland Cancer	
Primary Tumor (T)		
TX	Primary tumor cannot be assessed	
T0	No evidence of primary tumor	
T1	Tumor is ≤2 cm in greatest dimension without extraparenchymal extension[a]	
T2	Tumor is >2 cm but not >4 cm in greatest dimension without extraparenchymal extension[a]	
T3	Tumor is >4 cm in greatest dimension and/or has extraparenchymal extension[a]	
T4a	Moderately advanced disease Tumor invades the skin, mandible, ear canal, and/or facial nerve	
T4b	Very advanced disease Tumor invades the skull base and/or pterygoid plates and/or encases the carotid artery	
Regional Lymph Nodes (N)		
NX	Regional lymph nodes cannot be assessed	
N0	No regional lymph node metastasis	
N1	Metastasis in a single ipsilateral lymph node ≤3 cm in greatest dimension	
N2a	Metastasis in a single ipsilateral lymph node >3 cm but not >6 cm in greatest dimension	
N2b	Metastases in multiple ipsilateral lymph nodes with none >6 cm in greatest dimension	
N2c	Metastases in bilateral or contralateral lymph nodes with none >6 cm in greatest dimension	
N3	Metastasis in a lymph node >6 cm in greatest dimension	
Distant Metastasis (M)		
MX	Distant metastasis cannot be assessed	
M0	No distant metastasis (no pathologic M_0; use clinical M to complete stage group)	
M1	Distant metastasis	

[a]*Extraparenchymal extension* is clinical or macroscopic evidence of invasion of soft tissues. Microscopic evidence alone does not constitute extraparenchymal extension for classification purposes.
From Flint PW, Haughey BH, Lund VJ, et al. *Cummings Otolaryngology—Head and Neck Surgery.* 6th ed. Philadelphia, PA: Saunders; 2015, table 87-3, and Edge SB. *The American Joint Committee on Cancer: AJCC Cancer Staging Manual.* 7th ed. New York, NY: Springer; 2010.

MUCOEPIDERMOID CARCINOMA

- Most common salivary malignancy (adult and pediatric)
- Diagnostic similarity on FNA: necrotizing sialometaplasia (hard palate) and adenosquamous carcinoma
- Grading: low, intermediate, and high grades

- Correlates with clinical aggressiveness and adjuvant treatment
- MECT1-MAML2 t(11;19)(q21;p13) translocation

ADENOID CYSTIC CARCINOMA

- Second most common salivary malignancy in the parotid gland
- Patterns: tubular, cribriform, and solid
- Slowly progressive, infiltrative growth with distant metastases developing over years
- Tendency to display perineural invasion
- Differential diagnosis: polymorphous low-grade adenocarcinoma, pleomorphic adenoma, and basal cell adenoma
- MYB-NFIB t(6;9) translocation

POLYMORPHOUS LOW-GRADE ADENOCARCINOMA

- Arises mainly from minor salivary glands: most commonly from the hard/soft palate junction
- Second most common minor salivary gland carcinoma
- Differential diagnosis: pleomorphic adenoma and adenoid cystic carcinoma
- Low-grade malignancy with excellent prognosis

ACINIC CELL CARCINOMA

- Arises mainly in the parotid gland (90% of all acinic cell cases)
- Second most common childhood salivary gland malignancy
- Low-grade malignancy but approximately 33% will recur
- 10-15% will develop regional or distant metastases

MALIGNANT MIXED TUMORS

- True malignant mixed tumor (carcinosarcoma)
- Carcinoma ex pleomorphic adenoma
  - Any pleomorphic adenoma with carcinoma of any kind
  - Carcinoma form most commonly poorly differentiated adenocarcinoma not otherwise specified (NOS), salivary duct carcinoma, or undifferentiated carcinoma
  - Prognosis is dependent upon type of carcinoma
- Metastasizing pleomorphic adenoma

SALIVARY DUCT CARCINOMA

- One of the most aggressive salivary gland cancers
- Generally presents with a rapidly growing parotid mass
- Significant minority present with facial nerve paresis
- High grade by definition
  - 30-40% develop local recurrence
  - 50-75% develop distant metastases
- Significant minority are positive for ERBB2 (Her2/neu) receptors
- Typically negative for estrogen and progesterone receptors

CLASSIC HIGH-GRADE SALIVARY MALIGNANCIES

- High-grade mucoepidermoid carcinoma
- High-grade adenoid cystic carcinoma
- Salivary duct carcinoma
- SCC
- Adenocarcinoma NOS
- Undifferentiated carcinoma
- Implications

- Higher rate of locoregional recurrence
- Suggest role for postoperative radiation

LANDMARKS TO IDENTIFY THE FACIAL NERVE DURING PAROTIDECTOMY

- Tragal pointer (1-1.5 cm deep and inferior)
- Tympanomastoid suture line (6-8 mm deep)
- Retrograde dissection (marginal mandibular branch at the mandible superficial to facial vessels; buccal branch deep to the parotidomasseteric fascia, parallel to the parotid duct)
- Posterior belly of the digastric muscle (superior)

SURGICAL APPROACHES TO PARAPHARYNGEAL SPACE

- Transoral
- Transcervical +/- mandibulotomy
- Transcervial-transparotid
- Infratemporal fossa
- Transcervical-transmastoid

FACIAL NERVE MANAGEMENT

- If the facial nerve is fully intact before surgery then attempts should be made to preserve it via an R1 resection
- If the facial nerve is paretic or paralyzed before surgery then it should be resected to negative margins
- Reconstruction options
  - Primary neurorrhaphy
    - Nerve mobilization via mastoidectomy
  - Cable/interposition graft
    - Greater auricular nerve
    - Hypoglossal descendans/ansa cervicalis
    - Sural nerve

COMPLICATIONS OF PAROTIDECTOMY

- Seroma
- Hematoma
- Facial nerve paresis or paralysis
  - Immediate postoperative facial nerve dysfunction: 46%
  - Permanent facial nerve paralysis: 1-4%
  - Higher risk of paralysis in revision cases or for extended parotidectomy
- Sensory abnormalities: greater auricular nerve division
- Gustatory sweating (Frey syndrome)
  - Aberrant cross-innervation between postganglionic secretomotor parasympathetic fibers (parotid) to postganglionic sympathetic fibers (sweat glands of the skin)
  - Estimated incidence 35-60%
  - Diagnosis: minor starch/iodine test
  - Treatment: antiperspirant, glycopyrrolate lotion, tympanic neurectomy, and Botox
- First-bite syndrome
  - Most common after deep lobe parotidectomy with instrumentation in the parapharyngeal space
  - Characterized by severe cramping or spasm in the parotid with the first bite of a meal
  - Likely because of loss of sympathetic innervation, causing denervation supersensitivity activated by parasympathetic hyperactivation
  - Stimulates exaggerated myoepithelial cell contraction throughout the parotid
  - Treatment: pain medicine, acupuncture, and Botox injections; most patients improve over time, but few completely resolve
- Salivary fistula: treatment includes aspiration, pressure dressing, and wound care (may consider botulinum toxin)

RELATIVE INCIDENCE OF MALIGNANT SALIVARY GLAND NEOPLASMS

- Mucoepidermoid carcinoma (34%)
- Adenoid cystic carcinoma (22%)
- Adenocarcinoma (18%)
- Malignant mixed tumor (13%)
- Acinic cell carcinoma (7%)
- SCC (4%)
- Other (3%)

PROGNOSTIC VARIABLES

- Primary tumor site (submandibular and minor salivary are more aggressive)
- Primary tumor size (T classification)
- Age (>50 worse outcomes)
- Presenting symptoms (facial nerve paralysis and pain associated with metastases)
- Histologic type/grade (high grade)
- Local tissue invasion (perineural and bone)
- Positive resection margins
- High Ki-67 and low p27 expression
- Her2 (ERBB2) overexpression

INDICATION FOR ADJUVANT RADIATION

- Advanced stage
- Positive resection margins
- High-grade histologic types
- Local tissue invasion, perineural, or bone invasion

NEUTRON BEAM RADIATION

- Delivers more energy than conventional photon/electron radiation
- Historically considered for salivary tumors, which are thought to be radioresistant
- RTOG-MRG study on unresectable salivary cancers[18]
  - Only prospective randomized trial of radiation for salivary tumors
  - Compared fast neutron therapy with conventional photon RT (not IMRT)
  - Neutrons demonstrated significantly improved locoregional control but not overall survival
- Benefits of neutrons compared with modern IMRT techniques are controversial
  - Neutrons may have higher toxicities and side effects
  - Neutrons are less widely available

MELANOMA

RISK FACTORS ASSOCIATED WITH CUTANEOUS MELANOMA

- Inability to tan
  - Fair complexion
  - Blue/green eyes
  - Blond/red hair
  - Freckling
- History of blistering or peeling sunburns
- Immunosuppression
- Teenage outdoor summer jobs
- Tanning booth exposure
- Genetic/medical history
  - CDKN2A (p16) mutation
  - Family history of melanoma
  - History of prior melanoma
  - Actinic keratosis

- Nonmelanoma skin cancer
- Xeroderma pigmentosa
- Atypical (dysplastic) nevus
- Giant congenital melanocytic nevus
- Melanoma subtypes
  - Superficial spreading (70%)
  - Nodular (15-30%)
  - Lentigo maligna
  - Desmoplastic (<4%)
  - Unknown primary (2-8%)

DESMOPLASTIC MELANOMA

- Rare overall, but >50% of desmoplastic melanomas occur in the head and neck
- Distinct features
  - Majority of desmoplastic cases are amelanotic
  - Locally aggressive and highly infiltrative
  - Local recurrence in up to 50% of cases
  - Associated with neurotropic features: perineural and endoneural infiltration
  - Greater tumor thickness at time of diagnosis
- Subtypes
  - Pure desmoplastic melanoma: desmoplastic cells make up >90% of the lesion
    - 1% incidence of nodal metastasis: SLNB is not used for pure variants
  - Mixed desmoplastic melanoma: 22% incidence of nodal metastasis; SLNB is used for mixed variants

BIOPSY

- Recommended: complete excisional biopsy with narrow 1-2 mm margin
  - Allows for diagnosis
  - Allows for evaluation of important prognostic factors
    - Breslow depth
    - Ulceration
    - Mitotic rate
    - Angiolymphatic invasion and perineural invasion
- If not amenable to excisional biopsy, then a punch biopsy or incisional biopsy through the thickest or darkest portion is recommended
- Not recommended: shave biopsy, frozen section biopsy, and FNA
  - Prevents evaluation of tumor thickness, which dictates treatment
- Not recommended: excisional biopsy with wide margins (on initial view)
  - Removal of significant surrounding skin may compromise the ability to stage regional lymph node basins using SLNB
  - ABCD (concerning signs for melanoma)
    - A: asymmetry in appearance
    - B: border irregularity
    - C: color variation
    - D: diameter >6 mm
  - Melanoma staging (Table 5.10)

MOST IMPORTANT PREDICTORS OF SURVIVAL

- Stage I and II localized disease
  - Tumor thickness (most important prognostic indicator)
  - Tumor ulceration (second most important prognostic indicator)
  - Mitotic rate for T1 lesions only
- Stage III regional disease
  - Number of metastatic lymph nodes (most important)

Table 5.10 Melanoma Tumor-Node-Metastasis Classification

T Classification	Thickness	Ulceration Status
T1	≤1.0 mm	a: Without ulceration and mitosis $<1/mm^2$ b: With ulceration or mitosis $\geq 1/mm^2$
T2	1.01-2.0 mm	a: Without ulceration b: With ulceration
T3	2.01-4.0 mm	a: Without ulceration b: With ulceration
T4	>4.0 mm	a: Without ulceration b: With ulceration

N Classification	Number of Metastatic Nodes	Nodal Metastatic Mass
N1	One node	a: Micrometastasis[a] b: Macrometastasis[b]
N2	Two to three nodes	a: Micrometastasis[a] b: Macrometastasis[b] c: In-transit metastasis/satellite *without* metastatic nodes
N3	Four or more metastatic nodes, matted nodes, or an in-transit metastasis/satellite *with* metastatic nodes	

M Classification	Site	Serum
M1a	Distant skin, subcutaneous, or nodal metastases	Normal
M1b	Lung metastases	Normal
M1c	All other visceral metastases Any distant metastasis	Normal Elevated

[a]Micrometastases are diagnosed after sentinel lymph node biopsy.
[b]*Macrometastases* are defined as clinically detectable nodal metastases confirmed by therapeutic lymphadenectomy or when nodal metastasis exhibits gross extracapsular extension.
From Flint PW, Haughey BH, Lund VJ, et al. *Cummings Otolaryngology—Head and Neck Surgery*. 6th ed. Philadelphia, PA: Saunders; 2015, table 81-2.

- Tumor burden (microscopic vs. macroscopic nodal disease) (second most important)
- Primary tumor ulceration
- Stage IV distant disease
  - Elevated lactate dehydrogenase

REGIONAL DISEASE

- Satellite metastasis (N2C)
  - Defined as a nest of metastatic tumor >0.05 mm in diameter that is separate from the primary lesion by <2 cm
- In-transit metastasis (N2C)
  - Defined as metastatic tumor that is separate from the primary lesion by >2 cm but not in the lymph node basin
- Lymph node metastasis

RECOMMENDED SURGICAL MARGINS BY TUMOR THICKNESS (Table 5.11)

SENTINEL LYMPH NODE BIOPSY

- Nodal status is the most important prognostic factor for all melanoma patients
- 10-20% harbor occult microscopic nodal disease, with higher frequency correlating with higher Breslow depth
- Sentinel lymph node status is shown to represent accurately the status of the entire nodal basin

Table 5.11 Recommended Surgical Margins for Excision of Primary Cutaneous Melanoma

Tumor Thickness (mm)	Surgical Margin (cm)
In situ	0.5
<1.0	1.0
1.01-2.0	1.0-2.0
>2.0	2.0

From Flint PW, Haughey BH, Lund VJ, et al. *Cummings Otolaryngology—Head and Neck Surgery*. 6th ed. Philadelphia, PA: Saunders; 2015, table 81-4.

- Identifies the group that warrants therapeutic neck dissection, thereby sparing the remaining 80% an unnecessary neck dissection
- Cases with metastatic disease are not deemed candidates for SLNB
- Cases with previous surgical disruption of lymphatics can be considered, but accuracy is decreased

NATIONAL COMPREHENSIVE CANCER NETWORK INDICATIONS FOR SENTINEL LYMPH NODE BIOPSY[19,20]

- T2-T4 melanomas
- Some patients with T1b melanoma
- MSLT-1 showed that SLNB improved disease-free survival in intermediate and thick melanomas, but not overall survival

AMERICAN SOCIETY OF CLINICAL ONCOLOGY INDICATIONS FOR SENTINEL LYMPH NODE BIOPSY

- Thick melanomas (Breslow depth ≥4 mm)
- Intermediate thickness melanomas (Breslow depth 1-4 mm)
- Certain thin melanomas (0.75-1 mm) with adverse prognostic variables:
  - Ulceration
  - Extensive regression to 1.0 mm
  - Young age
  - Mitotic rate ≥1/mm^2
  - Angiolymphatic invasion
  - Deep positive margin

HISTOPATHOLOGIC MARKERS FOR MELANOMA

- S100, melan-A (MART-1), HMB-45

NONSURGICAL THERAPY FOR MELANOMA

- Radiation (may delay locoregional recurrence in high-risk patients)
- Immunotherapy
  - Interferon alpha-2b
  - Interleukin 2IL-2
  - Ipilimumab: monoclonal antibody activates T cells
  - PD-1 inhibitors Nivolumab and Pembrolizumab
  - Vemurafenib: inhibit mutated BRAF
  - Chemotherapy: dacarbazine (response rate 10-20% in stage IV)

THYROID MALIGNANCIES

EPIDEMIOLOGY

- Fastest increase in incidence of all major cancers in the United States
- Increasing incidence is almost completely attributable to papillary thyroid cancer
- Increasing incidence is also due largely to improved/increased detection methods
- Palpable thyroid nodules in 4-7% of US population
- Subclinical thyroid nodules on ultrasonography in 19-67% of US population
- Only 5% of thyroid nodules are malignant
- Younger and older patients are more likely to have a malignant thyroid nodule
- Patients younger than age 20 years have 20-50% incidence of malignancy when presenting with a single thyroid nodule

RECURRENT LARYNGEAL NERVE

- Right RLN
  - Exits the vagus nerve at the base of the neck
  - Loops around the right subclavian artery (fourth arch)
  - Returns deep to the innominate artery and back to the thyroid bed diagonally
  - "Nonrecurrent" RLN may rarely occur on the right side and enter from the lateral course
    - Associated with an aberrant retroesophageal subclavian artery (arteria lusoria)
- Left RLN
  - Exits the vagus nerve at the level of the aortic arch and ligamentum arteriosum (sixth arch), lateral to the obliterated ductus arteriosus

- Returns to the thyroid bed along the tracheoesophageal groove at a more medial and vertical course than the right RLN
- Crosses deep to the inferior thyroid artery 70% of the time

SUPERIOR LARYNGEAL NERVE (Fig. 5.20)

- Arises beneath the nodose ganglion of the upper vagus nerve
- Divides into internal and external branches 2 cm above the superior pole
  - Internal branch: travels medially, entering through the posterior thyrohyoid membrane to supply sensation to the supraglottis

  External branch: travels medially along, within, or deep to the inferior constrictor muscle to enter the cricothyroid muscle; travels with the superior thyroid artery, diverging 1 cm from the thyroid superior pole

PARATHYROID GLANDS

- 80% of patients have four parathyroid glands, with at least 10% having greater than four glands
- Superior parathyroid glands: at the level of the cricoid cartilage, medial to the intersection of the RLN and inferior thyroid artery
- Inferior parathyroid glands: lateral or posterior surface of lower thyroid pole

HISTOLOGY OF THYROID MALIGANCIES

- Papillary (79%)
- Follicular (13%)
- Hurthle cell (3%)
- Medullary (4%)
- Anaplastic thyroid cancer
- Lymphoma
- Metastatic cancer to thyroid

THYROID VASCULAR SUPPLY

- Inferior thyroid artery (branch of the thyrocervical trunk)
- Superior thyroid artery (branch of the external carotid artery)
- Superior, middle, and inferior thyroid veins (drain to the internal jugular or innominate veins)

GENETIC ALTERATIONS IN THYROID CANCER

- Papillary (RET, BRAF, and RAS)
- Follicular (RAS and PPARG)
- Poorly differentiated (RAS, BRAF, and TP53)
- Anaplastic (TP53, RAS, BRAF, and PIK3CA)
- Medullary (RET 95% in MEN-2)

RISK FACTORS FOR THYROID CANCER

- Age
- Sex (female): 3 times more likely to develop papillary thyroid carcinoma (PTC)
- Exposure to radiation: the only established environmental risk for thyroid cancer
  - Thyroid nodules with radiation history have 50% incidence of malignancy
  - Higher risk in exposure to children compared with adults
  - 1986 Chernobyl accident conferred a 60-fold increased risk in children
- Family history of thyroid cancer
  - Approximately 6% of patients with PTC have familial disease

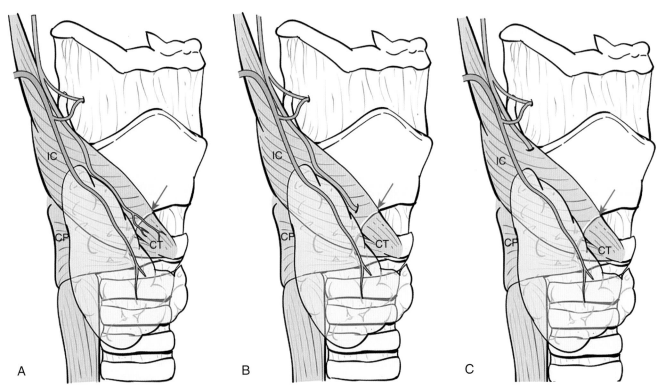

FIGURE 5.20 Variant Course of the External Branch of the Superior Laryngeal Nerve. (**A**) Type 1: the superior laryngeal nerve (SLN) runs superficial to the inferior constrictor muscle. (**B**) Type 2: the SLN dives into and runs deep to the inferior constrictor muscle. (**C**) Type 3: the SLN runs deep to the inferior constrictor muscle. (From Shah JP, Patel SG, Singh B. *Jatin Shah's Head and Neck Surgery and Oncology.* 4th ed. Philadelphia, PA: Mosby; 2012.)

- PTC occurs with increased frequency in certain families with breast, ovarian, renal, and central nervous system malignancies
- PTC: associated with Gardner and Cowden syndromes
- Medullary thyroid carcinoma (MTC): associated with MTC, MEN2A, and MEN2B syndromes

TNM STAGING FOR THYROID CANCER (Table 5.12)

- Excellent prognosis for younger PTC patients
- PTC patients younger than 45 years old cannot be greater than stage II

Table 5.12 **TNM Staging for Thyroid Cancer**	
Stage	**Description**
Primary Tumor (T)	
TX	Primary tumor cannot be assessed
T0	No evidence of primary tumor
T1	Tumor ≤2 cm in greatest dimension and limited to the thyroid
T1a	Tumor ≤1 cm in greatest dimension and limited to the thyroid
T1b	Tumor >1 cm but ≤2 cm in greatest dimension and limited to the thyroid
T2	Tumor >2 cm and ≤4 cm in greatest dimension and limited to the thyroid
T3	Tumor >4 cm in greatest dimension and limited to the thyroid *or* any tumor with minimal extrathyroid extension (eg, extension to sternothyroid muscle or perithyroid soft tissues)
T4a	Moderately advanced disease Tumor of any size that extends beyond the thyroid capsule to invade the subcutaneous soft tissues, larynx, trachea, esophagus, or recurrent laryngeal nerve
T4b	Very advanced disease Tumor invades prevertebral fascia or encases the carotid artery or mediastinal vessels
T4a	Intrathyroidal anaplastic carcinoma[a]: surgically resectable
T4b	Extrathyroidal anaplastic carcinoma[a]: surgically unresectable
Regional Lymph Nodes (N)	
NX	Regional lymph nodes cannot be assessed

Table 5.12 **TNM Staging for Thyroid Cancer—cont'd**	
Stage	**Description**
N0	No regional lymph node metastasis
N1	Regional lymph node metastasis
N1a	Metastasis to level VI (pretracheal, paratracheal, and prelaryngeal/Delphian lymph nodes)
N1b	Metastasis to unilateral, bilateral, or contralateral cervical (levels I through V) or retropharyngeal or superior mediastinal lymph nodes
Distant Metastasis (M)	
MX	Distant metastasis cannot be assessed
M0	No distant metastasis
M1	Distant metastasis

Grouping	**Age <45 Years**	**Age ≥45 Years**
Papillary/Follicular		
Stage I	Any T; any N M0	T1 N0 M0
Stage II	Any T; any N M1	T2 N0 M0
Stage III		T3 N0 M0
		T1 to T3 N1a M0
Stage IVA		T4a N0 M0
		T4a N1a M0
		T1 to T4a N1b M0
Stage IVB		T4b; any N M0
Stage IVC		Any T; any N M1
Medullary		
Stage I	T1 N0 M0	
Stage II	T2 N0 M0	
	T3 N0 M0	
Stage III	T1 to T3 N1a M0	
Stage IVA	T4a N0 M0	
	T4a N1a M0	
	T1 to T4a N1b M0	
Stage IVB	T4b; any N M0	
Stage IVC	Any T; any N M1	
Anaplastic		
Stage IVA	T4a; any N M0	
Stage IVB	T4b; any N M0	
Stage IVC	Any T; any N M1	

aAll anaplastic carcinomas are considered T4 tumors.
From Flint PW, Haughey BH, Lund VJ, et al. *Cummings Otolaryngology—Head and Neck Surgery*. 6th ed. Philadelphia, PA: Saunders; 2015, table 123-2, and Edge SB. *The American Joint Committee on Cancer: AJCC Cancer Staging Manual*. 7th ed. New York, NY: Springer; 2010.

AGE, METASTASIS, EXTENT OF DISEASE, AND SIZE OF TUMOR (AMES) FOR RISK STRATIFICATION

- Age (low risk includes men <41 years and women <51 years)
- Metastases
- Extent of tumor invasion
- Size of tumor (low risk includes <5 cm)

METASTASIS, AGE AT PRESENTATION, COMPLETENESS OF SURGICAL RESECTION, INVASION (EXTRATHYROIDAL), AND SIZE OF TUMOR (MACIS) SCORE

- Metastasis
- Age at diagnosis
- Completeness of surgical resection
- Invasion extrathyroid
- Size of tumor

Box 5.3 RISK STRATIFICATION FOR THYROID CANCER RECURRENCE

Low Risk (All of the Following Must Apply)
- No local or distant metastases
- All macroscopic tumor has been resected
- No tumor invasion of locoregional tissues or structures
- Tumor does not have aggressive histology (eg, tall cell, insular, and columnar cell carcinoma) or vascular invasion
- If ^{131}I is given, no ^{131}I uptake occurs outside the thyroid bed on the first posttreatment whole-body radioactive isotope scan

Intermediate Risk (Any of the Following)
- Microscopic invasion of tumor into the perithyroid soft tissues at initial surgery
- Cervical lymph node metastases or ^{131}I uptake outside the thyroid bed on the whole-body radioactive isotope scan done after thyroid remnant ablation
- Tumor with aggressive histology or vascular invasion

High Risk (Any of the Following)
- Macroscopic tumor invasion
- Incomplete tumor resection
- Distant metastases
- Thyroglobulinemia out of proportion to what is seen on the posttreatment scan

From Flint PW, Haughey BH, Lund VJ, et al. *Cummings Otolaryngology—Head and Neck Surgery*. 6th ed. Philadelphia, PA: Saunders; 2015, box 123-1.

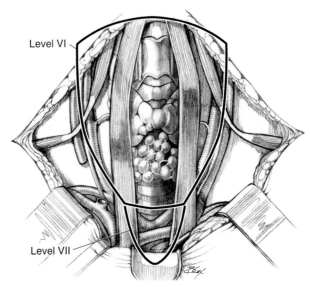

FIGURE 5.21 Boundaries of the central compartment of the neck (level VI). The compartment extends from the hyoid bone to the suprasternal notch, as well as the carotid arteries laterally. (From Pai SI, Tufano RP. Central compartment lymph node dissection. *Operat Tech Otolaryngol.* 2009;20:39-43.)

AMERICAN THYROID ASSOCIATION (ATA) RISK STRATIFICATION FOR RECURRENCE[21] (BOX 5.3)

METASTASIS TO THYROID

- Kidney
- Breast
- Lung
- Skin (melanoma and SCC)

FINE-NEEDLE ASPIRATION

- Highly sensitive and specific
- Decreased unnecessary surgery by 35-75%
- Yield of malignancies is tripled in thyroid surgeries after the advent of FNA
- 60-90% of nodules reveal a benign diagnosis
- 15% of aspirates are nondiagnostic or inadequate, warranting reaspiration
- Benign nodules require routine follow-up because of a 5% false-negative rate
- Follicular neoplasms cannot be classified by FNA because of the need for architecture

ULTRASOUND

- Provide key baseline information regarding nodule size and architecture
- Noninvasive and inexpensive way to track changes in nodules
- Ultrasound cervical lymph node mapping is recommended before all initial thyroidectomy because operative management may be altered in 20% of patients
  - Characteristics of suspicious lymph nodes
    - Loss of fatty hilum
    - Increased vascularity
    - Round node configuration
    - Solid nodule with hypoechogenicity
    - Microcalcifications

COMPUTED TOMOGRAPHY AND MAGNETIC RESONANCE IMAGING

- Usually unnecessary in evaluation of thyroid tumors
- Not as effective as ultrasound is in evaluation of thyroid nodules
- Useful for characterizing substernal extension, cervical and mediastinal lymphadenopathy, and trachea invasion
- Complements ultrasound by visualizing behind the sternum, trachea, and esophagus
- Recommended for bulky lymph node disease to facilitate surgical planning
- Iodinated contrast may preclude the use of postoperative radioactive iodine (RAI) for 2-3 months; however, this delay does not affect outcomes

PAPILLARY THYROID CARCINOMA MANAGEMENT

- Thyroglobulin-level monitoring
- Routine neck ultrasound monitoring
- Neck management
  - Elective lateral neck dissection is not recommended unless N+ disease is documented
  - Central neck dissection
    - Level VI boundaries: carotid to carotid and hyoid to innominate artery (Fig. 5.21)
    - Recommended for N+ disease
    - Recommended for palpable or visualized disease during surgery
    - Controversial for N0 disease
    - Compartmental dissection (not selective node plucking) is recommended (Fig. 5.22)
    - Higher incidence of inadvertent inferior parathyroidectomy

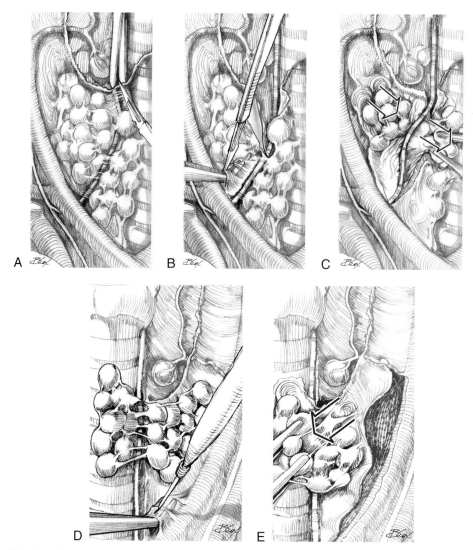

FIGURE 5.22 Management of the Recurrent Laryngeal Nerve in Central Neck Dissection. (**A**) After identification of the right RLN, the nerve is dissected inferiorly away from surrounding lymph node–bearing tissue. (**B**) The right RLN is transposed atraumatically to remove lymph node tissue both anteriorly and posteriorly. (**C**) The lymph node compartment is mobilized off the prevertebral fascia and esophagus, down to the innominate artery, to incorporate the superior mediastinal lymph nodes. (**D**) The left RLN loops around the aortic arch and travels deep to the innominate artery or brachiocephalic vein. (**E**) Because the esophagus is present immediately behind the left RLN, there are typically no lymph nodes posterior to it. En bloc resection of lymph nodes anterior and lateral to the left RLN are therefore sufficient, without mobilizing the nerve itself. (From Pai SI, Tufano RP. Central compartment lymph node dissection. *Operat Tech Otolaryngol.* 2009;20:39-43.)

- Incidence of recurrence over years
  - Thyroid bed recurrence: 5-6%
  - Regional lymphatic recurrence: 8-9%
  - Distant site recurrence: 4-11%
- Recommendation for RAI depends on risk profile and risk of recurrence
- Surveillance
  - Thyroglobulin
  - Routine surveillance U/S

FOLLICULAR THYROID CARCINOMA MANAGEMENT

- Cervical lymphadenopathy less common than PTC
- Classically hematogenous spread, rather than lymphatic spread
- Distant metastases more common than PTC
- FNA or frozen section cannot distinguish between follicular adenoma and carcinoma: requires diagnostic thyroidectomy
- Histology

- Minimally invasive follicular cancer
- Frankly invasive follicular cancer: greater likelihood of distant metastasis
- Factors of poor prognosis
  - Age >50 years, >4 cm in size, high grade, vascular invasion, extrathyroidal extension, and distant metastasis
- Recurrence rate is 30%, but much less for minimally invasive histology
- In contrast to PTC, mortality is directly related to recurrence

HURTHLE CELL CARCINOMA MANAGEMENT

- Tend to be more aggressive to follicular carcinoma
- Less amenable to RAI
- More likely than follicular carcinoma is to have cervical lymphadenopathy
- Overall survival is significantly worse than follicular thyroid carcinoma (FTC) or PTC
- Highest incidence of distant metastasis among well-differentiated thyroid cancers

MEDULLARY THYROID CANCER MANAGEMENT

- 5% of all thyroid carcinomas
- Arises from parafollicular C cells and secretes calcitonin
- Distant metastases are present in 50% of patients on diagnosis
- 30% are familial
  - Autosomal dominant, with nearly 100% penetrance
  - MEN2A: MTC, pheochromocytoma, and hyperparathyroidism
  - MEN2B: MTC, pheochromocytoma, mucosal neuromas, and Marfanoid body habitus
- Workup
  - Calcitonin: magnitude determines extent of disease
  - RET mutation testing: determines familial versus sporadic, tumor aggressiveness (based on mutation type), and need for family screening
    - Negative RET testing precludes need to test for multiple endocrine neoplasia (MEN) syndrome (eg, catecholamines, calcium, and abdominal MRI)
    - Negative RET testing suggests a greater likelihood that MTC is unifocal
  - Serum calcium: assesses for hyperparathyroidism
  - 24-hour urinary metanephrines and catecholamines: assesses for pheochromocytoma
  - Abdominal MRI: assesses for pheochromocytoma
  - Thyroid ultrasound with lymph node bed mapping
- Surgery
  - Any pheochromocytoma should be removed before thyroidectomy
  - Total thyroidectomy
  - Central neck dissection should be strongly considered
  - Lateral neck dissection should be strongly considered if central neck nodes are involved
  - When the primary lesion is >1 cm, ipsilateral lateral neck dissection should be considered because 60% will have nodal metastases
- Surveillance
  - Calcitonin and carcinoembryonic antigen monitoring
  - Flushing and diarrhea may appear with significant disease
  - Salvage surgery is preferred for recurrent or residual disease
  - RAI is not effective
  - External beam radiation is controversial
  - Targeted therapies are available for recurrent/metastatic disease (cabozantinib and vandetanib)

ANAPLASTIC THYROID CANCER MANAGEMENT

- Classically one of the most aggressive malignancies
- Median survival of 5 months; median 1-year overall survival of 20%
- Typically presents with long-standing neck mass that enlarges rapidly
  - Often accompanied by pain, dysphonia, dysphagia, and dyspnea
  - Most patients die of superior vena cava syndrome, asphyxiation, or exsanguination
- Workup
  - Advance care planning
  - Nutritional support
  - Airway management
  - Core biopsy or operative biopsy is necessary given tissue heterogeneity and the possibility of lymphoma
- Treatment
  - Surgical resection can be considered if grossly negative margins (R1 resection) can be achieved
  - Tumor debulking (R2 resection) does not improve locoregional control or survival

- Tracheostomy may overcome acute airway distress, but it is not typically recommended because it may increase suffering and lead to a prolonged hospital stay
- Postoperative radiation may improve locoregional control

ADJUVANT TREATMENT

- Thyroid stimulating hormone (TSH) suppression
  - Long-term levothyroxine administration to suppress TSH and, therefore, possible recurrence or progression of thyroid cancer
  - Goal TSH of <0.1 for intermediate-to-high-risk patients
  - Goal TSH of 0.1-0.5 for low-risk patients
- RAI
  - For higher risk PTC and FTC
  - Decreases risk of recurrence and disease-specific mortality
  - Indications
    - Any primary tumor >4 cm
    - Extrathyroidal extension
    - Distant metastases
    - High-risk features (poorly differentiated subtypes, vascular invasion, and multifocal disease)
    - Not recommended for primary tumors <1 cm
  - Dosage
    - Typically 100 mCi for residual thyroid bed uptake
    - Typically 100-200 mCi for regional or distant disease, or aggressive subtypes
    - No clear evidence on whether fixed amounts versus quantitative tumor dosimetry tailored to patient is superior
- External beam radiation; suggested indications:
  - Anaplastic thyroid cancer
  - Patient older than 45 with gross extrathyroid extension and high likelihood of microscopic residual disease
  - Patient with gross residual tumor unlikely to respond to further surgery or RAI

PARATHYROID DISORDERS

PARATHYROID HORMONE

- Intact parathyroid hormone (PTH) (1-84) is the major circulating form of biologically active PTH
- Half-life of 3-5 minutes
- Cleared by liver and kidney
- Targets and functions of PTH
  - Kidney
    - Increase resorption of calcium
    - Decrease resorption of phosphorus
    - Convert 25-hydroxyvitamin (25-OH) D3 (calcifediol) to 1,25-dihydroxyvitamin (1,25-OH) D3 (calcitriol)
  - Skeletal system: stimulate osteoclast activity via osteoblast modulation
  - Intestine: increase calcium absorption through vitamin D
- Calcitonin
  - Much smaller role than PTH in calcium homeostasis
  - Secreted by parafollicular cells in thyroid gland
  - Inhibits bone resorption

PARATHYROID GLAND

- Normal weight varies and can be between 30 and 60 mg
- Fat content varies and hovers around 50% and increases with age

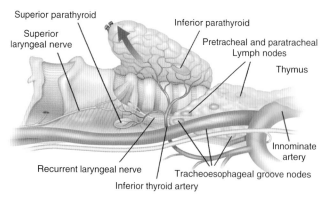

FIGURE 5.23 Parathyroid Location Relative to Adjacent Thyroid Neurovascular Structures. The thyroid gland is mobilized medially. The inferior parathyroid must be distinguished from neighboring pretracheal and paratracheal lymph nodes, as well as fat lobules and thyroid tissue. (From Friedman M, Kelley K, Maley A. Central neck dissection. *Operat Tech Otolaryngol.* 2011;22:169-172.)

- 85% of patients have four glands, whereas 3-6% have three glands
- Approximately 1% of patients have a hyperfunctioning fifth parathyroid gland; most fifth glands have been found in the mediastinum (thymus and aortic arch)
- 0.5-3% incidence of intrathyroidal parathyroid glands
- Location (Fig. 5.23)
  - Superior parathyroid
    - Cricothyroid junction approximately 1 cm cranial to the juxtaposition of the RLN and inferior thyroid artery
    - Paraesophageal location in 1% of cases
    - More consistent position compared with inferior parathyroid glands
    - Embryologically deep (dorsal) to the RLN
  - Inferior parathyroid
    - Inferior pole of the thyroid and along the thyrothymic ligament
    - Migratory pathway into the anterior-superior mediastinum
    - Up to 33% of missed parathyroid glands are found in the anterior-superior mediastinum
    - More variable position compared with superior parathyroid glands (longer migratory descent during development)
- Arterial supply
  - Inferior thyroid artery supplies the large majority of both superior and inferior parathyroid glands (>80%)
  - However, abundant plexus of vessels may provide additional vascularization
  - Superior thyroid artery may provide dominant arterial supply for superior parathyroid glands in up to 10-20% of patients
- Parathyroid carcinoma
  - May be difficult to distinguish from benign parathyroid adenoma
  - Histologically challenging, although increased mitotic figures is an indicator
  - Only reliable indicators are invasion of surrounding structures and metastasis
  - Typically indolent growth with recurrence is common
  - Morbidity is more typically associated with uncontrolled hormone secretion

KEY ELEMENTS OF BIOCHEMICAL DIAGNOSIS OF PRIMARY HYPERPARATHYROIDISM

- High calcium
- Elevated PTH
- Normal creatinine
- Low or low-normal phosphate
- Urinary calcium >125 mg/24 hours
- Normal 25-OH vitamin D and 1,25-OH vitamin D

SYMPTOMS OF HYPERCALCEMIA

- Kidney and urinary tract: nephrolithiasis and urolithiasis; most stones are calcium oxalate
- Skeletal system: osteitis fibrosis cystica (bone pain, pathologic fracture, and cystic bone change) osteoporosis; hyperparathyroidism-related bone loss occurs at cortical bone sites and spares trabecular bone
- Neuromuscular system: muscle weakness (40% incidence), fatigue, and aches; muscle weakness improves after parathyroidectomy in 80-90% of patients
- Neurologic: anxiety, psychosis, depression, deafness, dysphagia, and dysosmia; depression improves after parathyroidectomy in 50% of patients
- Gastrointestinal: peptic ulcer, pancreatitis, and cholelithiasis
- Cardiovascular: hypertension

CAUSES OF PARATHYROID HORMONE-MEDIATED HYPERCALCEMIA

- Primary hyperparathyroidism
  - Parathyroid adenoma
  - Parathyroid lipoadenoma
  - Parathyroid hyperplasia
  - Parathyroid carcinoma
- Secondary hyperparathyroidism
  - Insufficient calcium intake, decreased calcium absorption, and vitamin-D deficiency
  - Renal insufficiency or failure
- Tertiary hyperparathyroidism
  - Long-standing renal insufficiency or failure leading to autonomous parathyroid hyperfunctioning

HYPERCALCEMIA OF MALIGNANCY

- PTH-related protein secretion (lung, esophagus, head and neck, renal cell, ovary, bladder, and pancreatic)
- Ectopic PTH secretion by small cell lung cancer, small cell ovarian cancer, and squamous cell lung cancer
- Ectopic 1,25-OH D production by B-cell lymphoma and Hodgkin disease
- Lytic bone metastasis (multiple myeloma, lymphoma, breast cancer, and sarcoma)
- Tumor cytokines

FAMILIAL HYPERCALCEMIC HYPOCALCIURIA

- Autosomal dominant disorder
- Inactivating mutations in the calcium-sensing receptor of the parathyroid gland
- Low 24-hour urine calcium relative to their hypercalcemia
  - 24-hour calcium-to-creatinine clearance ratio
  - Familial hypercalcemic hypocalciuria: ratio <0.01
  - Hyperparathyroidism: ratio >0.01

HYPERPARATHYROIDISM WITH NORMAL CALCIUM LEVELS

- May have physiologic secondary hyperparathyroidism
- Before parathyroidectomy, must rule out:
  - Low calcium or vitamin-D intake
  - Calcium or vitamin D malabsorption
  - Inability to convert 25-OH vitamin D to 1,25-OH vitamin D
  - Hypercalciuria

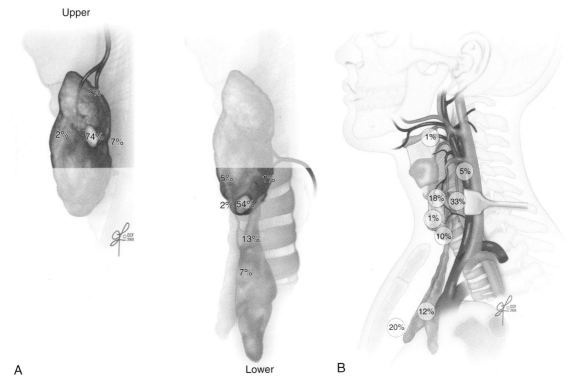

Upper

Lower

A   B

FIGURE 5.24 Superior and Inferior Parathyroid Distribution. (**A**) Normal distribution of the superior and inferior parathyroid glands. (**B**) Distribution of ectopic parathyroid glands. (From Randolph G. *Surgery of the Thyroid and Parathyroid Glands.* 2nd ed. Philadelphia, PA: Saunders; 2013, fig. 59-3.)4, Gregory W. Randolph. Surgery of the Thyroid and Parathyroid Glands. 2nd edi. Philadelphia: Elsevier Saunders; 2013.

- Lithium and thiazide diuretics may falsely elevate calcium and PTH, and patient must be off the drugs for at least 1 month before re-evaluation

IMAGING LOCALIZATION STUDIES FOR HYPERPARATHYROIDISM

- Ultrasound
  - Well-tolerated and inexpensive
  - Poor localization of enlarged parathyroid glands in retroesophageal, retrotracheal, retrosternal, and deep thoracic inlet locations
- Technetium 99m sestamibi scintigraphy
  - Parathyroid glands that are dense with mitochondria take up sestamibi more intensely (and clear sestamibi more slowly) compared with thyroid gland parenchyma
  - Reported 100% sensitivity and 90% specificity
  - Can identify double adenomas, but is inaccurate for smaller adenoma size and four-gland parathyroid hyperplasia
- Single-photon emission CT/CT
  - Provides greater anatomic localization
  - Helps aid in minimally invasive directed approach
  - Helps accurately locate ectopic glands (thymic, retroesophageal, mediastinal, and intrathyroid)
  - Helps in directed re-exploratory surgery
- Four-phase CT scan
  - Precontrast, immediate, early delayed, and late-delayed phases
  - Allows visualization of early enhancement and early washout of parathyroid candidates relative to thyroid tissue and lymph nodes
- CT imaging
  - Less effective than MRI
  - High false-positive rates
  - Subject to distortion from metal clips in reoperative cases

- MRI
  - Parathyroid adenomas have low T1-intensity and high T2-intensity
  - More effective for finding ectopic parathyroid candidates

SURGICAL APPROACH

- Systematic approach is crucial
- Abnormal gland identified and sent for frozen section analysis
- Half-life of PTH is 2-5 minutes
- Goal is >50% decrease in PTH and drop to normal PTH range
- If PTH remains elevated, a bilateral four-gland exploration is required
  - Ectopic areas should be examined, including thymic tissue, carotid sheath, paraesophageal space, and hemithyroidectomy if necessary
- Experience of surgeon
  - Experienced surgeons (>10 parathyroidectomies per year): 90% success rate
  - Inexperienced surgeons: 70% success rate, with 15% remaining hypercalcemic and 14% becoming permanently hypocalcemic
- Approaches
  - Bilateral cervical exploration
  - Directed unilateral cervical exploration
  - Minimally invasive techniques

CONSENSUS INDICATIONS FOR SURGERY FOR ASYMPTOMATIC PRIMARY HYPERPARATHYROIDISM[22]

- Serum calcium >1 mg/dL above the upper limit of normal
- Creatinine clearance reduced >60 mL/min
- Age <50 years old

- Bone mineral density (lumbar spine, femoral neck, hip, and distal radius)
  - For postmenopausal women and men >50 years and T-score <2.5
  - For premenopausal women and men <50 years and Z-score <2.5
- Surgery requested by patient, or patient unsuitable for surveillance
- 24-hour urine calcium >400 mg/dL (optional)
- Ectopic parathyroid locations (Fig. 5.24)
  - Mediastinum and thymus
  - Retroesophageal
  - Intrathyroidal
  - Carotid sheath
- Parathyroid carcinoma signs and symptoms
  - Higher serum calcium (70% incidence of calcium >14 mg/dL)
  - Higher PTH (70% incidence of 5 times upper limit of normal PTH)
  - Higher likelihood of a neck mass

MULTIPLE GLAND DISEASE

- Double parathyroid adenoma
  - Between 1% and 2% incidence
  - Up to 10% incidence in patients older than 60 years
- Sporadic diffuse hyperplasia
  - Up to 10-15% incidence
  - 40% of equivocal sestamibi scans found to have diffuse multigland hyperplasia
  - 3.5 gland parathyroidectomy performed after all hypercellular glands are found
- Familial hyperparathyroidism
  - Familial types are more likely to have multiglandular disease and persistent hyperparathyroidism after surgery
  - MEN I: high and early penetrance with four-gland hyperplasia
  - MEN IIA: less frequent multigland involvement and lower incidence of persistent hyperparathyroidism after surgery compared with MEN I
  - Non-MEN familial hyperparathyroidism: more aggressive than MEN or sporadic subtypes
- Renal failure–induced secondary hyperparathyroidism
  - Requires subtotal parathyroidectomy or total parathyroidectomy with autotransplantation

ELEVATED PTH AFTER CURATIVE PARATHYROIDECTOMY (NORMAL CALCIUM AND INTRAOPERATIVE PARATHYROID HORMONE)

- Up to 20% of patients
- Speculative causes are development of secondary hyperparathyroidism in response to rapidly changed calcium levels
  - Vitamin-D deficiency
  - Changes in renal function
  - Peripheral resistance to PTH

RE-EXPLORATION OF FAILED PARATHYROIDECTOMY

- A substantial number of cases are single adenomas that are in a "standard" location
- If ectopic adenoma, 16-38% are in the thymus, and up to 10% are intrathyroid

- 6% incidence of RLN paralysis in re-exploration, compared with 1% incidence for initial surgery
- Greater likelihood of permanent hypocalcemia
- Systematic approach
  - Anterior mediastinum (thyrothymic ligament and tracheoesophageal groove)
  - Retropharyngeal/retroesophageal region
  - Thyroid bed with thyroid lobectomy if warranted
  - Carotid sheath
  - Contralateral side

MEDICAL MANAGEMENT OF HYPERPARATHYROIDISM

- Adequate hydration
- Furosemide (loop diuretics)
- Bisphosphonates (alendronate): decrease calcium gut absorption and 1,25-OH vitamin D
- Estrogen
- Calcitonin
- Calcimimetics (cinacalcet): sensitizes PTH receptor to calcium

UNTREATED MILD HYPERPARATHYROIDISM

- Most patients show no significant progression of symptoms
- Disease progression in 27% of patients, including marked hypercalcemia, hypercalciuria, and loss of bone mineral density
- Impossible to predict which patients will progress
  - 33% of patients who develop hypercalcemic crisis had initial symptoms of mild hypercalcemia
  - Younger patients appear more prone to progressive hypercalcemia
- Risk of occult symptoms and end-organ damage increases over time

REFERENCES

1. Marx RE. A new concept in the treatment of osteoradionecrosis. *J Oral Maxillofac Surg*. 1983;41:351–357.
2. Bonner JA, Harari PM, Giralt J, et al. Radiotherapy plus cetuximab for squamous-cell carcinoma of the head and neck. *N Engl J Med*. 2006;354:567–578.
3. Cooper JS, Zhang Q, Pajak TF, et al. Long-term follow-up of the RTOG 9501/intergroup phase III trial: postoperative concurrent radiation therapy and chemotherapy in high-risk squamous cell carcinoma of the head and neck. *Int J Radiat Oncol Biol Phys*. 2012;84:1198–1205.
4. Bernier J, Domenge C, Ozsahin M, et al. Postoperative irradiation with or without concomitant chemotherapy for locally advanced head and neck cancer. *N Engl J Med*. 2004;350:1945–1952.
5. Bernier J, Cooper JS, Pajak TF, et al. Defining risk levels in locally advanced head and neck cancers: a comparative analysis of concurrent postoperative radiation plus chemotherapy trials of the EORTC (#22931) and RTOG (# 9501). *Head Neck*. 2005;27:843–850.
6. Pignon JP, le Maitre A, Maillard E, Bourhis J, Group, M-NC. Meta-analysis of chemotherapy in head and neck cancer (MACH-NC): an update on 93 randomised trials and 17,346 patients. *Radiother Oncol*. 2009;92:4–14.
7. Blanchard P, Baujat B, Holostenco V, et al. Meta-analysis of chemotherapy in head and neck cancer (MACH-NC): a comprehensive analysis by tumour site. *Radiother Oncol*. 2011;100:33–40.
8. Haddad R, O'Neill A, Rabinowits G, et al. Induction chemotherapy followed by concurrent chemoradiotherapy (sequential chemoradiotherapy) versus concurrent chemoradiotherapy alone in locally advanced head and neck cancer (PARADIGM): a randomised phase 3 trial. *Lancet Oncol*. 2013;14:257–264.
9. Cohen EEW, Karrison TG, Kocherginsky M, et al. Phase III randomized trial of induction chemotherapy in patients with N2 or N3 locally advanced head and neck cancer. *J Clin Oncol*. 2014;32:2735–2743.

10. Byers RM, El-Naggar AK, Lee Y-Y, et al. Can we detect or predict the presence of occult nodal metastases in patients with squamous carcinoma of the oral tongue? *Head Neck.* 1998;20:138–144.

11. Ho AS, Tsao GJ, Chen FW, et al. Impact of positron emission tomography/computed tomography surveillance at 12 and 24 months for detecting head and neck cancer recurrence. *Cancer.* 2013;119:1349–1356.

12. Goodwin Jr WJ. Salvage surgery for patients with recurrent squamous cell carcinoma of the upper aerodigestive tract: when do the ends justify the means? *Laryngoscope.* 2000;110:1–18.

13. Janot F, de Raucourt D, Benhamou E, et al. Randomized trial of postoperative reirradiation combined with chemotherapy after salvage surgery compared with salvage surgery alone in head and neck carcinoma. *J Clin Oncol.* 2008;26:5518–5523.

14. Fakhry C, Zhang Q, Nguyen-Tan PF, et al. Human papillomavirus and overall survival after progression of oropharyngeal squamous cell carcinoma. *J Clin Oncol.* 2014;32:3365–3373.

15. The Department of Veterans Affairs Laryngeal Cancer Study Group. Induction chemotherapy plus radiation compared with surgery plus radiation in patients with advanced laryngeal cancer. *N Engl J Med.* 1991;324:1685–1690.

16. Forastiere AA, Goepfert H, Maor M, et al. Concurrent chemotherapy and radiotherapy for organ preservation in advanced laryngeal cancer. *N Engl J Med.* 2003;349:2091–2098.

17. Forastiere AA, Zhang Q, Weber RS, et al. Long-term results of RTOG 91-11: a comparison of three nonsurgical treatment strategies to preserve the larynx in patients with locally advanced larynx cancer. *J Clin Oncol.* 2013;31:845–852.

18. Laramore GE, Krall JM, Griffin TW, et al. Neutron versus photon irradiation for unresectable salivary gland tumors: final report of an RTOG-MRC randomized clinical trial. Radiation Therapy Oncology Group. Medical Research Council. *Int J Radiat Oncol Biol Phys.* 1993;27:235–240.

19. Morton DL, Cochran AJ, Thompson JF, et al. Sentinel node biopsy for early-stage melanoma: accuracy and morbidity in MSLT-I, an international multicenter trial. *Ann Surg.* 2005;242:302–311, discussion 311–313.

20. Morton DL, Thompson JF, Cochran AJ, et al. Final trial report of sentinel-node biopsy versus nodal observation in melanoma. *N Engl J Med.* 2014;370:599–609.

21. American Thyroid Association (ATA) Guidelines Taskforce on Thyroid Nodules and Differentiated Thyroid Cancer, Cooper DS, Doherty GM, et al. Revised American Thyroid Association management guidelines for patients with thyroid nodules and differentiated thyroid cancer. *Thyroid.* 2009;19:1167–1214.

22. Bilezikian JP, Khan AA, Potts Jr JT. Third International Workshop on the Management of Asymptomatic Primary Hyperthyroidism. Guidelines for the management of asymptomatic primary hyperparathyroidism: summary statement from the third international workshop. *J Clin Endocrinol Metab.* 2009;94:335–339.

6 Pediatric Otolaryngology

OTOLOGY

PEDIATRIC OTOLOGIC DEVELOPMENT

- Pinna
  - Normal adult ear ranges from 5.5 to 6.5 cm
  - Grows rapidly during the first 2-3 years, reaching 90% adult size by age 8 years
  - Microtia is often associated with hypoplasia or aplasia of the middle ear
- Tympanic membrane (TM)
  - Adult dimensions at birth
- Eustachian tube
  - Patent during embryologic development (allowing amniotic fluid in middle ear space)[1]
  - Shorter length, less acute angle of orientation in pediatric population allows micro-organisms from the nasopharynx to gain access to the middle ear space
  - Approximately 50% of adult length at birth
  - Tensor veli palatini develops with time to open the tubal lumen more efficiently
- Middle ear, ossicles, and petrous temporal bone
  - Adult sized at birth
- Mastoid
  - Cortex is very thin, predisposing for subperiosteal spread of mastoiditis in children
  - Mastoid pneumatization continues through early childhood; infant's mastoid bone and marrow can bleed substantially during mastoidectomy, often requiring bone wax and diamond burr to stop bleeding
  - Styloid process is underdeveloped at birth, making the extratemporal portion of the facial nerve at risk from external trauma such as in forceps delivery

FUNCTIONS OF THE EUSTACHIAN TUBE

1. Ventilation of the middle ear and pressure equalization
2. Drainage by mucociliary clearance of secretions of the middle ear
3. Protection of the middle ear from sounds, pathogens, and secretions from the nasopharynx[2]

RELEVANT EUSTACHIAN TUBE ANATOMY

- As the child ages, the angle becomes less acute and the Eustachian tube lengthens; coupled with a more developed and mature immune system, older children (>7 years of age) are less susceptible to otitis media
- The medial one-third is bony; the lateral two-thirds are cartilaginous
- Most narrow at the junction of the bony and cartilaginous portion, forming the isthmus where the cartilaginous tube extends slightly into the lumen of the bony canal

- Torus tubarius: mucosal-lined fibrocartilaginous projection of the eustachian tube into the nasopharynx, identified behind the posterior aspect of the inferior turbinate and is an important landmark for balloon dilation[3]
- Rosenmüller fossa: depressed pocket extending posteriorly along the medial boarder of the eustachian tube, medial to torus

MUSCLES RELATED TO THE EUSTACHIAN TUBE[4]

1. Tensor veli palatini/dilator tubae: act of swallowing or yawning causes this muscle to contract and open up to allow pressure equalization
2. Tensor tympani
3. Levator veli palatine: elevates the soft palate
4. Salpingopharyngeus

TENSOR VELI PALATINI ANATOMY

- Three anchoring points
  - Pterygoid hamulus
  - Ostmann fat pad plays an important role in closing the Eustachian tube to prevent retrograde flow of nasal secretions
  - Medial pterygoid muscle
- Dilator tubae portion attaches to cartilaginous tube more perpendicularly[5]
- Tendon of the tensor tympani attaches to the medial aspect of the handle of the malleus

CONGENITAL MEMBRANOUS MALFORMATIONS OF THE INNER EAR

- Bony labyrinth is unaffected, and computed tomography (CT) of the inner ear is normal[6]
- Scheibe aplasia, also known as cocheosaccular dysplasia, is the most common membranous malformation
- Complete membranous labyrinthine dysplasia (rare), associated with Jervell and Lange-Nielsen and Usher syndromes
- Alexander dysplasia: cochlear basal turn dysplasia; high-frequency sensorineural hearing loss (SNHL)

CONGENITAL OSSEOUS AND MEMBRANOUS MALFORMATIONS OF THE INNER EAR

- Can be recognized radiographically
- Michel aplasia: characterized by the absence of the cochlea and labyrinth; cessation of the otic capsule at the third week of development[7]
- Cochlear anomalies (Fig. 6.1)

- Cochlear aplasia (arrest at fifth week): no hearing
- Common cavity (arrest at fourth week): severe-to-profound hearing loss
- Cochlear hypoplasia (arrest at sixth week): 15% of cochlear anomalies, and with variable hearing
- Incomplete partition type 2 has replaced "Mondini deformity" (arrest at seventh week of gestation): it is defined by a cochlea with 1.5 turns with cystic middle and apical turns; the most common cochlear malformation; associated with enlarged vestibular aqueduct (EVA); Pendred syndrome; predisposition to meningitis; variable degrees of SNHL
- Labyrinthine anomalies (40% of radiologically abnormal cochlea will have a lateral semicircular canal [SCC] abnormality)
  - Cochlear abnormalities are common in patients with SCC aplasia
  - Degree of hearing loss does not necessarily correlate with severity of labyrinthine deformity[8]
  - SCC dysplasia: 4 times as common as SCC aplasia, associated with conductive hearing loss (CHL)
  - SCC aplasia: found with CHARGE (coloboma of the eye, heart defects, atresia of the nasal choanae, retardation of growth and/or development, genital and/or urinary abnormalities, and ear abnormalities and deafness) association

- Aqueduct anomalies:
  - Normally 0.4-1.0 mm in diameter when measured halfway between the common crus and its external aperture
  - Enlarged vestibular aqueduct (Fig. 6.2) is the most common identified temporal bone abnormality in children imaged for SNHL; defined by vestibular aqueduct size of >1 mm at the midpoint and >2 mm in diameter at the operculum; progressive and sudden decrements in hearing with approximately 40% eventually developing profound SNHL; the likelihood of hearing loss progression increases as the size of the vestibular aqueduct increases; type of hearing loss can be SNHL, mixed, or purely conductive[9]
  - Enlarged cochlear aqueduct: usually 3-4 mm in diameter and ranges from 1 to 10 mm; significance is controversial
- Internal auditory canal (IAC) abnormalities
  - Narrow IAC: <3 mm; if facial function is present, then CNVIII will most likely be absent; magnetic resonance imaging (MRI) of the temporal bone should be ordered to determine further the presence of the cochlear nerve
  - Widened IAC: >10 mm is associated with a cerebrospinal fluid (CSF) gusher in the cochlear implantation and stapedectomy

JOINT COMMITTEE ON INFANT HEARING POSITION STATEMENT FOR NEONATAL HEARING SCREENING: BIRTH TO 28 DAYS

- Recommends universal newborn screening before hospital discharge; infants who pass the neonatal screening but have a risk factor should have at least one diagnostic audiology assessment by 24 to 30 months of age; if risk criteria are met, recommend additional testing later, even if the newborn screening was passed
  - Prematurity
  - Family history of childhood SNHL
  - Congenital infections/sepsis
  - Low Apgar scores
  - TORCH (*Toxoplasmosis gondii*, other viruses, rubella, *Cytomegalovirus* [CMV], and herpes simplex)
  - Craniofacial abnormalities
  - Low birth weight
  - Exchange transfusions for hyperbilirubinemia

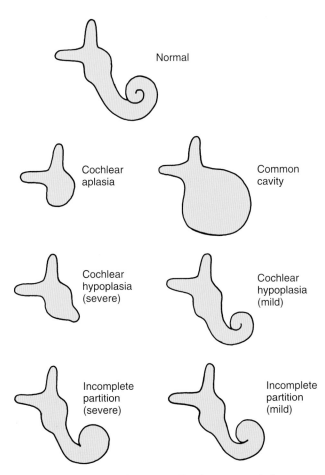

Normal

Cochlear aplasia

Common cavity

Cochlear hypoplasia (severe)

Cochlear hypoplasia (mild)

Incomplete partition (severe)

Incomplete partition (mild)

FIGURE 6.1 Cochlear Malformations. Drawings were made from coronal CT scans. (From Jackler RK, Luxford WM, House WF. Congenital malformations of the inner ear: a classification based on embryogenesis. *Laryngoscope.* 1987;97(suppl 40):2 and Flint PW, Haughey BH, Lund VJ, et al. *Cummings Otolaryngology—Head and Neck Surgery.* 6th ed. Philadelphia, PA: Saunders; 2015.)

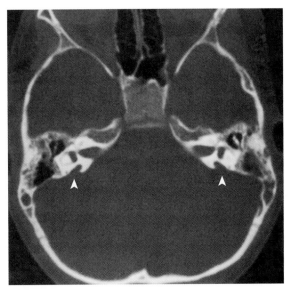

FIGURE 6.2 Bilateral enlargement of the vestibular aqueducts (*arrowheads*) as seen on an axial CT scan. (From Flint PW, Haughey BH, Lund VJ, et al. *Cummings Otolaryngology—Head and Neck Surgery.* 6th ed. Philadelphia, PA: Saunders; 2015.)

- Bacterial meningitis
- Ototoxic antibiotics (gentamicin/tobramycin)
- Hypoxemia
- Encephalopathy
- Loop diuretics (furosemide/Lasix)
- Mechanical/assisted ventilation
- Stigmata of a known syndrome associated with hearing loss

JOINT COMMITTEE ON INFANT HEARING POSITION STATEMENT FOR INFANTS (29 DAYS TO 2 YEARS) HEARING SCREENING (Table 6.1)

- Separate risk criteria for infants: different from newborns (may need earlier and more frequent testing)
  - Persistent otitis media with effusion (OME) for at least 3 months
  - Parent concern regarding hearing, speech, language, or developmental delay
  - Head trauma resulting in skull fracture

Table 6.1	**Monitoring Protocol for At-Risk Children**
Risk Factor	**Recommended Follow-Up**
In utero infection STDs (CMV), infections	Every 3-18 months Yearly until school aged
Meningitis	Every 3 months to 1 year 18 months Yearly until school aged
Craniofacial/temporal bone anomalies Syndromes (eg, Down, Usher, Pierre Robin, Alport, CHARGE, and Waardenburg) Cleft palate	Every 6 months until 18 months Yearly until school aged
Extracorporeal membrane oxygenation	Every 6 months until 18 months Yearly until school aged
Head trauma (especially basilar or temporal fracture)	Every 6 months until 18 months Yearly until school aged If there is a TM rupture, monitor for cholesteatoma
Hyperbilirubinemia	Every 6 months until 18 months (IF transfused) Yearly until school aged
NICU stay >5 days	Follow-up at 9-12 months Repeat test after 1 year
Ototoxic medications Aminoglycosides (-mycin drugs) Lasix	Immediately following course 6 months after completion Repeat every 6 months until 18 months Yearly until school aged
Mechanical ventilation Greater than 5 days	Follow-up at 9-12 months Repeat test after 1 year
Chronic otitis media	Audiology/ENT referral
Speech/language delay	Within 6 months before starting speech therapy
Family history of congenital/ progressive hearing loss	Repeat every 6 months until 18 months Yearly until school aged
Failed newborn hearing screen	Referral to audiology

ENT, Ear, nose, and throat; *NICU*, neonatal intensive care unit; *STDs*, sexually transmitted diseases.
All babies with any of the risk factors should receive an A-ABR—to rule out auditory neuropathy. Therefore, basically, any NICU baby needs to have an A-ABR. OAEs are fine for well-baby nurseries.

- Family history of delayed-onset hearing loss
- Neonatal intensive care unit (NICU) stay >5 days
- Extracorporeal membrane oxygenation history
- Presence of neurodegenerative disorders
- Meningitis
- Chemotherapy medications with potential ototoxicity
- Childhood infections associated with SNHL (meningitis and CMV)

METHODS OF AUDIOLOGIC EVALUATION (NEWBORN TO 48 MONTHS)

1. Auditory brainstem response (ABR), also known as a brainstem auditory evoked response test
   a. For hearing screens: automated ABR (A-ABR) or screening (S-ABR) systems test for the presence or absence of wave V at soft stimulus
      i. Stimulus is usually click stimuli at 35-40 dB, with no operator interpretation.
      ii. Results are given as Pass or Refer for each ear.
      iii. It is a highly effective screening with sensitivity/specificity of 96-98%, but it does not rule out minimal or mild hearing loss.
   b. Diagnostic ABR: Used when hearing loss is suspected because of an abnormal A-ABR screening result (OR absent otoacoustic emissions (OAEs) screening result; see OAE section).
      i. Used to determine frequency-specific hearing thresholds, as well as type of hearing loss (sensorineural, conductive, or mixed)
      ii. Child must be completely asleep throughout testing; often requires sedation after 6 months of age
      iii. An ABR is not a "functional" test of hearing, but it is an estimated hearing test in which the child does not actively participate; there is no cortical processing; results should always be confirmed or supported by behavioral testing when possible (see Behavioral auditory testing section).
2. OAEs for hearing screens or as part of an audiologic test battery (Note: can only be used as a screen for well babies, not NICU babies)
   a. OAEs test cochlear outer hair cell function; if present, cochlear outer hair cell function is normal and normal-to-near-normal hearing is assumed; there are two types of OAEs:
      i. Transient evoked OAE (TEOAE)
         (1) Click stimuli at 80-86 dB; typically only tests a small range of frequencies
         (2) May be present/pass even with mild hearing loss (about 30 dB)
      ii. Distortion product OAE (DPOAE)
         (1) More frequency-specific compared with TEOAE and can test a wider range of frequencies
         (2) May be present even with mild hearing loss (about 30 dB)
   b. Factors that may adversely affect testing:
      i. Debris or cerumen in the external auditory canal (EAC)
      ii. Poor probe fit because of stenotic canal
      iii. Middle ear effusion (MEE) or any conductive component
      iv. Patient compliance—patient must be relatively quiet and still throughout testing
   c. OAE testing may miss auditory neuropathy spectrum disorder: in this case, children will have present OAEs, but an abnormal ABR
3. Behavioral auditory testing
   a. For infants/children of 6 months and older corrected age
   b. A functional test: the child participates in the task, and testing involves cortical processing of sound

c. Generally three types of test methods depending on age/developmental status:
  i. Visual reinforcement audiometry (VRA)
    (1) Child must be at least 6 months corrected age
    (2) Child should have good head control and be able to make an orienting movement to sound stimuli (turn head left and right in response to sound)
    (3) Child should be able to see visual stimuli approximately 3 feet away
  ii. Conditioned play audiometry
    (1) For children usually 2-2.5 years (corrected age) and older
    (2) Child responds to an auditory stimulus with a conditioned play paradigm (drop a block in a bucket when you hear the sound)
    (3) Play activity can vary from child to child, but the child must be able to self-regulate, which requires a longer attention span
  iii. Standard audiometry
    (1) For children 4-5 years and older into adulthood
    (2) Standard "raise your hand when you hear the beep" task
d. Behavioral testing should minimally include tonal **AND** speech stimuli; a full audiologic evaluation should also include immittance testing (tympanometry and acoustic reflex thresholds) and OAEs

NOTE: If there are parental or primary care provider concerns at any point during child development, results of screening should be corroborated with behavioral testing. Likewise, if screening, diagnostic, or behavioral testing was normal in the past but new concerns have arisen or there is regression in speech, language, or auditory skills, refer the patient to an audiologist.

HOW DO YOU APPROACH A CASE IN WHICH A 3-MONTH-OLD FAILS TWO NEWBORN HEARING SCREENING TESTS?

- History
  - Prematurity
  - Low Apgar scores; 0-4 at 1 minute and 0-6 at 5 minutes
  - NICU stay and length
  - Mechanical ventilation >5 days
  - Weight <1500 g
  - Intrauterine infections (eg, CMV, rubella, syphilis, herpes, and toxo)
  - Elevated hyperbilirubinemia, >20, requiring exchange transfusions
  - Meningitis
  - Use of intravenous (IV) antibiotics (eg, aminoglycosides) and/or loop diuretics
  - Renal abnormalities
  - Family history of congenital or early onset hearing loss
  - Consanguinity
- Physical exam
  - Appearance: craniofacial dysmorphism, preauricular tags/pits, microtia/atresia, and café-au-lait spots
  - Otoscopic exam (may be simple MEE)
- Workup/testing
  - Diagnostic audiometric testing such as ABR to confirm sensorineural versus CHL
  - Genetic testing/referral (connexin 26/30 or other genes based on clinical suspicion)
  - Imaging (CT temporal bone)
  - Ophthalmology evaluation
  - Electrocardiogram (EKG) (rule out prolonged QT interval in Jervell and Lange-Nielsen syndrome [JLNS])
  - Urinalysis, blood urea nitrogen, creatinine, and, if clinically indicated, renal ultrasound
  - Congenital CMV testing (urine/saliva analysis)

WHAT PERCENTAGE OF PEDIATRIC HEARING LOSS IS DUE TO GENETIC FACTORS?

- 50% is due to genetic causes
  - Genetic cause most often the etiology, especially after environmental factors are ruled out
  - 80% recessive causes, of which 70% are nonsyndromic
  - AR accounts for 75-80%; AD approximately 20%; sex-linked approximately 2-5%; and mitochondrial <1%
- Remaining 50% may be environmental (eg, perinatal infections), multifactorial, or unknown

CONNEXIN 26

- Nonfunctional gap junction protein
- Mutations in the GJB2 account for 30-50% of recessive deafness
- Product of the GJB2 gene
- Most common cause of hereditary autosomal recessive nonsyndromic SNHL
- Found in 50% of nonsyndromic severe-to-profound SNHL

IMAGING IN PEDIATRIC SENSORINEURAL HEARING LOSS

- Most of the time both CT and MRI are not required to evaluate a child with congenital hearing loss
- Concordance between CT and MRI is ~70-80%[12]
- Asymmetric unilateral SNHL
- Progressive SNHL
- Temporal bone fracture and hearing loss with head trauma
- Planning and evaluation cochlear implantation; cochlear nerve aplasia can present similarly to other causes of auditory neuropathy; MRI can distinguish cochlear nerve presence, which has prognostic value in cochlear implantation
- Recurrent meningitis
- Suspected auditory neuropathy

AUDITORY NEUROPATHY

- Presence of OAEs and/or cochlear microphonics and absent ABR responses
- Undergo trial of binaural amplification; if no progress with speech and language development, then consider cochlear implantation
- Intact outer hair cell function, but absent or severely abnormal ABR
- Lesion may be located at or between inner hair cells and the auditory nerve
- 20-30% of patients ultimately develop loss of outer hair cell function and SNHL
- Several etiologies including genetic, anatomic, and environmental causes
- Patients should use American Sign Language or another form of manual communication in addition to spoken language

INCOMPLETE PARTITION TYPE 2 (MONDINI APLASIA)

1. Defined as cochlea with 1.5 turns, absent interscalar septum between middle and apical turns, "Mondini" malformation historically has referred to the incomplete cochlea, with <2.5 turns
2. Associated with EVA

3. Associated with dilated vestibule
4. Linked to mutations in the Pendred syndrome (PDS) (SLC26A4)[13]

SYNDROMES ASSOCIATED WITH SCHEIBE MALFORMATION

1. Usher syndrome
2. Refsum disease
3. Down syndrome
4. Waardenburg[14]

AUTOSOMAL DOMINANT SYNDROMES ASSOCIATED WITH SENSORINEURAL HEARING LOSS

1. Alport syndrome
2. Pierre Robin syndrome
3. Branchio-oto-renal (BOR) syndrome
4. Neurofibromatosis (NF)
5. Crouzon disease
6. Stickler syndrome
7. Duane Syndrome
8. Waardenburg syndrome
9. Treacher Collins syndrome[15]

BRANCHIO-OTO-RENAL SYNDROME

- Characterized by external, middle, and inner ear anomalies; branchial sinuses; pits; tags; and renal dysplasia
- Mutations in the EYA1 gene and less commonly in the SIX-1 gene
- Autosomal dominant disorder with nearly 100% penetrance
- Branchial cleft anomalies: cervical fistulas, sinuses, and cysts
- Otologic malformations: conductive, sensorineural, or mixed hearing loss (nearly 90%); preauricular pits or tags (82%); auricular malformations (32%); middle and inner ear anomalies
  - 2% of children with severe/profound SNHL are affected with BOR
- Individuals with ear pits and branchial defects warrant renal ultrasound[16]

CENTRAL NEUROFIBROMATOSIS (NEUROFIBROMATOSIS TYPE 2)

- Autosomal dominant, with high penetrance but variable expressivity: 50% sporadic mutations
- NF 2 is linked to mutation of a tumor suppressor gene on chromosome 22
- Bilateral acoustic neuromas (vestibular schwannomas) often before age 20; may be unilateral
- Presenting features in young adulthood of tinnitus, vestibular dysfunction, and worsening hearing loss
- Café-au-lait spots and cutaneous neurofibromas are fewer in number than in NF type I
- NF 2 results in other cranial, spinal, and peripheral nerve schwannomas, intracranial meningiomas, and optic gliomas
- Radiosurgery can retard the growth of a tumor, but resection after radiation is more difficult
- Auditory brainstem implants have been used with some hearing and spatial attention, but with limited language and speech skills[17]

STICKLER SYNDROME

- Autosomal dominant, mutation of type II and type XI collagen genes

- Severe myopia, which may lead to retinal detachment or cataracts
- Joint hypermobility and enlargement with early-onset arthritis
- Pierre Robin sequence: micrognathia is common and may result in a cleft palate
- Hearing loss may be SNHL, conductive, or mixed

WAARDENBURG SYNDROME

- 4 different types of Waardenburg have been classified based on phenotype and genetic mutation (MITF gene/PAX3 gene)
- Type 1: unilateral or bilateral SNHL, white forelock, iris pigment anomalies (heterochromia iridis), dystopia canthorum, and broad nasal root
- Type 2 is identical to type 1, but without dystopia canthorum: SNHL is more common in type 2 than in type 1
- Type 3: features of type 1 with upper limb abnormalities
- Type 4: type 1 features and Hirschsprung disease

TREACHER COLLINS SYNDROME (MANDIBULOFACIAL DYSOSTOSIS) (Fig. 6.3)

- Autosomal dominant
- CHL is secondary to ossicular abnormalities but can be accompanied by SNHL, aural atresia, and ear canal stenosis
- Hypoplastic mandible and cleft palate
- Downward slanting palpebral fissures and coloboma of the lower eyelids
- Bilateral symmetrical facies and eyelid coloboma distinguish Treacher Collins from similar but unilateral findings of Goldenhar

AUTOSOMAL RECESSIVE SYNDROMES ASSOCIATED WITH SENSORINEURAL HEARING LOSS

1. Usher syndrome
2. PDS
3. JLNS

PENDRED SYNDROME

- PDS is early-onset and often progressive SNHL or mixed
- Associated with an organification defect in the thyroid
- Bi-allelic mutations in the PDS or SLC26A4 gene occur in 15-20% of patients[18]
- Most common syndromic form of SNHL
- Recessive inheritance typically, but several pedigrees raise the possibility of dominant inheritance with variable expression
- Bilateral EVA and bilateral incomplete partition type 2 cochlear defect visible on temporal bone imaging resulting in mild to profound SNHL and usually progressive hearing loss
- Can develop euthyroid goiter in childhood or as young adult; thyroid dysfunction, so endocrine testing is important
- A gene encodes the protein *pendrin*, a chloride/bicarbonate exchange protein; abnormal ion exchange causes abnormal cochlear potential
- Pendrin genetic testing is the preferred diagnostic tool: perchlorate discharge test demonstrates an abnormal organification of nonorganic iodine; however, because of radioactive exposure, it is used infrequently

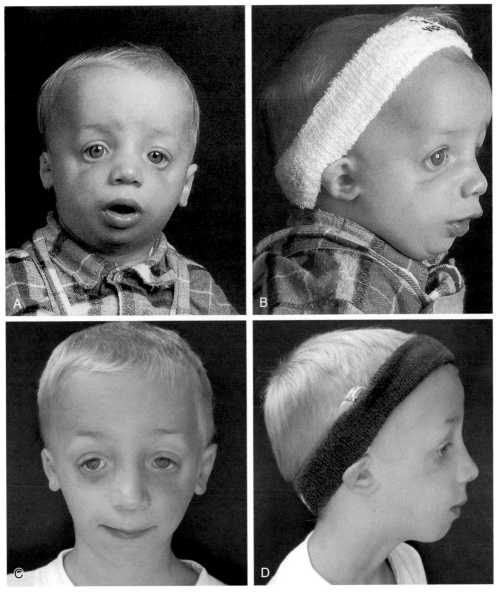

FIGURE 6.3 (**A**) Characteristic facial appearance of a 10-month-old child with mandibulofacial dysostosis (Treacher Collins syndrome). (**B**) Oblique view of the same patient. Note the absent external ear canal, which is bilateral, and the headband, which holds bone conduction hearing aids. (**C**) Frontal view of the same patient at age 6 years. (**D**) Oblique view of the same patient at age 6 years. (From Flint PW, Haughey BH, Lund VJ, et al. *Cummings Otolaryngology—Head and Neck Surgery.* 6th ed. Philadelphia, PA: Saunders; 2015.)

JERVELL AND LANGE-NIELSEN SYNDROME

- Recessively inherited severe-to-profound hearing loss in conjunction with a cardiac conduction defect that leads to syncopal episodes and sudden death
- Autosomal recessive
- Severe-to-profound bilateral congenital SNHL
- Heart disease: prolonged QT interval, ventricular arrhythmias, syncopal episodes, and death
- High rate of cardiac and fatal events despite β-blockers, which do lower mortality[19]
- Prevalence is low in children with congenital SNHL
- EKG is important in young infants with severe-to-profound hearing loss to rule out cardiac conductive anomalies

USHER SYNDROME

- Characterized by SNHL and progressive retinitis pigmentosa (RP)

- Autosomal recessive
- 50% of concomitant deafness and blindness
- Three clinically distinct subtypes, which differ with severity or progression of hearing loss, onset and severity of retinal degeneration, and manifestation of vestibular dysfunction
  - Type I: congenital bilateral profound hearing loss, clinically apparent RP in first 10 years of life, significantly impaired vestibular dysfunction (may present as delayed crawling or walking)[20]
  - Type II: moderate, often progressive, down-sloping SNHL, normal vestibular function, and onset of RP in the first/second decade[21]
  - Type III: progressive Hodgkin lymphoma (HL), variable vestibular dysfunction, and variable onset of RP[22]
- Diagnosed with electroretinography; requires ophthalmology consultation

X-LINKED RECESSIVE SYNDROMES ASSOCIATED WITH SENSORINEURAL HEARING LOSS

- 1% hereditary hearing loss is sex-linked
  a. Norrie syndrome: SNHL, congenital or progressive blindness
  b. Oto-palato-digital syndrome: CHL, hypertelorism, small nose, midface hypoplasia, cleft palate, short stature, and digital anomalies
  c. Wildervanck syndrome: SNHL or mixed hearing loss, Klippel-Feil malformation (fused cervical vertebrae), and abducens paralysis
  d. Alport syndrome: progressive SHNL and renal disease

ALPORT SYNDROME

- Predominantly X-linked, but can be autosomal recessive (COL4A3 and COL4A4 genes)
- Results from abnormal basement membrane structure with basilar membrane, stria vascularis, and renal glomerulus
- Hearing loss is often not detected until patient is a teenager, with symmetric progressive high-frequency SNHL in late childhood/early adolescence
- "Red diaper"➔hematuric nephritis, family history of hematuria, and chronic renal failure
- Eye lesions (anterior lenticonus with bulging lens) and retinopathy[23]

NORRIE SYNDROME

- X-linked recessive and caused by mutation in the protein norrin
- Congenital/rapidly progressive blindness because of pseudoglioma development and cataracts
- Ear findings: progressive SNHL with onset in the second/third decade
- SNHL and congenital or progressive blindness

OTO-PALATO-DIGITAL SYNDROME

- X-linked gene FLNA
- Hypertelorism, flat midface, small nose, cleft palate, short stature, broad fingers, toes of variable length, and wide space between the first and second toe
- CHL: potentially amenable to surgical correction CHL for ossicular malformation

WILDERVANCK SYNDROME

- X-linked dominant inheritance recessive
- Encompasses Klippel-Feil malformation
- SNHL or mixed hearing loss because of bony inner ear malformation
- CNVI paralysis with eye retraction on lateral gaze (ie, Duane syndrome)

OTOLOGY AND MIDDLE EAR DISEASE

RISK FACTORS FOR PEDIATRIC ACUTE OTITIS MEDIA

- Early onset of infections: younger than 8 months of age
- Daycare attendance: grouping of six or more infants or children

- Family history of severe or recurrent infections in siblings
- Craniofacial abnormalities (Down syndrome, cleft palate, and Crouzon's)
- Breastfeeding <3 months' duration
- Tobacco exposure-smoking in the household of parents, grandparents, or other caregivers
- Immunodeficiency: human immunodeficiency virus (HIV) and low immunoglobulin G (IgG), IgA
- Male gender (boys > girls)
- Allergies: dietary, medications, lotions, and creams (suspected)

MOST COMMON ETIOLOGIC AGENTS IN PEDIATRIC ACUTE OTITIS MEDIA

- *Streptococcus pneumoniae*
- *Haemophilus influenzae*
- *Moraxella catarrhalis*
- Group A *Streptococcus*

COMPLICATIONS AND SEQUELAE OF OTITIS MEDIA

- Intratemporal
  - CHL
  - TM perforation
  - Speech and language delay
  - Chronic suppurative otitis media
  - Atelectasis of the middle ear
  - Adhesive otitis media
  - Tympanosclerosis
  - Cholesteatoma
  - Vestibular and balance problems
  - Mastoiditis and petrositis
  - Facial paralysis
  - Adhesive otitis media ossicular fibrosis, discontinuity, and/or fixation
- Intracranial
  - Meningitis
  - Brain abscess (epidural or subdural)
  - Lateral sinus thrombosis
  - Otic hydrocephalus

INDICATIONS FOR TYMPANOSTOMY TUBE PLACEMENT

- Chronic OME for >3 months bilaterally or >6 months unilaterally
  - May proceed earlier if:
    - Persistent, severe acute otitis media
    - Suspected antimicrobial resistance
    - Significant hearing loss
    - Speech/language delay
    - Developmental delay
    - Severe TM retraction
    - Disequilibrium/vertigo/tinnitus
- Recurrent MEE with excessive cumulative duration (6-12 months)
- Patulous eustachian tube
- Hyperbaric oxygen therapy
- Infectious complication of otitis media

COMPLICATIONS OF TYMPANOSTOMY TUBES

- Otorrhea, recurrent
- Granuloma formation at the tube site
- TM perforation development

- Early extrusion (<6 months)
- Plugged (nonfunctioning) tympanostomy tube
- Cholesteatoma
- Tympanosclerosis
- Migration of the tube into the middle ear

INDICATIONS FOR MYRINGOTOMY AND TYMPANOSTOMY TUBE PLACEMENT AND CULTURE (ACUTE OTITIS MEDIA)

1. Facial paralysis
2. Mastoiditis
3. Meningitis or other intracranial complication
4. Complication in immunosuppressed patients not responding to antibiotics

BACTERIOLOGY OF ACUTE MASTOIDITIS (WITHOUT CHOLESTEATOMA)

1. *S. pneumoniae*
2. *H. influenzae*
3. *Streptococcus pyogenes*
4. *Staphylococcus aureus*

INDICATIONS FOR BONE-CONDUCTING HEARING AIDS

1. Atresia and/or microtia (inability to use traditional hearing aids)
2. CHL with an air-bone gap of >30 dB
3. Mixed hearing loss with an air-bone gap of >30-35 dB, but with mild-to-moderate SNHL
   a. Baha sound processor can compensate for SNHL of up to 65 dB HL
4. Single-sided deafness with normal hearing in their good ear
   a. Improved speech understanding by overcoming head shadow effect and giving 360-degree sound awareness
5. Inability to fit a traditional hearing aid or contralateral routing of signals because of skin allergy with ear mold or chronic draining ears

DIFFERENTIAL DIAGNOSIS OF AURAL POLYP IN A CHILD

1. Foreign body (prior tympanostomy tube history)
2. Otitis externa
3. Cholesteatoma
4. Histiocytosis X (eosinophilic granuloma)
5. Malignant lesion (eg, rhabdomyosarcoma)

HEAD AND NECK

HISTORY AND EXAM FINDINGS FOR A CHILD WITH A NEW-ONSET NECK MASS (Fig. 6.4)

- History
  - Time of onset and duration
  - Change in size (eg, enlargement or fluctuation in size)
  - Fevers
  - Recent infection, for example, upper respiratory infection (URI)
  - Drainage
  - Skin changes (erythema, violaceous, and ecchymosis)
  - Airway distress and/or signs of obstruction (eg, stertor, stridor, and snoring)
  - Dysphagia or drooling
  - Fevers
  - Previous surgery in the body part
  - Recent trauma
  - Sick contacts, flu, or tuberculosis (TB) exposure
  - Exposure to cats, ticks, mosquitos, and/or insects
  - Travel history: regional or international
  - Immunization history: absence of routine vaccinations
  - History of radiation exposure
  - Weight loss and night sweats (TB symptoms)
- Physical exam
  - Location
  - Size
  - Head tilt or torticollis
  - Skin changes and overlying skin color
  - Tenderness to palpation
  - Fluctuance to ballottement
  - Mobility in relation to skin (dermal) or subcutaneous (muscle/fascia)
  - Movement with swallowing
  - Range of neck motion
  - Inability to handle secretions, stridor, or other signs of respiratory distress
  - Presence of fistula or sinus

DIFFERENTIAL DIAGNOSIS OF A CHILD WITH A NEW-ONSET NECK MASS, BY LOCATION

- Midline neck mass
  - Thyroglossal duct cyst (TGDC)
  - Dermoid cyst
  - Lymphadenopathy/lymphadenitis
  - Sialocele of the floor of the mouth, "plunging ranula"
  - Thyroid mass
- Lateral neck mass
  - Lymphadenopathy/lymphadenitis
  - Branchial cleft cyst, sinus, and fistula
  - Lymphatic or vascular malformation
  - Mycobacterial infection, including atypical
  - Hemangioma
  - Fibromatosis coli (sternocleidomastoid [SCM] tumor of infancy)
  - Neoplastic (see below)

DIFFERENTIAL DIAGNOSIS OF A CHILD WITH A NEW-ONSET NECK MASS, BY ETIOLOGY

- Infectious/inflammatory
  - Lymphadenopathy, lymphadenitis, phlegmon, and abscess
  - Mycobacterial infection, including atypical
  - Cat scratch/*Bartonella henselae*
  - Toxoplasmosis
  - Fungal
  - Kawasaki disease
    - Fever >5 days
    - Conjunctivitis
    - Oral ulcers and strawberry tongue
    - Erythematous rash
    - Edema, erythema, and peeling of the hands and feet
    - Nonpurulent cervical lymphadenopathy
    - Echocardiogram
    - Treatment w/immunoglobulins and aspirin
- Neoplastic
  - Lymphoma (Hodgkin's)
  - Rhabdomyosarcoma
  - Neuroblastoma
  - Salivary gland tumor

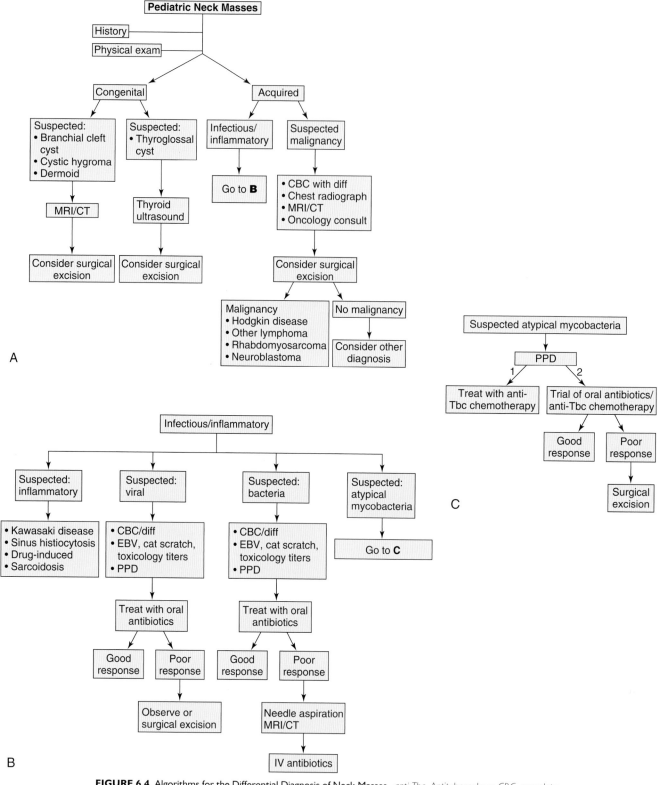

FIGURE 6.4 Algorithms for the Differential Diagnosis of Neck Masses. *anti-Tbc*, Antituberculous; *CBC*, complete blood count; *PPD*, purified protein derivative. (From Flint PW, Haughey BH, Lund VJ, et al. *Cummings Otolaryngology— Head and Neck Surgery*. 6th ed. Philadelphia, PA: Saunders; 2015.)

- • Thyroid mass/carcinoma (CA)➔ papillary CA is more common than medullary CA
  - • Nasopharyngeal (NP) CA
- • Congenital
  - • Branchial cleft cyst
  - • TGDC

- • Lymphatic or vascular malformation
- • Hemangioma
- • Teratoma
- • Dermoid cyst and thymic cyst
- • Laryngocele
- • Fibromatosis coli (SCM tumor of infancy; Fig. 6.5)

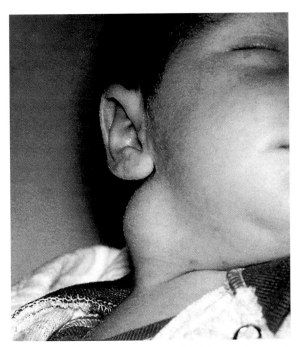

FIGURE 6.5 Infant with Congenital Torticollis. Note the firm mass in the midportion of the SCM muscle. (From Flint PW, Haughey BH, Lund VJ, et al. *Cummings Otolaryngology—Head and Neck Surgery.* 6th ed. Philadelphia, PA: Saunders; 2015.)

BRANCHIAL CLEFT CYSTS AND SINUSES

- Incomplete closure of the branchial arch apparatus between the cleft and pouch
- Lined with stratified squamous epithelium
  - Contains other dermal structures such as hair follicles, sebaceous glands, and sweat glands
  - Five mesodermal arches (first to fourth and sixth) contain own arterial and nerve supply

BRANCHIAL CLEFT ANOMALY BASICS

- First branchial anomaly, Work Type 1: may course medially or laterally to the facial nerve
  - Ectodermal in origin and duplications of membranous EAC
  - Located in the periparotid and preauricular area, parallel to the EAC
  - Expression of material from the ear canal helps confirm the embryologic origin of the lesion
  - Tract may open into the medial canal or middle ear space
  - Extremely rare
- First branchial anomaly, Work Type 2: may be intimately involved with the facial nerve (medial or lateral)
  - Composed of both ectoderm and mesoderm
  - Considered duplication of membranous and cartilaginous EAC
  - Otoscopy should be performed to determine if fistula/sinus tract may end near the EAC, near the bony/cartilage junction
  - Expression of material from the ear canal helps confirm the embryologic origin of the lesion
  - More common than type 1
- Second branchial anomaly
  - Most common overall branchial anomaly (cysts, sinuses, and fistulas)
  - Cyst and/or sinuses may be found along the anterior border of the SCM in the lower one-third of the neck

- Tract passes superiorly and laterally to the common carotid artery, superficially to CNIX and CNXII
- Tract splits the internal/external carotid artery
- May enter the pharynx close to the middle constrictor or open into the tonsillar fossa
- Tonsillectomy: the time of neck surgery is dependent on whether the fistula tract opens into the tonsillar fossa region
- Third branchial anomaly
  - Very rare
  - Along the anterior border of the SCM in the lower neck, the tract goes laterally and superiorly (superficial) to the common carotid, superficially to CNXII, but deeply to the CNIX and internal carotid artery
  - Passes through the thyrohyoid membrane
  - Opens into the upper piriform sinus
  - Direct laryngoscopy with cauterization of the piriform sinus is now advocated as the first-line treatment, but if this fails, then comprehensive surgical resection is required
- Fourth branchial anomaly
  - Very rare and usually on the left
  - On the left side, it starts along the anterior border of the SCM, tracks inferiorly deep to the common carotid, and loops around the aortic arch
  - On the right side, the tract loops around the right subclavian artery before ascending in the neck
  - Opens into the apex of the piriform sinus of the hypopharynx

NERVE, MUSCLE, CARTILAGE, AND ARTERY DERIVATIVES OF THE BRANCHIAL ARCHES

- First arch (first mandibular) structures
  - Nerve: trigeminal (V)
  - Artery: internal maxillary
  - Cartilage (Meckel): malleus (except manubrium), incus (except long process), sphenomandibular ligament, anterior malleolar ligament, mandible, premaxilla, maxilla, zygoma, and part of the temporal bone
  - Muscle: muscles of mastication, tensor tympani, tensor veli palatini, anterior belly of the digastric muscle; mylohyoid
- Second arch structures
  - Nerve: facial (VII)
  - Artery: stapedial
  - Cartilage (Reichert): manubrium of the malleus, long process of the incus, stapes (except foot plate), lesser cornu, upper body of the hyoid, and stylohyoid ligament
  - Muscle: muscles of facial expression, auricularis, stapedius, posterior belly digastric, and stylohyoid
- Third arch structures
  - Nerve: glossopharyngeal
  - Artery: common and internal carotid
  - Cartilage: greater cornu and lower body of the hyoid
  - Muscle: stylopharyngeus
- Fourth arch structures
  - Nerve: superior laryngeal nerve
  - Artery: subclavian on the right and arch of the aorta on the left
  - Cartilage: thyroid and cuneiform cartilages
  - Muscle: pharyngeal and laryngeal muscles
- Sixth arch structures
  - Nerve: recurrent laryngeal nerve
  - Artery: pulmonary artery on the right and ductus arteriosus on the left
  - Cartilage: cricoid, arytenoid, and corniculate cartilages
  - Muscle: pharyngeal and laryngeal muscles

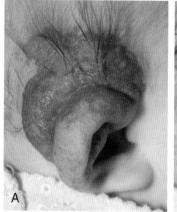
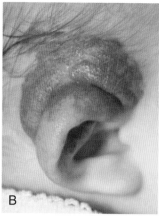
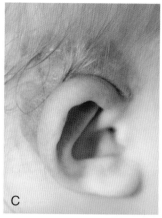
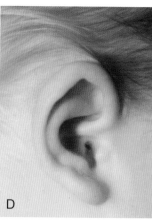

FIGURE 6.6 Superficial Segmental Hemangioma Treated with Propranolol. (**A**) Pretreatment with postauricular ulceration. (**B**) After 1 month of corticosteroid treatment. (**C**) After 1 month of propranolol treatment. (**D**) After 4 months of propranolol treatment. (From Flint PW, Haughey BH, Lund VJ, et al. *Cummings Otolaryngology—Head and Neck Surgery*. 6th ed. Philadelphia, PA: Saunders; 2015.)

CLINICAL DIFFERENCES BETWEEN HEMANGIOMAS AND VASCULAR MALFORMATIONS

- Hemangioma of infancy (Fig. 6.6)
  - Usually absent at birth but appears during infancy
  - Proliferates for 6-9 months and then involutes (partially or completely) over 3-5 years
  - Glucose transporter 1 (GLUT-1) staining positive
  - Separate from congenital hemangioma
  - Present at birth
  - GLUT-1 staining negative
  - Two types
    - Rapidly involuting congenital hemangioma
    - Noninvoluting congenital hemangioma
  - Lesions described as focal versus segmental; superficial versus deep versus mixed
  - MRI: enhancement and flow voids are present on T1 and T2
  - Complications: airway compromise, cutaneous ulceration, visual obstruction, high-output cardiac failure, and psychosocial consequences
- Vascular malformation
  - Present at birth, but some appear later in childhood
  - Sudden enlargement can be seen with infection, trauma, or adolescence
  - Divided into high-flow (arteriovenous malformation) and low-flow (lymphatic, venous, and capillary) lesions
  - MRI or CT diagnostic
  - Lymphatic malformation is the most common
  - Lymphatic malformation can distort the facial skeleton such as the mandible; arteriovenous malformation can cause bony destruction

MANAGEMENT OF HEMANGIOMAS

- Many require only observation, EXCEPT for those compressing and/or compromising the airway, impairing vision, or causing skin ulceration or bleeding
- Propranolol is currently the mainstay of management
- Other treatment options:
  - Oral or intralesional steroids
  - Surgical excision: cold knife or laser; ideally best to wait until after the proliferation stage

- Interferon-α2a: rarely used because of the risk of spastic diplegia
- Pulsed-dye laser: ideal for superficial hemangioma; can be combined with surgical excision
- Management of subglottic hemangioma
  - Usually present with biphasic stridor, diagnosed by laryngoscopy and bronchoscopy (lesion is most often on the left posterolateral subglottis)
  - 50% will have a cutaneous hemangioma
  - Propranolol is the first-line therapy, possibly combined with systemic steroids
  - Airway compromise despite first-line therapy: intralesional steroids, interferon-α2a, and surgery (eg, open excision vs. tracheotomy)

KASABACH-MERRITT SYNDROME

- Platelet-trapping coagulopathy resulting in an enlarging hemangioma-like tumor[24]
- May be associated with tufted angioma or kaposiform hemangioendothelioma
- Not associated with hemangioma of infancy
- Thrombocytopenia resulting in bleeding, with scattered petechiae when platelet levels fall below 10,000 mm^3
- Chemotherapy (interferon-2 alpha) is reserved for patients with life-threatening coagulopathy

MANAGEMENT OF VASCULAR MALFORMATIONS

- Lymphatic malformations (Fig. 6.7)
  - Classified as macrocystic versus microcystic, infrahyoid versus suprahyoid and unilateral versus bilateral
  - Large suprahyoid microcystic malformations are more problematic
  - MRI or CT for diagnosis and characterization of lesions
  - Sclerotherapy (doxycycline, alcohol, and OK-432,) is useful for macrocystic lesions
  - Surgical excision is most effective for localized macrocystic lesions
  - Cranial nerve or great vessel injury is possible with extensive microcystic lesions
  - Laser (CO$_2$, Nd:YAG) or radiofrequency ablation for oral cavity and tongue

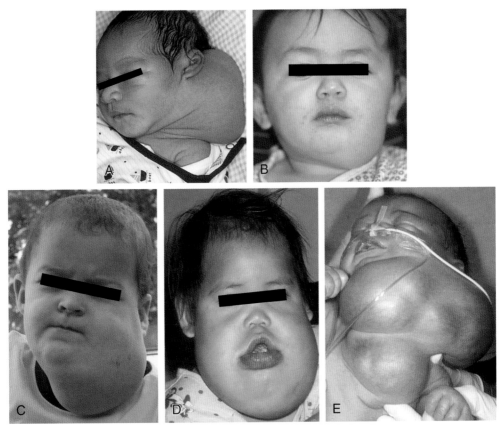

FIGURE 6.7 Head and Neck Lymphatic Malformation Stages. (**A**) Stage 1, unilateral infrahyoid. (**B**) Stage 2, unilateral suprahyoid. (**C**) Stage 3, unilateral suprahyoid and infrahyoid. (**D**) Stage 4, bilateral suprahyoid. (**E**) Stage 5, bilateral suprahyoid and infrahyoid. (From Flint PW, Haughey BH, Lund VJ, et al. *Cummings Otolaryngology—Head and Neck Surgery*. 6th ed. Philadelphia, PA: Saunders; 2015.)

- Venous malformations
  - May be present in muscle tissue under skin or mucosa; will enlarge with Valsalva and have a bluish hue
  - CT scan may show phleboliths
  - May have associated coagulopathy
  - Treatment with sclerotherapy and/or surgery
- Capillary malformations
  - Persistently dilated skin capillaries
  - Serial pulse-dye laser therapy
  - If involving the upper face and eyelid, need brain MRI and ophthalmology evaluation to assess for Sturge-Weber syndrome
- Arteriovenous malformations
  - High-flow vascular malformations
  - Pulsatile mass or diffuse area of increased blood flow
  - Diagnosed with MR or CT angiography
  - Four clinical stages: dormancy, expansion, destruction, and heart failure
  - Treatment: observation versus surgical excision with preoperative embolization

STURGE-WEBER SYNDROME

- Capillary malformation that involves the eye and skin (CNV1), as well as the leptomeninges
- Presents as port wine stain of the upper face and eyelid
- Requires brain MRI and ophthalmology evaluation
- Associated with seizures, developmental delay, and focal neurologic deficits

FOUR MOST COMMON CONGENITAL MIDLINE MASSES

1. TGDC (Fig. 6.8)
   - The majority of TGDC present at or below the hyoid bone in the midline, but less commonly can occur superiorly
   - The tract leads into the base of the tongue, and infections are polymicrobial, consistent with oral pathogenic flora
   - Ultrasound is the preferred diagnostic modality because there is no radiation exposure, and it can discern the makeup of the mass and identify normal thyroid tissue
   - Although rare, papillary adenocarcinoma has been found in the cyst
2. Dermoid cyst
   - It is possible to differentiate between a TGDC via needle aspirate; a dermoid cyst has sebaceous contents, whereas a TGDC is more fluid/cyst filled
3. Lymphadenopathy
4. Hemangioma

SISTRUNK PROCEDURE

- In the patient with an acute infection, the infection should be treated initially with antibiotics. I and D if an abscess with the cyst has developed; surgery should be undertaken after resolution of active, acute infection
- TGDC excision: excision of the cyst, usually with the cuff of surrounding tissue, and excision of the central portion of the hyoid bone

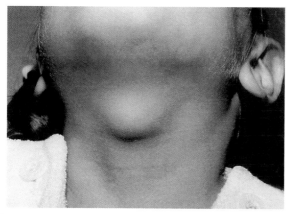

FIGURE 6.8 TGDCs are often found in the midline of the neck at or near the hyoid bone. (From Flint PW, Haughey BH, Lund VJ, et al. *Cummings Otolaryngology—Head and Neck Surgery.* 6th ed. Philadelphia, PA: Saunders; 2015.)

- Excision of the central hyoid bone reduces the recurrence rate to ~5% , down from ~40%; a small wedge resection of the tissue tract into the base of the tongue is advocated by some surgeons to reduce recurrence further

ATYPICAL MYCOBACTERIAL INFECTION (Fig. 6.9)

- Also known as the nontuberculous mycobacteria; must be distinguished from mycobacterium tuberculosis
- Nontender node enlarging slowly over weeks to months in the jugulodigastric or submandibular area, possibly with fluctuance; less often involves the periparotid or submandibular regions
- Classically, it involves the skin with violaceous hue; therefore, diagnosis can be made on clinical grounds, and it may spontaneously drain
- Fever is rare, and there are few systemic effects with no pulmonary involvement; however, chest x-ray (CXR) should be obtained
- Purified protein derivative may be negative or with an intermediate reaction (5-15 mm induration) in atypical infection; cultures may take several weeks to grow and may also be negative in culture-positive specimens
- Infectious Disease consultation
  - Antimycobacterial drug therapy may be offered
  - Clarithromycin/azithromycin may also be effective
- Invariably is resolved spontaneously in the immunocompetent patient
- May lead to chronic draining fistula for 3-6 months
- Curettage treatment may be safely offered
- Superficial parotidectomy/submandibular gland excision for refractory infections

PEDIATRIC ACUTE SIALADENITIS

- Reduced salivary flow is a common initiator
- Ductal metaplasia can occur
- Rule out autoimmune disease
  - Sjögren syndrome
  - Sarcoidosis
- Rule out obstruction
  - Stricture
  - Stone
- Rule out functional disease
  - Medication
  - Metabolic (ie, diabetes)

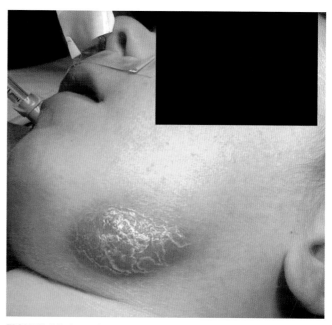

FIGURE 6.9 Atypical Mycobacterial Infection in an Advanced Stage with Skin Erosion. (From Flint PW, Haughey BH, Lund VJ, et al. *Cummings Otolaryngology—Head and Neck Surgery.* 6th ed. Philadelphia, PA: Saunders; 2015.)

- Rule out infectious etiology
- Microbiology
  - *S. aureus*
  - *Streptococcus viridans*
  - *S. pneumoniae*
  - *Escherichia coli*
- First initiate conservative therapy with hydration, sialogogues, and glandular massage
- If this fails or bacterial infection is suspected, then add antibiotics

CONSIDERATIONS FOR PEDIATRIC PAROTID MASSES

- Pleomorphic adenoma is the most common benign epithelial tumor
- Hemangioma is the most common mesenchymal benign mass
- Mucoepidermoid CA (low grade and well differentiated) is the most common malignant tumor

DIFFERENTIAL DIAGNOSIS OF A PEDIATRIC BASE OF THE TONGUE MASS

1. TGDC
2. Lingual thyroid gland
3. Vallecular cyst
4. Dermoid cyst
5. Teratoma
6. Malignant neoplasm

TESTS TO CONSIDER IN THE PEDIATRIC PATIENT WITH A BASE OF THE TONGUE MASS

- CT or MR scan: define depth and extent of the mass
- Thyroid ultrasound: assess for the presence of a normal thyroid; thyroid can be within TGDC or at the tongue base (lingual thyroid)
- Thyroid technetium scan if there is a possible lingual thyroid

MOST COMMON HEAD AND NECK MALIGNANCIES IN CHILDREN UNDER I YEAR OLD

1. Retinoblastoma
2. Neuroblastoma
3. Germ cell neoplasms
4. Rhabdomyosarcoma

MOST COMMON HEAD AND NECK MALIGNANCIES IN CHILDREN BETWEEN I AND 5 YEARS OLD

1. Retinoblastoma
2. Rhabdomyosarcoma
3. Non-Hodgkin lymphoma (NHL)
4. HL

MOST COMMON HEAD AND NECK MALIGNANCIES IN CHILDREN BETWEEN 6 AND 10 YEARS OLD

1. HL
2. Rhabdomyosarcoma
3. NHL
4. Thyroid cancer

MOST COMMON HEAD AND NECK MALIGNANCIES IN CHILDREN BETWEEN I I AND 18 YEARS OLD

1. Thyroid cancer
2. HL
3. NHL
4. Melanoma

PEDIATRIC THYROID CANCER

- Associated with radiation exposure
- Usually papillary thyroid CA
- Management with subtotal or total thyroidectomy: neck dissection for nodal involvement

PEDIATRIC SALIVARY GLAND CANCER

- Most commonly mucoepidermoid CA, and usually low grade
- Acinic cell CA second most common in children
- Treatment is surgical with possible adjuvant therapy

NASOPHARYNGEAL CARCINOMA

- Often presents as neck mass with nasal obstruction
- May have unilateral otitis media and/or rhinorrhea
- Increased incidence in African (black) and Asian teenagers
- Treatment with chemotherapy and radiation

DIFFERENTIAL DIAGNOSIS OF SMALL BLUE CELL MALIGNANCIES OF CHILDHOOD

1. Neuroblastoma
2. Lymphoma
3. Rhabdomyosarcoma
4. Peripheral primitive neuroectodermal tumors

PRESENTATION AND ASSESSMENT FOR LYMPHOMA

- Third most common childhood cancer
- History
  - Painless neck swelling
  - Rapid enlargement may cause tenderness
  - Stage B (see below) symptoms, which confer worse prognosis
  - Fever above 38.0°C for 3 consecutive days
  - Unexplained weight loss of 10% or more in 6 months
  - Drenching night sweats
- Physical exam
  - Painless supraclavicular or cervical mass
  - Lymphadenopathy firm on palpation, "rubbery"
  - Explore other lymph node basins
  - Spleen is the most common extranodal site
- Lab work
  - Complete blood count
  - Erythrocyte sedimentation rate
  - C-reactive protein
  - Liver function tests
- Imaging
  - CXR
  - CT neck and chest
  - CT or MRI of abdomen and pelvis
  - Positron emission tomography (PET) has been found to be more accurate than CT for staging: used to track disease response to therapy
- Surgery
  - Mainly for biopsy for diagnosis
  - Specimen should be sent fresh to the pathologist to facilitate flow cytometry, immunohistochemical staining, molecular genetic testing, and electron microscopy
  - Resection is rarely indicated
- Bone marrow biopsy
- Lumbar puncture

WORLD HEALTH ORGANIZATION CLASSIFICATION OF HODGKIN LYMPHOMA

- Most commonly found in teenage children
- An association between HL and Epstein-Barr virus (EBV) infection, may have evidence of prior exposure and in situ hybridization showing EBV genomes and pathognomonic Reed–Sternberg cells[25]
- Classic HL
  - 90% of HL, comprised of lymphocyte-depleted, nodular sclerosing, mixed cellularity, and lymphocyte-rich subtypes
    - Mixed cellularity: pleomorphic lymphocytes, more numerous Reed–Sternberg (RS) cells
    - Nodular sclerosis: most common classic variant, fibrosis comprising neoplastic and inflammatory cells resulting in nodules
    - Lymphocyte-depleted: few lymphocytes with many RS cells, associated with HIV, rare in children; when disease is localized and nonbulky, is usually treated by limited cycles of chemotherapy and minimal radiation
    - Lymphocyte predominant: many small B lymphocytes; can be treated with radiation alone or sometimes surgical excision and observation

ANN ARBOR STAGING OF HODGKIN LYMPHOMA

- HL treatment is dependent on staging via Ann Arbor
  - Stage 1: involvement of a single lymph node region (stage I) or single extralymphatic site (stage IE)
  - Stage 2: involvement of two or more lymph node regions (stage II) or extralymphatic sites (stage IIE) on the same side of the diaphragm
  - Stage 3: involvement of two or more lymph node regions (stage III) or extralymphatic sites (stage IIIE) on both sides of the diaphragm, the spleen (stage IIIS), or both (stage IIISE)
  - Stage 4: diffuse or disseminated involvement of one or more extralymphatic organs and tissues with or without associated lymph node involvement (stage IV)
    - A: no systemic symptoms
    - B: weight loss, fever, or night sweats

TREATMENT OF HODGKIN LYMPHOMA

- Combined chemotherapy and radiation therapy favored approach
  - Reduces side effects compared with sole radiation therapy or chemotherapy alone
  - Long-term disease survival of 85-100% in early-stage disease
  - Disease survival of 60% in advanced-stage disease[26]

NON-HODGKIN LYMPHOMA

- Critical distinction is that almost all pediatric NHLs are high grade[27]
- Most important prognostic factors are the amount of tumor burden, the stage, and the serum lactate dehydrogenase level
  - Low grade
    - Small lymphocyte
    - Follicular, small cleaved
    - Follicular, small cleaved and large cell mixed
  - Intermediate grade (diffuse)
    - Small cleaved cell
    - Mixed small and large cell
    - Large cell
  - High grade
    - Large cell
    - Lymphoblastic
    - Small cell noncleaved, Burkitt lymphoma

ST. JUDE STAGING OF NON-HODGKIN LYMPHOMA

- Stage I: single tumor (extranodal) or single anatomic area (nodal) with exclusion of the mediastinum and abdomen
- Stage II: single tumor (extranodal) with regional node involvement
  - Two or more nodal areas on the same side of the diaphragm
  - Two single (extranodal) tumors with or without regional node involvement on the same side of the diaphragm
  - Primary gastrointestinal tumor with or without involvement of associated mesenteric nodes only
- Stage III: two single tumors (extranodal) on opposite sides of the diaphragm
  - Two or more nodal areas above and below the diaphragm
  - All primary intrathoracic tumors
  - All extensive primary intraabdominal disease
  - All paraspinal or epidural tumors regardless of other tumor sites

- Stage IV: any of the abovementioned criteria with initial central nervous system (CNS) and/or bone marrow involvement

BURKITT LYMPHOMA

- Most common pediatric NHL cytogenetic evidence of the C-myc rearrangement is the "gold standard" for diagnosis of Burkitt lymphoma
- B-cell lineage, classic "starry sky" pattern of ingested apoptotic cells on histology
- Endemic and sporadic variants: EBV positivity 90-95% in endemic cases and 15-20% in sporadic cases

RHABDOMYOSARCOMA OF THE HEAD AND NECK (Table 6.2)

- 4.5% of all pediatric malignancies and the most common sarcoma of the head and neck[28]
- 35% of all cases occur in the head and neck
- Parameningeal tumor sites include the nasopharynx and nasal cavities, paranasal sinuses, infratemporal and pterygopalatine fossae, as well as the middle ear; increased likelihood of cranial nerve palsy and intracranial extension[29]
- Nonparameningeal sites include all other sites within the head and neck, such as the parotid and submandibular area, and represent more favorable prognostic sites
- Primary site in the head and neck is the orbit (most common, 25-35% of cases); PET CT is the imaging modality of choice
- Metastatic sites
  - Lungs
  - Bone
  - Bone marrow
- Treatment is multimodal (surgery/chemo/external beam radiation therapy)
  - When feasible, complete excision improves survival and reduces adjuvant radiation and chemotherapy
  - Distant metastases may still be surgical candidates

RHABDOMYOSARCOMA HISTOPATHOLOGY

- Embryonal: most common in infants and children; spindle-shaped cells with interspersed large rhabdomyoblasts
  - Botryoidal and pleomorphic variants
  - Higher incidence in Beckwith-Wiedemann syndrome
- Alveolar: poorer prognosis; worse with PAX3/FOX01 translocation gene; most common in adolescents; small round cells in a dense configuration resembling pulmonary alveoli

NEUROBLASTOMAS OF THE HEAD AND NECK

- Most common extracerebral solid tumors of infancy and childhood
- Embryonal tumors of the sympathetic nervous system
- Along the sympathetic chain from the neck to the pelvis
- Paraganglia from the adrenal medulla and other retroperitoneal and pelvic sites
- 40% of diagnoses occur before patients are 1 year old; 80% before 5 years old
- Primary sites in the head and neck (2-5% of neuroblastomas)
- Can present with impingement of head and neck structure, such as jugular foramen cranial nerves or upper-aerodigestive structures
- Neck (sympathetic chain): may result in ipsilateral ptosis (Horner syndrome)

Table 6.2 Tumor-Node-Metastasis Pretreatment Staging Classification

Stage	Site	T	Size	Node	Metastases
1	Nonparameningeal	T1 or T2	*a* or *b*	N0 or N1 or Nx	M0
2	Parameningeal	T1 or T2	*a*	N0 or Nx	M0
3	Parameningeal	T1 or T2	*a*	N1	M0
			b	N0 or N1 or Nx	M0
4	Any	T1 or T2	*a* or *b*	N0 or N1 or Nx	M1

Data adapted from Rhabdomyosarcoma: Review of Children's Oncology Group (COG) Soft-Tissue Committee Experience and Rationale for Current COG Studies.[30]
T: T1, confined to anatomic site of origin; T2, extension and/or fixative to surrounding tissue.
Size: *a* ≥5 cm in diameter; *b* >5 cm in diameter.
Nodes: N0, regional nodes not involved; N1, regional nodes involved; Nx, regional status unknown.
Metastases: M0, no distant metastases; M1, metastases present (includes positive cytology in CSF).

- Orbit: may result in proptosis and periorbital ecchymoses ("panda eyes")
- Metastatic lesions can occur in the head and neck
- Urine or serum catecholamines and metabolites (homovanillic acid, vanillylmandelic acid, and dopamine)
- Staging system reflects tumor burden, surgical resectability, and pattern of metastases
- Management consists of surgical removal and chemotherapy
- Excisional biopsy with removal of adjacent enlarged nodes is typically performed for head and neck neuroblastoma
- Salvage therapy can be performed after chemotherapy
- Radiation therapy used, but is not curative

NOSE AND PARANASAL SINUS DISEASE

DIFFERENTIAL OF CHILD WITH MIDLINE NASAL MASS

1. Dermoid cyst (most common)
2. Glioma
3. Encephalocele
4. Hemangioma

FURSTENBERG SIGN

- Enlargement of a nasal mass with crying, straining, and compression of the jugular veins, consistent with encephalocele that communicates with CSF (not glioma)

THREE TYPES OF CONGENITAL NEUROECTODERMAL NASAL MASSES (Fig. 6.10)

- Glioma
  - Heterotopic glial tissue without patent CSF communication, but may have fibrous stalk
  - Can be extranasal (commonly at glabella) or intranasal
  - Furstenberg sign: negative
  - Not associated with meningitis
  - 60% extranasal, 30% internal, and 10% combined
  - Management is surgical excisional biopsy
  - Extranasal approaches: lateral rhinotomy, external rhinoplasty, transglabellar subcranial, bicoronal, and midline nasal
  - Intranasal approaches: endoscopic excision
- Encephalocele: extracranial herniation of cranial contents through a defect in the skull
  - Pulsatile, bluish compressible lesions that transilluminate
  - Furstenberg sign: positive
  - Meningocele: meninges only
  - Meningoencephalocele: meninges plus brain tissue
  - Management is surgical excision
  - Small cranial bone defect and smaller lesions may be treated endoscopically
  - Larger lesions often require a combined craniotomy approach
- Dermoid: frontal nasal inclusion cysts of tracts related to a defect of the anterior embryological neuropore
  - Midline nasal pit or mass that may occur from the nasal tip to the cranial space
  - Protruding hair from the sinus opening is pathognomonic
  - Firm, lobulated, and noncompressible mass
  - Intracranial extension 4-45% of cases
  - Recurrent meningitis suggests intracranial tract
  - Management is surgical: external rhinoplasty, lateral rhinotomy, transflabellar, subcranial, paracanthal, and bicoronal
  - Intracranial extension: craniotomy

CLASSIFICATION OF CONGENITAL NASAL ENCEPHALOCELES

- Encephaloceles 5 times more common in lumbosacral area
- Sincipital: 25% of all cases
  - Nasofrontal: glabellar mass causing telecanthus and inferior displacement of nasal bones
  - Nasoethmoidal: dorsal nasal mass causing superior displacement of nasal bones and inferior displacement of alar cartilages
  - Naso-orbital: orbital mass causing proptosis and visual disturbance
- Basal: less common intranasal masses, often not discovered until later in childhood
  - Transethmoidal (most common subtype): unilateral nasal mass or hypertelorism
  - Sphenoethmoidal: unilateral nasal mass or hypertelorism
  - Trans-sphenoidal: NP mass, associated with cleft palate
  - Spheno-orbital: unilateral exophthalmos or diplopia

EMBRYOLOGIC SPACES AND STRUCTURES RELATED TO NASAL GLIOMAS, ENCEPHALOCELES, AND DERMOIDS

- Anterior neuropore: most distal end of the ectoderm-derived neural tube
- Prenasal space: behind the nasal bones but in front of the nasal and septal cartilages
- Foramen cecum: defect in the anterior skull base at the apex of the prenasal space that normally closes after a dural diverticulum retracts from the prenasal space into the cranium
  - May not close (encephalocele) or may close prematurely (glioma)
- Fonticulus nasofrontalis: fontanelle between inferior frontal bones and nasal bones

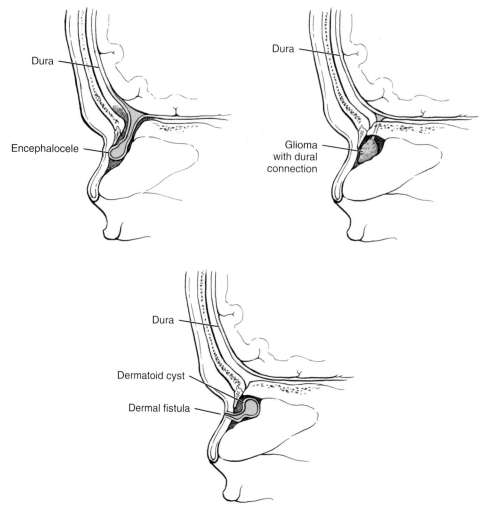

FIGURE 6.10 Schematic View of the Common Midline Nasal Masses. (From Flint PW, Haughey BH, Lund VJ, et al. *Cummings Otolaryngology—Head and Neck Surgery*. 6th ed. Philadelphia, PA: Saunders; 2015.)

HISTORY AND PHYSICAL EXAMINATION FOR AN INFANT OR A CHILD WITH NOISY BREATHING

- History
  - Onset of stridor (What is the age of onset? Sudden or gradual?)
  - Character of stridor (inspiratory, expiratory, and biphasic)
  - Strength of cry and characteristic of vocalization (eg, strong or weak cry)
  - Frequency (Constant or episodic? Hourly or daily?) and progression (Better or worse?)
  - Triggers: What events make the stridor better or worse?
  - Exacerbating and relieving factors (Medications, temperature, humidification, or exercise?)
  - Ability to feed (Presence of coughing, choking, or cyanosis? Volume and length of bottle/breast feeds?)
  - Activity level (Strength to feed, play, exercise, and climb stairs?)
  - Presence of gastroesophageal reflux disease (GERD) symptoms (Postprandial vomiting, restless sleep, or opisthotonus)
  - History of perinatal events (NICU stay? Less than 36 weeks? Prior endotracheal and length of intubation?)

- Physical examination
  - General appearance, color cyanosis of lips, fingers, work of breathing (respiratory rate: infants >40/min; toddlers >30/min)
  - Inspection of thorax and neck for retractions, accessory muscle use
  - Listening for the character of stridor (biphasic, inspiratory, expiratory)
  - Pulse oximetry (below 90% on room air or supplemental oxygen)
  - Signs of distress and impending respiratory failure (Slow prolonged inspirations?)
  - Nasal patency in infants (Can a 5 Fr. feeding tube pass bilaterally?)
  - Auscultation of mouth, neck, and chest (Location and intensity of stridor, wheezes; airflow; rales?)
  - Location of stridor by its auditory pattern
    - Inspiratory: supraglottis and glottis
    - Biphasic: glottis, subglottis, and upper trachea
    - Expiratory: mid to lower trachea
  - Craniofacial anomalies (midface hypoplasia; retrognathic mandible; skeletal dysplasia; macroglossia; short or fused cervical spine, or microstomia)
- Clinical evaluation (the "workup")

- What should be done depends on clinical stability of child's airway (Should the child be intubated or extubated? Which setting should be used, ICU, hospital, or outpatient?)
- Medical imaging may be of limited utility if the acuity of the child is worrisome or perilous (will often need personnel for clinical monitoring)
- CXR film (anteroposterior [AP]/lateral): look for pulmonary aeration/atelectasis, tracheal air column, cardiac location, and cardiomegaly)
- AP/lateral neck film (Are soft-tissue masses present? What is the position of tongue and patency of the nasopharynx?)
- Flat plate of the abdomen: air in the stomach; small bowel loops; situs inversus
- CT scan of head, neck, and thorax (teratoma; vascular malformation; tracheal/bronchial anomalies)
- MR scan of head, neck, thorax, and abdomen (lymphatic malformation)
- Observation versus airway endoscopy "the gold standard"; observation for critically ill or unstable patients may be prudent, depending on the imaging and clinical findings; airway endoscopy requires skilled pediatric intensivists, anesthesiologists, and otolaryngologists
- Flexible fiberoptic laryngoscopy (when practical considering equipment and clinical setting)
  - Assess nasal cavities, nasopharynx, oropharynx, hypopharynx, tongue base, and supraglottic larynx
  - Assess vocal fold appearance and mobility
- Direct laryngoscopy and bronchoscopy
  - Allows for airway visualization as well as ability to secure the airway (if not intubated already)
  - Identification and removal of supraglottic lesions: cysts, papilloma, fibroma, and lymphatic malformations
  - Ability to assess for tracheal developmental anomalies (stenosis, complete rings, mediastinal compression, and bronchial lesions)

INDICATIONS FOR LARYNGOSCOPY AND BRONCHOSCOPY FOR PEDIATRIC STRIDOR

- Severe stridor with impending respiratory failure (may require initial intubation)
- Progressive and worsening stridor
- Any event of stridor associated with: cyanosis, apneic episodes, dysphagia, severe choking, progressive failure to thrive (FTT), or radiologic abnormality identifying or suggesting airway lesion
- Stridor not explained by outpatient fiberoptic nasopharyngo-laryngoscopy (NPL) examination
- History or clinical findings suggestive of ingested or aspirated foreign body

NEONATAL TRACHEOSTOMY SAFETY FACTORS (DURING AND AFTER SURGERY)

- Lowering fraction of inspired oxygen (FiO$_2$) before entry into trachea
- Vertical tracheal incision
- Stay sutures in tracheal rings labeled "left" and "right" taped to chest until first trach change
- "Maturing" sutures connecting trachea to inferior/superior skin incision
- Flex neck and snuggly place Velcro or twill tape tracheotomy ties (able to admit fingertip only)
- Postoperative observation in Pediatric intensive care unit (PICU)
- Smaller tracheotomy tube at the bedside
- No trach change or manipulation of sutures or ties until stoma matures (postoperative day [POD] 3 to 7)

- Daily change of dressing under the tracheotomy ties to avoid moisture and skin breakdown
- Monitor neck skin twice a day (BID) at minimum
- Consult "wound care" nurse early if any concern for ulceration
- Monitor nutritional status/body weight of neonates

ONE-MONTH-OLD INFANT WITH INSPIRATORY STRIDOR SINCE BIRTH, WORSE WITH CRYING AND WHEN SUPINE: WHAT ARE THE MOST LIKELY DIAGNOSES?

- Laryngomalacia (most likely)
- Vocal cord paresis
- Congenital subglottic stenosis
  - GERD

THREE-MONTH-OLD INFANT WITH WORSENING BIPHASIC STRIDOR ×2 WEEKS: WHAT IS THE LIKELY LEVEL OF OBSTRUCTION AND MOST LIKELY DIAGNOSIS?

- Glottis or subglottis
- Most likely subglottic hemangioma

PEDIATRIC AIRWAY ABNORMALITIES THAT ARE WORSE WHEN SUPINE

- Laryngomalacia
- Tongue-base lesions or collapse (eg, vallecular cysts, micrognatia, or Pierre Robin sequence)
- Vascular compression
- Mediastinal mass

GASTROESOPHAGEAL REFLUX DISEASE–RELATED LARYNGEAL DISORDERS IN PEDIATRICS

- Apnea or apparent life-threatening events
- Croup
- Cough
- Hoarseness or dysphonia
- Aspiration
- Laryngomalacia
- Subglottic edema

CLINICAL CHARACTERISTICS OF LARYNGOMALACIA

- Inspiratory stridor: noticed shortly after birth, worse with crying, feeding, or in supine position
- May exhibit GER: arching of back and frequent spit-ups
- Most cases will improve with time as long as the child feeds well and gains weight
- Severe cases may result in FTT, apneic events, and cyanotic episodes
- Symptoms may be worse in the patient with neuromuscular disorders

ANATOMICAL CHARACTERISTICS OF LARYNGOMALACIA (Fig. 6.11)

- Floppy or flaccid laryngeal tissues: mucosa of the arytenoids and aryepiglottic folds, and cartilage of the epiglottis

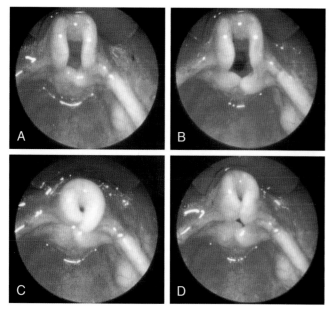

FIGURE 6.11 Laryngomalacia. Progressive airway obstruction on inspiration. Note the progressive curling of the omega-shaped epiglottis and prolapse of the arytenoids on inspiration. (From Benjamin B. The pediatric airway. In: *Slide Lecture Series, American Academy of Otolaryngology—Head and Neck Surgery.* 1992 and Flint PW, Haughey BH, Lund VJ, et al. *Cummings Otolaryngology—Head and Neck Surgery.* 6th ed. Philadelphia, PA: Saunders; 2015.)

- Narrowed or "Omega-shaped" epiglottis
- Shortened aryepiglottic folds
- Poor visualization of vocal folds because of supraglottic collapse

INDICATIONS FOR INTERVENTION IN SEVERE LARYNGOMALACIA

- Indications
  - FTT, weight loss from poor feeding
  - Airway obstruction resulting in apnea and/or cyanosis
  - Pulmonary hypertension and cor pulmonale
  - Severe chest deformity
- Interventions
  - Medical treatment of GERD (H2 blockers; proton pump inhibitors)
  - Direct suspension laryngoscopy with bronchoscopy: division of aryepiglottic fold and removal of redundant arytenoid mucosa
  - Partial epiglottectomy
  - Epiglottopexy
  - Tracheostomy: when severe and unresponsive to prior interventions

LARYNGEAL AND LARYNGOTRACHEOESOPHAGEAL CLEFTS

- Failure of fusion of the posterior cricoid lamina
- Benjamin-Inglis Classification is most commonly used
  - Type I: interarytenoid cleft (above the level of the vocal folds)
    - Medical management is often adequate
  - Type II: partial or complete cricoid cleft, extends below the level of the vocal cords and through the cricoid lamina
  - Type III: total cricoid cleft with extension into the cervical trachea (Fig. 6.12)

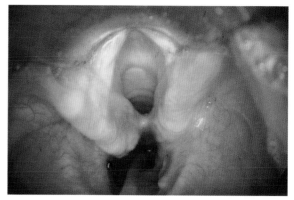

FIGURE 6.12 Laryngotracheal Cleft: Benjamin-Inglis Type 3. (From Benjamin B. The pediatric airway. In: *Slide Lecture Series, American Academy of Otolaryngology—Head and Neck Surgery.* 1992 and Flint PW, Haughey BH, Lund VJ, et al. *Cummings Otolaryngology—Head and Neck Surgery.* 6th ed. Philadelphia, PA: Saunders; 2015.)

  - Type IV: laryngotracheoesophageal cleft into the intrathoracic trachea/carina

FACTORS THAT SUPPORT SURGICAL REPAIR OF LARYNGEAL CLEFT

- Recurrent aspiration and "wet" tracheal cough
- Recurrent pneumonias and hospitalizations
- Airway aspiration and intermittent airway obstruction

DIFFERENTIAL DIAGNOSIS OF PEDIATRIC VOCAL FOLD PARALYSIS

Unilateral
  - Iatrogenic (most common)
    - Thoracic surgery (eg, prior aortic arch surgery or patent ductus arteriosus [PDA] ligation)
    - Tracheoesophageal (TE) fistula repair
  - Idiopathic
Bilateral
  - Neurologic disease
    - Meningomyelocele
    - Arnold-Chiari malformation
    - Hydrocephalus
    - Neonatal subdural hemorrhage or hematoma
  - Birth trauma
    - Cervical traction-type injury (eg, forceps delivery)
  - Malignant disease (intracranial, cervical, or thoracic)
  - Genetic syndrome (Mobius)

ARNOLD-CHIARI MALFORMATION

- Herniation of the cerebellum through the foramen magnum of the skull
- Pressure injury on the vagus nerves may result in bilateral vocal cord paralysis
- Diagnosed by MRI brain
- Early evaluation and neurosurgical decompression are most often recommended

ETIOLOGY, SYMPTOMS, AND PATTERN OF SPREAD FOR RECURRENT RESPIRATORY PAPILLOMATOSIS

- Etiology: human papillomavirus (HPV) infection (common types 6 and 11) resulting in proliferation of benign squamous papillomas within the respiratory tract

- Vertical transmission from cervical HPV in the young mother during delivery (risk 1 in 231 to 400)
- Types
  - Juvenile onset: more aggressive disease, typically diagnosed before the age of 5 years
  - Aggressive disease associated with more surgical procedures per year/more involved anatomical sites
  - Adult onset: less aggressive, slower progression, with higher likelihood of becoming disease free
- Symptoms
  - Hoarseness: principal presenting symptom
  - Stridor: second presenting symptom
  - Acute respiratory distress
  - Extralaryngeal spread
    - Oral cavity
    - Trachea
    - Bronchi
    - Lungs
    - May cause destruction of lung parenchyma (blebs, cysts, and cavitating lesions)
  - Higher risk of malignant carcinomatous transformation

TREATMENT MODALITIES FOR RECURRENT RESPIRATORY PAPILLOMATOSIS

- Surgical debulking with preservation of normal structures as much as possible
  - Microlaryngoscopy with forceps or powered microdebrider: currently the favored technique of pediatric otolaryngologists
  - Laser: direct line of sight for carbon dioxide (CO_2) beam or fiber
    - Controlled destruction with excellent hemostasis
    - Possible increased scar formation
    - Laser smoke may contain active viral DNA
  - Tracheostomy: for severe airway obstruction
  - Avoid unless absolutely necessary
  - If unavoidable, goal is for decannulation as soon as disease is managed
  - Associated with increased risk of distal spread
- Adjuvant medical therapy: 20% of patients will require some medical treatments[31]
  - Criteria for use:
    - More than four surgeries per year
    - Distal multisite spread of disease
    - Rapid regrowth of papilloma with airway compromise
  - Cidofovir
    - Broad-spectrum antiviral agent
    - Currently the most frequently used adjuvant therapy
    - Suggested indications
      - More than six surgeries per year
      - Decreasing interval between surgeries
      - Extralaryngeal spread
  - Photodynamic therapy
  - Indole-3-carbimol nutritional supplement: found in cruciferous vegetables
  - Mumps vaccine
  - Avastin (bevacizumab) is currently being investigated
  - HPV therapeutic vaccines
  - Interferon therapy: use has decreased because of side effects and the emergence of other therapies

SUBGLOTTIC HEMANGIOMA (Fig. 6.13)

- Twice as common in females than in males
- Typically present in the first 6 months of life with inspiratory or biphasic stridor: barking cough that responds temporarily to oral steroids ("recurrent croup")
- Grows rapidly in first 6 months, stabilizes for ~1 year, and then slowly involutes
- Diagnosis by direct laryngoscopy

TREATMENT OPTIONS FOR AIRWAY HEMANGIOMA

1. Observation with close monitoring Propranolol (first-line therapy)
   a. Pretreatment cardiac evaluation is recommended
2. Systemic or intralesional steroids
3. Laser excision
4. Microdebrider excision
5. Laryngotracheoplasty (may be useful for circumferential or bilateral hemangiomas)
6. Tracheotomy

CAUSES OF SUBGLOTTIC STENOSIS

- Congenital (term newborn cricoid diameter <3.5 mm)
  - Membranous soft tissues: bilateral
  - Circumferential fibrous connective tissue
  - Cartilaginous (more common than membranous)
  - Cricoid cartilage deformity "elliptical cricoid ring"
- Acquired (more common than congenital)
  - Intubation
  - Other laryngeal trauma: prior airway surgery, inhalational injury, or external trauma
  - Chronic inflammatory, infectious, or autoimmune processes: granulomatosis with polyangiitis (Wegener), tuberculosis, systemic lupus erythematosus, relapsing polychondritis, and sarcoidosis
  - Neoplasm: chondroma, hemangioma, and CA

CLASSIFICATION SYSTEM OF LARYNGEAL AND SUBGLOTTIC STENOSIS

- Laryngeal
  - Grade I: <70%
  - Grade II: 70-90%
  - Grade III: >90%, identifiable lumen
  - Grade IV: no lumen
- Subglottic stenosis (Myer Cotton)
  - Grade I: <50%
  - Grade II: 51-70%
  - Grade III: 71-99%
  - Grade IV: complete stenosis

REDUCTION IN THE AREA OF A SUBGLOTTIC AIRWAY WHEN THE RADIUS OF A FULL-TERM INFANT IS REDUCED BY 1 MM

- Reduces the cross-sectional area of the subglottis by approximately 50-60% ($A = \pi r^2$)

APPROACH TO REPAIR OF SUBGLOTTIC STENOSIS

- Technique depends on the length and severity of stenosis, maturity of scar, shape of scar (concentric, elliptical), and comorbidities
- Tracheotomy may have already been placed depending on the severity
- Grade 1 or low grade 2 subglottic stenosis → no repair, steroids, and nebulizers for exacerbations
- Grade 2/3 → endoscopic or open repair
- Grade 3/4 → open repair
- Endoscopic approach → laser resection with radial cuts and balloon dilation

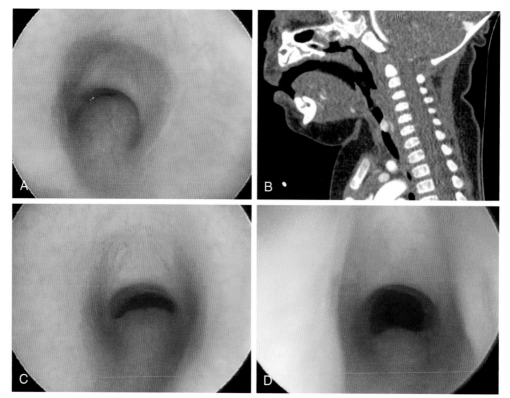

FIGURE 6.13 Endoscopic and Computed Tomography Appearance of Focal Tracheal Hemangioma. (**A**) Before propranolol therapy. (**B**) CT angiogram of tracheal hemangioma. (**C**) After 1 month of propranolol therapy. (**D**) After 4 months of propranolol therapy. (From Flint PW, Haughey BH, Lund VJ, et al. *Cummings Otolaryngology—Head and Neck Surgery*. 6th ed. Philadelphia, PA: Saunders; 2015.)

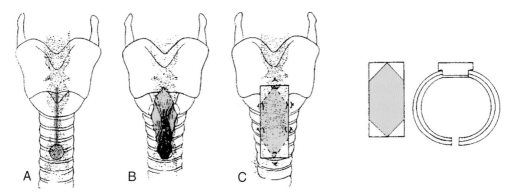

FIGURE 6.14 Anterior Cartilage Graft. (**A**) Vertical incision is made into the thyroid cartilage from a point immediately below the anterior commissure through the upper tracheal rings, with care taken to remain in the midline. (**B**) Intraluminal scar and lining mucosa are incised along the length of the stenotic segment. (**C**) Costal cartilage is shaped into a modified boat (inset) and placed in position with the lining of the perichondrium facing internally. (From Flint PW, Haughey BH, Lund VJ, et al. *Cummings Otolaryngology—Head and Neck Surgery*. 6th ed. Philadelphia, PA: Saunders; 2015.)

- Open approaches
  - Anterior cricoid split (for relatively healthy infants with subglottic stenosis)
  - Single-stage laryngotracheal reconstruction (anterior/posterior grafts) with decannulation (Fig. 6.14)
  - Multistage reconstruction with stenting and serial dilations before decannulation

CONTRAINDICATIONS TO OPEN-AIRWAY REPAIR

- Significant and poorly controlled GERD reflux
- Ventilation requirements (ie, still needs intubation or tracheotomy)

SURGICAL TREATMENT OF SUBGLOTTIC STENOSIS

- Endoscopic: indicated for symptomatic grade I/II lesions
  - Laser (radial cuts): carbon dioxide
  - Endoscopy and dilation (eg, balloon dilation)
  - Microlaryngeal: suspension and microdebrider or cup forceps "cold" techniques
  - Consider adjuvant treatments (eg, steroids and mitomycin C)
- Grade III/IV lesions
  - Tracheostomy
  - Anterior cricoid split: typically used in neonates and infants with good pulmonary function

- May augment with cartilage graft (eg, auricular and thyroid ala)
- Laryngotracheal reconstruction
- Anterior ± posterior cricoid split with augmentation with cartilage (eg, rib, thyroid ala, and hyoid bone)
  - 1 stage: tracheotomy is removed or avoided, and patient is kept intubated for several days to a week for stenting
  - 2 stage: tracheotomy is kept, and stent is placed above the trach
- Cricotracheal resection: severe grade III or grade IV subglottic/tracheal stenosis starting at least 1cm distal to the vocal cords

INDICATIONS FOR ANTERIOR CRICOID SPLIT FOR NEONATES

1. Two or more failed extubations secondary to small cricoid ring or extensive submucosal fibrosis with a healthy cricoid
2. Weight >1500 g
3. No assisted ventilation for 10 days
4. Minimal or no supplemental oxygen requirement (FiO_2 <30%)
5. No congestive heart failure for 1 month
6. No acute URI
7. No antihypertensive medications for 10 days

INDICATIONS FOR LARYNGOTRACHEAL RECONSTRUCTION WITH CARTILAGE GRAFTS

- Glottic or subglottic stenosis (grade II or III)
- No significant tracheomalacia or tracheal obstruction

INDICATIONS FOR LONG-TERM STENTING IN PEDIATRIC AIRWAY RECONSTRUCTION

- Extensive circumferential scarring
- Prior failed airway reconstruction
- Lack of airway rigidity
- Craniofacial or vertebral anomalies (avoid potentially difficult reintubation)

VARIOUS STENTS USED IN PEDIATRIC AIRWAY RECONSTRUCTION

- Endotracheal tube
- Montgomery T-tube
- Aboulker fluoroplastic stent
- Cotton-Lorenz fluoroplastic stent

TRACHEAL CAUSES OF STRIDOR

1. Tracheomalacia
2. Vascular compression from an aberrant great vessel
3. Segmental stenosis
4. Complete tracheal rings
5. Tracheoesophageal fistula (TEF)
6. Hemangioma
7. Tracheal cyst

MOST COMMON CONGENITAL VASCULAR ANOMALIES THAT CAN CAUSE TRACHEOMALACIA (Fig. 6.15)

- Innominate artery compression
  - Common form of incomplete vascular ring

- Abnormally distal takeoff from aortic arch causing anterior compression of the trachea 1-2 cm above the carina
- Double aortic arch
  - Most common true vascular ring
- Right aortic arch with aberrant left subclavian artery and left ligamentum arteriosum
- Pulmonary artery sling
  - Left pulmonary artery arises from the right pulmonary artery and passes between the esophagus and trachea, compressing the right main-stem bronchus and distal trachea

TRACHEOESOPHAGEAL FISTULA PRESENTATION, INVESTIGATIONS, TYPES, AND INTERVENTIONS

- Most patients are diagnosed shortly after birth
  - Respiratory distress
  - Cyanosis during nursing
  - Excessive drooling
  - Inability to pass a feeding tube
  - CXR may show gastric bubble
  - Contrast radiographic studies may present a risk of significant pulmonary aspiration
  - Endoscopy the mainstay for diagnosis
- Types
  - Esophageal atresia (EA) and distal TEF (85%)
  - Isolated EA (8%)
  - H-type TEF (4%)
  - EA with proximal TEF (3%)
  - EA with proximal and distal TEF (<1%)
- Management
  - Immediate gastrostomy tube placement
  - Surgical correction at 3 months of age
  - May require dilation of esophageal strictures
  - Risk of recurrent laryngeal nerve injury

VATER ASSOCIATION

- V: vertebral/vascular anomalies
- A: anal atresia
- T: tracheal anomalies, for example, TE fistula
- E: esophageal anomalies, for example, distal stenosis or agenesis
- R: renal/radial bone anomalies
- VACTERL association
  - C: cardiac anomalies (PDA and valve problems)
  - L: Limb anomalies (extra digits and shortened limbs)

SURGICAL MANAGEMENT OF TRACHEAL STENOSIS: PROCEDURES AND COMPLICATIONS

- Endoscopic approach
  - Cold knife lysis
  - Laser excision
  - Dilation (balloon dilation is the most common)
  - Stents
- Open approaches
  - Patch tracheoplasty: rib cartilage and pericardium
  - Segmental resection with primary anastomosis
  - Anterior wedge resection (for localized stenosis, eg, stenosis at the tracheotomy site)
  - Tracheal autograft
  - Slide tracheoplasty
  - Transplant (autograft or allograft)

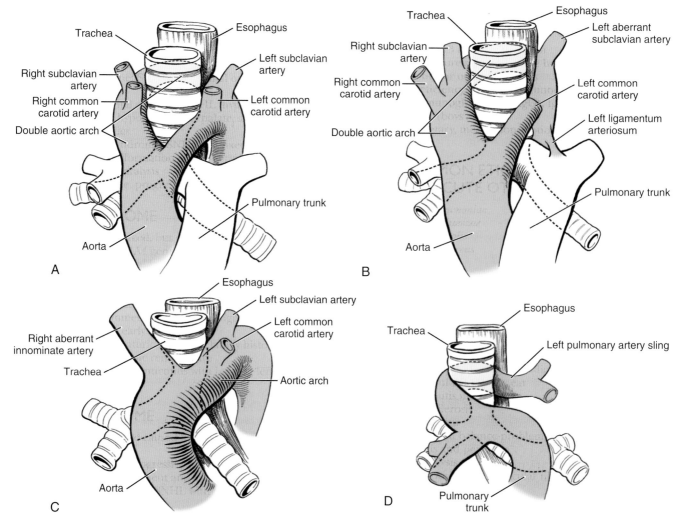

FIGURE 6.15 (A) Double aortic arch. **(B)** Right aortic arch with aberrant left subclavian artery and left ligamentum arteriosum. **(C)** Aberrant innominate artery. **(D)** Left pulmonary artery sling. (From Flint PW, Haughey BH, Lund VJ, et al. *Cummings Otolaryngology—Head and Neck Surgery*. 6th ed. Philadelphia, PA: Saunders; 2015.)

- Complications
  - Granulation tissue
  - Restenosis
  - Recurrent injury to the laryngeal nerve
  - Dehiscence of repair
  - Tracheobronchomalacia
  - TE fistula
  - Aspiration

DISCUSS AERODIGESTIVE FOREIGN BODIES (Table 6.3)

- Most commonly in boys under 3 years old
- Reliable history and witnessed aspiration or ingestion are most important for diagnosis
- AP/PA and lateral x-rays are useful initial studies: inspiratory and expiratory films or lateral decubitus films may be useful for possible airway foreign body
- Reasonable suspicion of airway foreign body mandates bronchoscopy
- Suspicion of aerodigestive battery foreign body mandates emergent removal
- Mid to distal esophageal foreign bodies in asymptomatic older children may be observed for 8 to 16 hours to see if the object will pass

ANATOMICAL AREAS WHERE ESOPHAGEAL FOREIGN BODIES ROUTINELY BECOME LODGED

1. Upper esophageal sphincter cricopharyngeus
2. Aortic arch
3. Left main-stem bronchus
4. Lower esophageal sphincter

CONSIDERATIONS FOR CAUSTIC INGESTION

- Concentration and duration of contact affect the extent of injury
- Acid causes coagulation necrosis: a more superficial injury
- Alkalis produce liquefaction necrosis: a deeper injury
- Depending on the depth of injury, consider antibiotics and steroids to reduce scarring and stricture formation
- NG tube is controversial: if needed, ideally it is placed under direct visualization
- General pediatric and GI consultation
- Complications➔ tongue scarring with fixation; soft palate scarring with NP reflux; hypopharyngeal, laryngeal, or esophageal strictures

Table 6.3 Overview of the Management of Aerodigestive Foreign Bodies

	Airway Foreign Body	Esophageal Foreign Body
History	Witnessed aspiration Cough, dyspnea, wheezing, and stridor Refractory asthma	Witnessed ingestion Vomiting, drooling, dysphagia, odynophagia, emesis, food refusal, and chest pain
Physical examination	Decreased lung sounds, wheezing, and crackles Tachypnea and hypoxemia	Drooling, poor feeding, and choking
Imaging	PA and lateral radiographs (radiopaque foreign body, unilateral emphysema or hyperinflation, and localized atelectasis or infiltrate)	PA and lateral radiographs (radiopaque foreign body, widened prevertebral shadow, loss of lordosis)
Treatment	If adequate suspicion, proceed immediately to rigid bronchoscopy for removal	*Young symptomatic children:* FB present >24 h or sharp metallic or caustic objects should undergo endoscopic removal *Asymptomatic children:* recent ingestion (<24 h), and no esophageal disorders can be observed for 8-16 h

FB, Foreign body; *PA,* posteroanterior.
From Flint PW, Haughey BH, Lund VJ, et al. *Cummings Otolaryngology—Head and Neck Surgery.* 6th ed. Philadelphia, PA: Saunders; 2015, table 207-1.

- Severe burn➔ G-tube and peroral string placement for subsequent retrograde bougie esophageal dilation

AGENTS RESPONSIBLE FOR CAUSTIC INGESTION AND THEIR DAMAGE PATTERN

- Acid: pH <7, causes coagulative necrosis and creates a coagulum that prevents deeper tissue injury
- Base: pH >7, causes liquefactive necrosis, penetration into tissues, and deeper injury
- Bleaches: pH ~7, usually mild irritant and does not cause significant tissue injury

INITIAL MANAGEMENT STRATEGY FOR CAUSTIC INGESTIONS (Fig. 6.16)

- Presence of oral injury cannot accurately predict presence or absence of more distal involvement
- Vomiting should not be induced
- Oral dilution with water or milk (limit to 15 mL/kg)
- IV fluids and nothing by mouth (NPO)
- "Blind" nasogastric tube (NGT) placement is contraindicated
- Chest and abdominal x-ray to assess for free air in the mediastinum or abdomen
- Antibiotics use is controversial
- Antireflux medication use is controversial
- Esophagoscopy timing is controversial (<12 hours an evolving lesion may be missed; >48 hours may risk perforation)
  - Grade 0: no injury
  - Grade I: mucosal edema and hyperemia
  - Grade IIa: superficial, noncircumferential, whitish membranes, shallow ulcers, hemorrhage, and friable exudates
  - Grade IIb: deep, circumferential lesions with stricture formation
  - Grade IIIa: small, scattered areas of necrosis
  - Grade IIIb: extensive necrosis
  - Grade IV: perforation
- If evaluation starts >48 hours after ingestion, an esophagram may be obtained as an initial assessment instead of esophagoscopy
- Treatment
  - Observation for grade I and II lesions
  - Consider steroids for grade II
  - Stenting with NGT if there is a risk of stricture
  - If stricture or risk of stricture is found, repeat assessment with dilation in 2-3 weeks

- May require long-term serial dilations
- Esophagectomy with intestinal interposition graft for severe stricture and perforation
- Mortality rates are high

DIFFERENTIAL DIAGNOSIS OF PEDIATRIC UPPER-AIRWAY INFECTIONS (Table 6.4)

- Laryngotracheitis (croup)
  - Caused by parainfluenza; also influenza, respiratory syncytial virus (RSV), measles, adenovirus, varicella, and HSV I
  - URI prodrome, slow onset, affects patients aged 6 months to 3 years, variable/minimal fever, hoarse with "barking" cough, and can develop respiratory difficulty with inspiratory stridor
  - Diagnosis: clinical; radiographic "steeple sign" on AP views
  - Treatment: expectant
  - Humidification
  - Racemic epinephrine
  - Steroids
  - Direct laryngoscopy, bronchoscopy, and possible intubation if medical therapy fails: use a tube 0.5 mm smaller than estimated, and extubate when air leak detected
- Supraglottitis (epiglottitis)
  - Caused by *Haemophilus influenzae* type B, also Group A beta-hemolytic *Streptococcus, Staphylococcus,* pneumococcus, *Klebsiella,* and *H. parainfluenzae*
  - Mild URI prodrome, rapid onset of high fever, toxic symptoms, drooling, dysphagia; affects children 1-8 years old
  - Diagnosis: history, clinical presentation, do not agitate the child; radiographics only if diagnosis is in question
  - Management: OR intubation, rigid/flexible bronchoscopy; IV antibiotics (ceftriaxone, cefotaxime, and ampicillin/sulbactam); extubation usually within 48 hours once swelling is down and air leak is present
- Bacterial tracheitis
  - Caused by *S. aureus,* also *S. pyogenes, H. influenzae, M. catarrhalis*
  - URI prodrome, rapid onset in children 6 months to 8 years old; high fever, hoarseness with cough, dysphagia, and toxic symptoms
  - Management: OR intubation, bronchoscopic suction and cultures of airway exudates; extubation when normothermic, decreased secretions, and air leak present

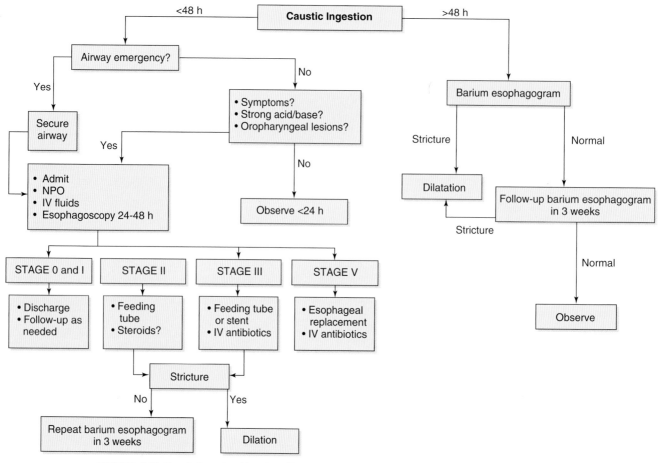

FIGURE 6.16 Caustic Ingestion Algorithm. (From Flint PW, Haughey BH, Lund VJ, et al. *Cummings Otolaryngology—Head and Neck Surgery.* 6th ed. Philadelphia, PA: Saunders; 2015.)

Table 6.4 Differential Diagnosis of Upper-Airway Infections in Children

	Laryngotracheitis (Viral Croup)	Supraglottis (Epiglottitis)	Bacterial Tracheitis	Retropharyngeal Abscess
Age	6 months to 3 years	1-8 years	6 months to 8 years	1-5 years
Onset	Slow	Rapid	Rapid	Slow
Prodrome	URI symptoms	None or mild URI	URI symptoms	URI symptoms
Fever	Variable or none	High	High	Usually high
Hoarseness and barky cough	Yes	No	Yes	No
Dysphagia	No	Yes	Yes	Yes
Toxic appearance	No	Yes	Yes	Variable
Radiographs	Subglottic narrowing	Rounded enlarged epiglottis	Subglottic narrowing; diffuse haziness; tracheal wall irregularities	Widened prevertebral space

URI, Upper respiratory infection.
From Flint PW, Haughey BH, Lund VJ, et al. *Cummings Otolaryngology—Head and Neck Surgery.* 6th ed. Philadelphia, PA: Saunders; 2015, table 197-1.

- Retropharyngeal abscess
  - Caused by mixed bacteriae: Streptococci, *S. aureus, H. influenzae,* Bacteroides, peptostreptococci, and fusobacteria
  - URI prodrome in children usually <6, fever, sore throat, progressive dysphagia, and drooling
  - Diagnosed on the lateral soft-tissue x-ray: subcutaneous gas and widening of prevertebral tissues (>2× diameter of C2 body 90% sensitive); CT scan
  - Management: secure airway, IV antibiotics, and possible OR drainage (transoral vs. transcervical)

CRANIOFACIAL

CLEFT LIP/PALATE: CLASSIFICATION AND ETIOLOGY

- Unilateral or bilateral (Fig. 6.17)
  - Complete: involves entire lip/premaxilla
  - Incomplete: remaining small bridge of tissue is the Simonart bar/band
  - Etiology

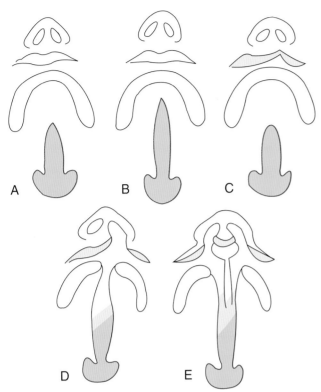

FIGURE 6.17 Classification of Cleft Palate. The division between primary palate (prolabium, premaxilla, and anterior septum) and secondary palate is the incisive foramen. (**A**) Incomplete cleft of the secondary palate. (**B**) Complete cleft of the secondary palate (extending as far as the incisive foramen). (**C**) Incomplete cleft of the primary and secondary palates. (**D**) Unilateral complete cleft of the primary and secondary palates. (**E**) Bilateral complete cleft of the primary and secondary palates (Kernahan DA, Stack RB. A new classification for cleft lip and cleft palate. Plast Reconstr Surgery Transplant Bull. 1958; 22:435-41.). (From McCarthy JG, Cutting CB, Hogan VM. Introduction to facial clefts. In: Mathes SJ, ed. *Plastic Surgery*. Philadelphia, PA: Saunders; 1990:2243 and Flint PW, Haughey BH, Lund VJ, et al. *Cummings Otolaryngology—Head and Neck Surgery*. 6th ed. Philadelphia, PA: Saunders; 2015.)

- Multifactorial: combination of genetics, environmental influences, and other
- Genetics
- 30% cleft lip and palate is associated with syndrome, and 50% cleft palate is associated with syndrome
- Incidence of cleft lip varies by ethnic group
- Incidence of cleft palate does not vary by ethnicity
- Teratogens: alcohol, tobacco smoke, phenytoin, and retinoic acid
- Prenatal multivitamins and folic acid may decrease risk

ANATOMICAL ANOMALIES IN CLEFT LIP DEFECT

- Orbicularis oris muscle with abnormal direction and insertion
- Prolabial skin deficient
- Shortened columella, which deviates to the noncleft side
- Floor of the nose may be absent
- Central portion of the alveolar arch may be deficient
- Widened nasal tip is deflected to the noncleft side
- Septum and anterior nasal spine are displaced to the noncleft side

MILESTONES FOR CLEFT LIP/PALATE REPAIR

- Lip adhesion: 2-4 weeks with second stage at 3 months (not as commonly done currently)
- Lip repair: 2-3 months
- Palate repair: 8-12 months

- Correction of velopharyngeal insufficiency (VPI): 4 years
- Orthodontics: >4 years
- Lip revision: >4 years
- Nasal reconstruction
  - Tip: 6-10 years
  - Dorsum: 15-17 years

SURGICAL REPAIR OF CLEFT LIP AND PALATE

- Lip adhesion: if done, performed at 2-4 weeks of age, with definitive repair at 4-6 months of age
- Cleft lip repair: if no contraindications and no previous lip adhesion, repair is performed at 10-12 weeks
  - Millard rotation advancement technique
  - Tennison-Randall (single) triangular flap interdigitation
  - Bardach (double) triangular flap interdigitation
  - Bilateral cleft repair (Millard)
  - Straight-line closure (rarely used anymore)
- Cleft palate repair: performed 9-12 months up to 18 months of age if child is growing and gaining weight; restoration of the soft palate sling incorporating the tensor and levator palate
  - Von Langenbeck
  - V-Y pushback
  - Bardach two-flap palatoplasty
  - Schweckendiek: closure of soft palate only
  - Furlow double Z-plasty (for soft palate repair)

THREE CHARACTERISTICS OF SUBMUCOUS CLEFT PALATE

1. Bifid uvula
2. Zona pellucida (translucent zone in the midline of the soft palate)
3. Notched posterior hard palate

VELOCARDIOFACIAL SYNDROME

- Autosomal dominant, but most patients present « de novo »
- Deletion of 22q11
- Characterized by abnormal facies, VPI, cleft lip/palate, and cardiac anomalies
- Long face, malar flatness, mandibular micrognathia, and microcephaly
- Palatal clefting ranges from bifid uvula to submucosal cleft palate to true cleft palate: VPI and middle ear disease are common
- Cardiac anomalies are common
- Medialized internal carotid arteries may be present: requires contrast imaging before pharyngeal surgery

PATTERNS OF VELOPHARYNGEAL CLOSURE (MAY ASSIST IN SURGICAL PLANNING IN CASES OF VELOPHARYNGEAL INSUFFICIENCY)

1. Coronal (55%, most common)
2. Sagittal (10-15%, least common)
3. Circular (10-20%)
4. Circular with Passavant ridge (15-20%)

MANAGEMENT OF VELOPHARYNGEAL INSUFFICIENCY

- Medical
  - Speech therapy
  - Prosthetics
  - Palatal lift
  - Obturator

- Surgical: sphincter pharyngoplasty is ideal for coronal or circular closure patterns
  - Superiorly based pharyngeal flap is ideal for sagittal or circular closure patterns
  - Furlow palatoplasty (Double Z-plasty) increases the thickness and length of the palate
  - Posterior pharyngeal wall augmentation is ideal for a small midline gap

CHOANAL ATRESIA

- Incidence 1:5000-8000 births
- Two-thirds are unilateral, usually on the right
- 50% of unilateral and 75% of bilateral are associated with other anomalies
- Four parts to the anatomic deformity
  - Narrow nasal cavity
  - Lateral bony obstruction from the pterygoid plate
  - Medial bony obstruction from the vomer
  - Membranous obstruction
- 29% bony atresia; 71% mixed bony-membranous
- Endoscopy and CT confirm the diagnosis
- Severity of presentation depends on unilateral or bilateral atresia
  - Bilateral: increased respiratory effort, retractions, and cyanosis
  - Unilateral: may present later in life with unilateral thick rhinorrhea
- General management approach
  - Unilateral atresia: non-urgent repair, can wait until ~1 year of age
  - Bilateral atresia: establish airway and gastric feeding
  - Oral airway
  - May require intubation
- Surgical repair approaches
  - Transnasal (preferred with improved endoscopic techniques)
  - Stenting and use of Mitomycin C remain controversial
  - Transpalatal
  - Transseptal

SYNDROMES ARE ASSOCIATED WITH CHOANAL ATRESIA

- 50% of unilateral cases and 75% of bilateral cases are associated with a syndrome
  - CHARGE association
  - Crouzon
  - Apert
  - Treacher Collins
  - Velocardiofacial

CLASSIFICATION OF MICROTIA (Fig. 6.18)

- Type I: mild deformity with major structures present to some degree
- Type II: moderate deformity with major structures present but with deficiency of tissue
- Type III: severe deformity, "peanut ear," few or no recognizable landmarks, and lobule may be present
- Type IV: anotia; no auricle or lobule

GENERAL MANAGEMENT APPROACH FOR MICROTIA

- Observation
- Prosthetic
  - Adhesive
  - Implant
- Reconstruction
  - Rib cartilage
  - Performed when patient is between 5 and 10 years old
  - Medpor

SYNDROMES ASSOCIATED WITH MICROTIA/ AURAL ATRESIA

1. Goldenhar
2. Treacher Collins
3. BOR
4. Crouzon

GENERAL MANAGEMENT APPROACH FOR CONGENITAL AURAL ATRESIA

- Soft Band Bone conduction hearing aid in children can be used starting at age 6-12 months
- Surgical options: BAHA Attract versus Connect versus atresiaplasty
- BAHA is Food and Drug Administration approved for children aged 5 years and older: in Europe, it is approved for children aged 3 years and older
  - Excellent closure of the air-bone gap
  - Does not interfere with associated microtia repair, although plastics repair of the outer ear is typically done first
- Atresiaplasty: age and timing of repair is controversial

GRADING CONGENITAL AURAL ATRESIA (JAHRSDOERFER SYSTEM)

- 10-point system based on high-resolution CT findings
  - Mastoid pneumatization
  - Oval window open
  - Round window status
  - Malleus-incus complex present
  - Incus-stapes connection
  - Facial nerve normal
  - Middle ear space
  - External ear appearance
  - Presence of the stapes (worth 2 points if normal; 1 point if abnormal but present)
- 6 points or greater indicates favorable candidate for atresiaplasty
- Higher points have better hearing outcomes

COMPLICATIONS IN AURAL ATRESIA REPAIR

- Facial nerve injury
- SNHL
- External auditory meatal stenosis
- Lateralization of TM

FACIAL NERVE FINDINGS IN MIDDLE EAR ATRESIA

- May cover the oval window and stapes
- More acute angle is taken at the second genu, crossing more anterolateral to the middle ear instead of inferiorly
- Dehiscence of facial nerve bony canal

CONSIDERATIONS FOR OTOPLASTY

- Normal auriculocephalic angle is 25-35 degrees: >40 degrees is considered abnormal

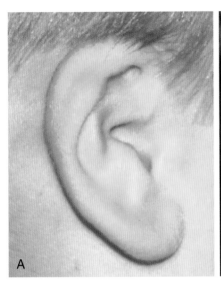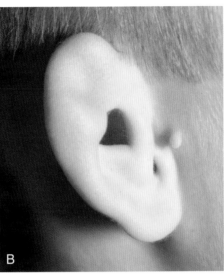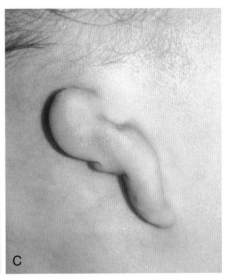

FIGURE 6.18 (A) Type I microtia with constricted ear and minimal tissue deficiency. **(B)** Type II microtia with absence of major portions of the ear. **(C)** Type III microtia with markedly deformed and small cartilaginous remnant. (From Flint PW, Haughey BH, Lund VJ, et al. *Cummings Otolaryngology—Head and Neck Surgery*. 6th ed. Philadelphia, PA: Saunders; 2015.)

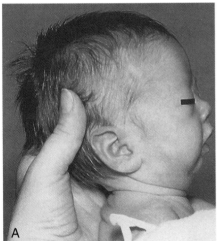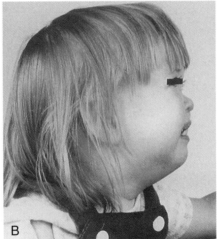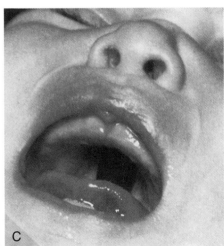

FIGURE 6.19 (A) A newborn with Pierre Robin sequence. **(B)** The same child at age 2 years. Note the partial mandibular catch-up growth. **(C)** U-shaped cleft palate in a patient with Pierre Robin sequence. (From Flint PW, Haughey BH, Lund VJ, et al. *Cummings Otolaryngology—Head and Neck Surgery*. 6th ed. Philadelphia, PA: Saunders; 2015.)

- Normal distance of helical rim scalp 15-20 mm
- Cartilaginous growth almost complete at age 5 years
- Most common abnormalities are treated with otoplasty
  - Insufficient furl at the antihelix
  - Misshapen conchal bowl
- Reconstruct at age 5 or 6 years (before the child starts school)
- Cartilage sparing technique: Mustarde sutures to recreate the antihelical fold
- Cartilage sculpting technique: reshaping/scoring/splitting cartilage to weaken and recreate the antihelical fold
- Furnas sutures: decrease the conchomastoid angle

SYNCHONDROSES OF THE PEDIATRIC SKULL BASE

- Spheno-occipital synchondrosis: principal growth center; persists into adolescence

- Sphenoethmoidal
- Sphenofrontal
- Intersphenoidal
- Frontoethmoidal

PIERRE ROBIN SEQUENCE (Fig. 6.19)

- Triad of:
  - Retrognathia
  - Glossoptosis
  - Cleft palate
- Pathology: retrognathia prevents the tongue from settling into the oral cavity, preventing secondary palate fusion
- Commonly associated with a syndrome (eg, Stickler and velocardiofacial)
- Airway interventions
  - Prone positioning
  - NP airway

- Tongue-lip adhesion
- Endotracheal intubation
- Tracheostomy
- Neonatal mandibular distraction osteogenesis (may allow avoidance of tracheostomy)

SINUS

MOST COMMON SYMPTOMS OF CHRONIC PEDIATRIC SINUSITIS

- Cough
- Rhinorrhea
- Nasal congestion
- Postnasal drip

DISCUSS CHRONIC PEDIATRIC SINUSITIS

- Inflammation of the nose and paranasal sinuses
- Two or more symptoms
  - Nasal blockage or obstruction
  - Nasal congestion and discharge (anterior and posterior)
  - Cough
  - Facial pain or pressure
- Need objective findings on endoscopy and/or CT
- Symptoms last 12 weeks or longer without relief
- May be difficult to differentiate from adenoid hypertrophy or adenoiditis
- Surgical treatment for failed maximum medical therapy
  - Adenoidectomy
  - Sinus irrigation
  - Balloon dilation
  - Functional endoscopic sinus surgery

COMORBID CONDITIONS ASSOCIATED WITH CHRONIC PEDIATRIC SINUSITIS

- Allergic rhinitis
- Asthma
- GERD
- Immunodeficiency and immunoglobulin deficiency
- Primary ciliary dyskinesia, which is diagnosed by mucosal biopsy (nasal or preferably tracheal) with examination of cilia
- Cystic fibrosis
  - Increased viscosity of secretions
  - Nasal polyposis (one of the few causes of polyposis in children)

LUND-MACKAY SYSTEM

- Each sinus (anterior ethmoid, posterior ethmoid, maxillary, frontal, and sphenoid) is scored: 0 (no opacification), 1 (partial opacification), and 2 (total opacification)
- Osteomeatal complex is scored: 0 (not occluded) and 2 (total occluded)
- Right and left sinuses are scored separately and added together
- Lund score ranges from 0 to 24 total

BACTERIOLOGY OF CHRONIC PEDIATRIC SINUSITIS

- Aerobes: alpha-hemolytic streptococci, *S. aureus*, *S. pneumoniae*, *H. influenzae*, and *M. catarrhalis*
- Anaerobes: infrequently identified

VIRUSES MOST COMMONLY ASSOCIATED WITH ACUTE SINUSITIS

- Rhinovirus
- Coronavirus
- Influenza
- RSV
- Parainfluenza

BACTERIOLOGY OF ACUTE SINUSITIS

- *S. pneumoniae*
- *H. influenzae*
- *M. catarrhalis*
- *S. aureus*
- α-Hemolytic Strep

INDICATIONS FOR COMPUTED TOMOGRAPHY SCANNING FOR PEDIATRIC ACUTE SINUSITIS

1. Concern for the presence of a complication of sinusitis
2. Severe illness or toxic condition that does not improve with medical therapy after 48-72 hours
3. Immunocompromise
4. Cystic fibrosis

WHAT FACTORS PREDISPOSE TO FUNCTIONAL ENDOSCOPIC SINUS SURGERY FAILURE REQUIRING REVISION IN PEDIATRICS?

1. Adhesions
2. Maxillary sinus stenosis or missed ostium
3. Sinonasal polyposis
4. History of allergic rhinitis
5. Male gender

SYNDROMES AND ASSOCIATIONS WITH HEAD AND NECK MANIFESTATIONS (NOT PREVIOUSLY DESCRIBED)

ACHONDROPLASIA

- Most common skeletal dysplasia
- Autosomal dominant, and most cases are spontaneous
- Associated with a narrow foramen magnum with the potential for brainstem compression, apnea, otitis, and hearing loss
- Over 50% have persistent OME and require insertion of middle ear tubes
- Disorder of endochondral bone formation: abnormal bones formed from cartilage
- Shortened limbs, frontal bossing, sunken bridge of the nose, midface hypoplasia, maxillary hypoplasia, nasal bone and septal hypoplasia, class 3 malocclusion, and cell-mediated immune deficiencies
- Normal cognitive function

DOWN SYNDROME

- Extra chromosome on no. 21 or no. 22
- Macroglossia/fissured tongue
- Brachycephaly
- Flat occiput

- Upslanting palpebral fissures
- Epicanthic folds
- Narrow ear canals
- Abnormally small ears
- Small nose
- Hypotonia
- Increased association with leukemia
- Increased incidence of subglottic stenosis
- Midface hypoplasia
- Large fissured lips
- Dental abnormalities
- Short neck
- Atlantoaxial subluxation and instability

APERT (ACROCEPHALOSYNDACTYLY), CROUZON (CRANIOFACIAL DYSOSTOSIS), AND PFEIFFER SYNDROMES

- Autosomal dominant, and most cases of Apert are spontaneous
- Findings
  - Craniosynostosis
  - Hypertelorism
  - Exophthalmos
  - Midface hypoplasia
  - Mandibular prognathism
  - Parrot-beaked nose
  - Syndactyly and cervical fusion seen in Apert syndrome
  - Pfeiffer is different from Apert: a different type of hand malformation and digital broadening in Pfeiffer syndrome
- Cognitive function ranges from normal to severe mental retardation

GOLDENHAR SYNDROME (PART OF THE OCULOAURICULOVERTEBRAL SPECTRUM)

- Most cases occur sporadically, and are autosomal recessive or dominant
- Characterized by hemifacial microsomia
  - Unilateral microtia/atresia with conductive loss
  - Facial asymmetry
  - Retrognathia/micrognathia
  - Asymmetric mandibular hypoplasia
  - Microstomia
  - May have a cleft lip/palate
- Also with vertebral anomalies and epibulbar dermoids

HURLER SYNDROME

- Autosomal recessive, as is the case with most mucopolysaccharidoses
- Leads to visceromegaly
- Mucopolysaccharidosis type I: deficiency of α-L-iduronidase
- Facies: coarse facial features and forehead prominence
- Dwarfism
- Mixed hearing loss
- Macroglossia
- Short neck
- Mental retardation
- Skeletal disorders with joint stiffness
- May develop severe obstructive sleep apnea (OSA)
- Progressive neurologic dysfunction

HUNTER SYNDROME

- Similar to Hurler, but is an X-linked disorder
- Incurable syndrome with multiple organ system mucopolysaccharidosis infiltration, usually dying as a teenager from cardiomyopathy

- Mucopolysaccharidosis type II: iduronate sulfatase deficiency
- Facies: prominent supraorbital ridges, large flattened nose, low-set ears, and large jowls
- Short stature
- May develop severe OSA
- Potential difficult airway
  - Short neck
  - Tracheal deposits of glycosaminoglycan leading to airway obstruction

BECKWITH-WIEDEMANN SYNDROME

- Macroglossia, omphalocele, visceromegaly, and cytomegaly of the adrenal cortex
- Result of genomic imprinting
- "Overall growth syndrome," with sporadic occurrence
- Macroglossia may cause airway obstruction or chronic alveolar hypoventilation
- Tongue reduction is effective for those unable to keep the tongue in the mouth

CHARGE SYNDROME

1. Coloboma (75-90%)
2. Heart defects (50-85%)
3. Atresia of the choanae (35-65%)
4. Retardation of growth and/or development
5. Genital hypoplasia/genitourinary defects (50-70%)
6. Ear anomalies and/or deafness (over 90%)

ADENOTONSILLAR PATHOLOGY

ADENOID HYPERTROPHY

- Most common cause of nasal-airway obstruction in children, but not the most common etiology in the neonate
  - Daycare, chronic allergies, and secondary-smoke exposure cause chronic inflammation
  - Best to assess the degree of obstruction with nasopharyngoscopy; lateral neck film is acceptable but is not as comprehensive and has the risk of radiation exposure
- Blood supply
  - Major bleeding after adenoidectomy is rare and can be indicative of an underlying bleeding disorder
  - Pharyngeal branch of the internal maxillary (major supply)
- Innervation: CNIX and CNX; very little pain should be expected after adenoidectomy
- Chronic adenoiditis predisposes to bacterial sinusitis
- Typical child has 6-8 viral URI/year[32]
- Techniques for removal: (1) suction cautery, (2) coblation, and (3) microdebrider

BLOOD SUPPLY TO THE TONSIL

1. Facial artery (tonsillar branch, ascending palatine branch)
2. Dorsal lingual branch of the lingual artery
3. Internal maxillary artery (descending palatine and greater palatine artery)
4. Ascending pharyngeal artery

COMMON CAUSES OF TONSILLITIS AND PHARYNGITIS

- Viral URI (rhinovirus, influenza, parainfluenza, and adenovirus)
- EBV (infectious mononucleosis)

- Transmitted via mucous membrane contact
  - Diagnosis with monospot, heterophile agglutination test
  - Can develop hepatosplenomegaly, so contact sports must to be avoided[33]
  - May develop a rash with amoxicillin
  - Nonsteroidal antiinflammatory drugs (NSAIDs) for pain
  - Consider steroids for obstructive tonsillar hypertrophy
- Group A β-hemolytic Streptococcus
  - 15-30% of children who present with tonsillitis
  - Streptococcal carrier may convert to active infection or spread the infection to another person
  - Diagnosis with rapid antigen detection test and/or throat culture
  - If rapid detection test is negative, proceed with throat culture
  - Antibiotics for a 10-day course
  - Consider tonsillectomy for repeat infections
  - Complications
    - Scarlet fever: generalized, nonpruritic, erythematous macular skin rash lasting 3-7 days, with strawberry tongue, fevers, and arthralgias
    - Rheumatic fever is now rare today; bacterial vegetation grows on mitral and tricuspid valves, resulting in heart murmur, relapsing fevers, and valve regurgitation or stenosis
    - Acute poststreptococcal glomerulonephritis results in generalized edema, hypertension, and hematuria/proteinuria
    - Pediatric autoimmune neuropsychiatric disorders associated with streptococcal infections (PANDAS)
- PFAPA (periodic fever, aphthous stomatitis, pharyngitis, and adenitis) syndrome
  - Constellation of symptoms, fevers lasting several days, constitutional symptoms
  - Critical to exclude autoimmune disorders and immunodeficiency (HIV) before arriving at PFAPA diagnosis
  - High fevers every 3-8 weeks
  - Associated with pharyngitis, aphthous stomatitis, and cervical adenitis
  - Treat with NSAIDs and consider steroids and tonsillectomy
  - Adenotonsillectomy is highly effective at resolving this condition[34]

PERITONSILLAR ABSCESS AND ITS MANAGEMENT

- Symptoms: severe unilateral sore throat, odynophagia, severe pain when ipsilateral soft palate is probed with a tonsil blade, drooling, muffled voice, trismus, and referred otalgia
- Exam: uvular deviation, drooling, and muffled voice
- Initial management of peritonsillar abscess
  - Hydration
  - Pain control
  - Antibiotics
  - Steroids to improve trismus
  - Incision and drainage or needle aspiration
  - Quinsey tonsillectomy
- Subsequent management for recurrence
  - CT scan
  - Repeat incision and drainage
  - Quinsey tonsillectomy
- Complications
  - Dehydration
  - Airway obstruction
  - Sepsis

- Spread to other neck spaces
- Great vessel injury (external and internal carotid artery)

CAUSES OF SUBACUTE OR CHRONIC UNILATERAL TONSILLAR HYPERTROPHY

- Ideopathic
- Neoplastic: lymphoma
- Infectious
  - Mycobacterium tuberculosis
  - Atypical mycobacteria
  - Actinomycosis
  - Fungal

GENERAL CRITERIA FOR ABNORMAL POLYSOMNOGRAM IN PEDIATRIC OBSTRUCTIVE SLEEP APNEA

- Apnea hypopnea index (AHI) >1
  - Mild: 1-5
  - Moderate: 5-10
  - Severe: >10
- Oxygen desaturation to below 92%
- Peak end tidal CO_2 >53 mm Hg
- Elevated end tidal CO_2 >50 mm Hg >10% of total sleep time

COMMON FACTORS INFLUENCING PEDIATRIC OSA

- Hypertrophied adenotonsillar tissue
- Obesity
- Craniofacial abnormalities particularly involving the mandible or maxilla (midface)
- Neuromuscular disease

HIGH-RISK GROUPS FOR PEDIATRIC OSA

- Obesity, body mass index >30
- Craniofacial abnormalities: achondroplasia, Pierre Robin sequence, and hemifacial microsomia
- Neuromuscular disease: cerebral palsy
- Down syndrome
- Mucopolysaccharidoses: Hunter or Hurler syndromes

DIFFERENCES IN ADULT AND PEDIATRIC OBSTRUCTIVE SLEEP APNEA

- FTT and enuresis seen in pediatrics
- Academic, social, emotional, and behavioral changes seen in pediatrics (poor school performance, hyperactivity, attention deficit, and aggression)

INDICATIONS FOR TONSILLECTOMY

- Infection
  - Recurrent acute infections 7 in 1 year, 5 per year for 2 years, and 3 per year for 3 or more years
  - Recurrent acute infections with complications (cardiac valve disease and febrile seizures)
  - Streptococcus carrier
  - Peritonsillar abscess
  - Mononucleosis with obstructing tonsils unresponsive to therapy
  - Chronic tonsillitis associated with halitosis, persistent sore throat, and cervical adenitis (controversial)
- Obstruction

- Sleep disordered breathing
- OSA
- Cor pulmonale
- FTT and dysphagia
- Craniofacial growth abnormalities
- Speech/occlusion abnormalities (controversial)
- Other
  - Suspicion of malignancy
  - PFAPA (periodic fever and aphthous ulcers)

CRITERIA THAT SHOULD SUGGEST AN OVERNIGHT STAY AFTER TONSILLECTOMY BECAUSE SOME PATIENTS HAVE WORSE AIRWAY OBSTRUCTION AFTER SURGERY

- Severe pediatric OSA (AHI >10)
- Cerebral palsy
- Under 3 years of age
- Weight under 15 kg
- Craniofacial abnormalities
- Medical comorbidity (eg, diabetes, seizures, Down syndrome, asthma, cardiac disease)
- Emesis or hemorrhage during or after surgery
- Long distance (over 1 hour) between home and the nearest hospital

SYMPTOMS, SIGNS, AND MANAGEMENT OF POSTOBSTRUCTIVE PULMONARY EDEMA

- Clinical:
  - Hypoxemia
  - Increased work of breathing
  - Pink frothy oral or tracheal secretions
  - Bilateral end expiratory wheezing and rales
  - CXR findings showing increased pulmonary markings and fluid overload
- Treatment
  - Oxygen therapy
  - Continuous positive airway pressure and possible intubation
  - IV fluid restriction
  - Diuretics
  - Consider steroids

INDICATIONS FOR FOLLOW-UP POLYSOMNOGRAM AFTER SURGERY FOR PEDIATRIC OBSTRUCTIVE SLEEP APNEA

- Persistent sleep-disordered breathing
- Preoperative apnea/hypopnea index (AHI >20)
- Preoperative complication of severe OSA (eg, pulmonary hypertension)
- Age <1 year

INDICATIONS FOR ADENOIDECTOMY (WITH DOCUMENTED ADENOID HYPERTROPHY)

- Infection
  - Recurrent/chronic adenoiditis or sinusitis
  - Second set of tympanostomy tubes
  - Chronic otitis media with or without effusion after 4 years of age
- Obstruction
  - Chronic nasal obstruction or obligate mouth breathing

- OSA or sleep-disordered breathing
- Craniofacial growth abnormalities
- "Slack jaw" or "adenoid" faces
- Dental occlusion abnormalities
- Hyponasal speech
- Before VPI surgery, in the setting of a pharyngeal flap, or to alleviate secondary nasal obstruction
- Suspected neoplasm

COMPLICATIONS OF ADENOTONSILLECTOMY

- Primary postoperative hemorrhage within 24 hours
- Secondary postoperative hemorrhage, between POD 1 to 14
- Bleeding history is most important in determination of preoperative risk; coagulation testing before tonsillectomy and adenoidectomy is not cost effective[35]
- Dehydration (minimal voiding in 12-24 hours)
- Tylenol with codeine hypermetabolizer leading to metabolically induced narcotic overdose
- Postoperative pulmonary edema: loss of auto-PEEP from chronic obstruction and loss of hypercapnic respiratory drive (may be seen with severe OSA)
- Mandibular dislocation
- Velopharyngeal insufficiency (may occur after adenoidectomy)
- NP stenosis (rare)
- Nontraumatic atlantoaxial subluxation (Grisel syndrome)
  - Results from C1-C2 subluxation with prevertebral inflammation
  - Complication following adenoidectomy, oftentimes inflammation and infection related to electrocautery[36]
  - Prolonged neck pain and stiffness for 2 weeks or more; head rotated away from the side where the atlas has shifted
  - Diagnosis confirmed with CT of the cervical spin
  - Treat with antiinflammatory medication and soft diet
  - May need neck immobilization (cervical collar)

RISK FACTORS FOR VELOPHARYNGEAL INSUFFICIENCY AFTER ADENOIDECTOMY

- VPI that fails to resolve in 8 weeks; patient should undergo speech therapy
- Occult submucous cleft
- Neuromuscular disorders (CNS)
- History of nasopharyngeal regurgitation before surgery

REFERENCES

1. Cotton RT, Gluckman JL, Seiden AM, Tami TA, Pensak ML. *Otolaryngology: The Essentials*. 1st ed. New York, NY: Thieme; 2001.
2. Schilder AGM, Bhutta MF, Butler CC, et al. Eustachian tube dysfunction: consensus statement on definition, types, clinical presentation and diagnosis. *Clin Otolaryngol*. 2015;40(5):307–411.
3. Miller BJ, Elhassan HA. Balloon dilatation of the Eustachian tube: an evidence-based review of case series for those considering its use. *Clin Otolaryngol*. 2013;38(6):525–532.
4. Tewfik TL, Singh H. *Eustachian tube dysfunction [eMedicine]*; 2016. http://emedicine.medscape.com/article/874348-overview. Accessed March 30, 2016.
5. Mansour S, Magnan J, Haidar H, Nicolas K, Louryan S. *Comprehensive and Clinical Anatomy of the Middle Ear*. Heidelberg: Springer; 2013.
6. Niparko JK. *Cochlear Implants: Principles and Practices*. Philadelphia, PA: Lippincott Williams & Wilkins; 2000.
7. Gross M, Eliashar R, Eiidan J. Michel's aplasia. *Otol Neurotol*. 2005;26(3):547.
8. Yu KK, Mukherji S, Carrasco V, et al. Molecular genetic advances in semicircular canal abnormalities and sensorineural hearing loss: a report of 16 cases. *Otolaryngol Head Neck Surg*. 2003;129(6):637–646.

9. Zhou G, Gopen Q, Kenna MA. Delineating the hearing loss in children with enlarged vestibular aqueduct. *Laryngoscope.* 2008;118(11):2062–2066.

10. Bhattacharyya N. *Auditory brainstem response audiometry [eMedicine]*; 2016. http://emedicine.medscape.com/article/836277-overview. Accessed March 30, 2016.

11. Jasper KM, Gaudreau P, Cartee TV, Reilly BK. Collodion baby: a unique challenge for newborn hearing screening. *Am J Otolaryngol.* 2016;37(3):263–264.

12. Wetmore RF, Muntz HR, McGill TJI. *Pediatric Otolaryngology: Principles and Practice Pathways.* New York, NY: Thieme; 2012:292–293.

13. Fitoz S, Sennarogablu L, Incesulu A, et al. SLC26A4 mutations are associated with a specific inner ear malformation. *Int J Pediatr Otorhinolaryngol.* 2007;71(3):479–486.

14. Cureoglu S, Schachern PA, Paperella MM. Scheibe dysplasia. *Otol Neurotol.* 2003;24(1):125–126.

15. Lee KJ. *Essential Otolaryngology: Head and Neck Surgery.* 8th ed. New York, NY: McGraw-Hill; 2003.

16. Graham JM, Scadding GK, Bull PD. *Pediatric ENT.* Berlin and New York, NY: Springer; 2003.

17. Colletti L. Beneficial auditory and cognitive effects of auditory brainstem implantation in children. *Acta Otolaryngol.* 2007;127(9):943–946.

18. Phelps PD, Coffey RA, Trembath RC, et al. Radiological malformations of the ear in Pendred syndrome. *Clin Radiol.* 1998;53(4):268–273.

19. Goldenberg I, Moss AJ, Zareba W, et al. Clinical course and risk stratification of patients with Jervell and Lange-Nielsen syndrome. *J Cardiovasc Electrophysiol.* 2006;17(11):1161–1168.

20. Kaplan J, Gerber S, Bonneau D, et al. A gene for Usher syndrome type 1 (USH1A) maps to chromosome 14q. *Genomics.* 1992;14(4):979–987.

21. Kimberling WJ, Weston MD, Moller C, et al. Localization of Usher syndrome type 2 to chromosome 1q. *Genomics.* 1990;7(2):245–249.

22. Mathur P, Yang J. Usher syndrome: hearing loss, retinal degeneration and associated abnormalities. *Biochim Biophys Acta.* 2015;1852(3):406–420.

23. Savige J, Colville D. Opinion: ocular features aid the diagnosis of Alport syndrome. *Nat Rev Nephrol.* 2009;5(6):356–360.

24. El-Dessouky M, Azmy AF, Raine PA, Young DG. Kasabach-Merritt syndrome. *J Pediatri Surg.* 1998;23(2):109–111.

25. Weiner MA, Leventhal BG, Marcus R, et al. Intensive chemotherapy and low-dose radiotherapy for the treatment of advanced-stage Hodgkin's disease in pediatric patients: a Pediatric Oncology Group Study. *J Clin Oncol.* 1991;9(9):1591–1598.

26. Smith RS, Chen Q, Hudson MM, et al. Prognostic factors for children with Hodgkin's disease treated with combined-modality therapy. *J Clin Oncol.* 2003;21(10):2026–2033.

27. Sandlund JT, Downing JR, Crist WM. Non-Hodgkin's lymphoma in childhood. *N Engl J Med.* 1996;334(19):1238–1248.

28. Huh WW, Skapek SX. Childhood rhabdomyosarcoma: new insight on biology and treatment. *Curr Oncol Rep.* 2010;12(6):402–410.

29. Reilly BK, Kim A, Pena MT, et al. Rhabdomyosarcoma of the head and neck in children: review and update. *Int J Pediatr Otolaryngol.* 2015;79(9):1477–1483.

30. Lawrence Jr W, Anderson JR, Gehan EA, Maurer H. Pretreatment TNM staging of childhood rhabdomysarcoma: a report of the Intergroup Rhabdomyosarcoma Study Group. Children's Cancer Study Group. Pediatric Oncology Group. *Cancer.* 1997;80:1165–1170.

31. http://www.ncbi.nlm.nih.gov/pubmed/18496162/

32. Wald ER, Guerra N, Byers C. Upper respiratory tract infections in young children: duration of and frequency of complications. *Pediatrics.* 1991;87(2):129–133.

33. Chetham MM, Roberts KB. Infectious monocucleosis in adolescents. *Pediatr Ann.* 1991;20(4):206–213.

34. Licameli G, Jeffrey J, Luz J, et al. Effect of adenotonsillectomy in PFAPA syndrome. *Arch Otolaryngol Head Neck Surg.* 2008;134(2):136–140.

35. Cooper JD, Smith KJ, Ritchey AK. A cost-effective analysis of the coagulation testing prior to tonsillectomy and adenoidectomy in children. *Pediatr Blood Cancer.* 2010;55(6):1153–1159.

36. Tschopp K. Monopolar electrocautery in adenoidectomy as a possible risk factor for Grisel's syndrome. *Laryngoscope.* 2002;112:1445–1449.

Laryngology | 7

LARYNGEAL AND PHARYNGEAL FUNCTION

Three functions of the larynx
1. Voice
2. Respiration
3. Deglutition

The only laryngeal abductor (Fig. 7.1) is the posterior crico-arytenoid (PCA).
- Attaches the cricoid to the muscular process of the arytenoid
- Pulls the muscular process posteriorly and caudally, rotating the vocal process laterally and upward

The only internal muscle of the larynx not supplied by the recurrent laryngeal nerve (RLN) is the cricothyroid (supplied by the external branch of the superior laryngeal nerve [SLN]).

Primary function of the internal branch of the SLN
- Sensation to the supraglottis

What is the myoelastic-aerodynamic theory?[1]
- Interaction of aerodynamic forces and the mechanical properties of the laryngeal tissues are responsible for inducing vocal fold vibration and generating vocal sound

What are the three components of sound creation?
1. Power source: the lungs
2. Vibrator/vibratory source: the larynx
3. Resonator: *supraglottal vocal tract*, including the supra-glottic larynx, pharynx, oral cavity, and potentially the nasal cavity

What is the best method for assessing vocal fold vibration?
- Laryngeal stroboscopy at multiple frequencies and intensities

What are the functions of the extrinsic muscles of the larynx in voice production?
1. Alter the position of the larynx, which in turn can affect the length of the vocal tract resonator
2. Stabilize the larynx within the neck when singing[2]

What are the functions of the intrinsic muscles of the larynx in voice production?
1. Adduction and abduction
2. Fine changes in tension of the vocal folds

What are the three histologic layers of the vocal fold?
1. Cover
2. Transition zone or vocal ligament
3. Body

What are the components of the vocal fold cover?
1. Squamous epithelium
2. Superficial layer of the lamina propria (Reinke space)
    - Composed of fibroblasts that produce proteins and glycoproteins
    - Forms an extracellular matrix of loose connective tissue

What are the components of the vocal fold transition zone or vocal ligament?
1. Intermediate layer of the lamina propria (comprised of elastin)
2. Deep layers of the lamina propria

What are the components of the vocal fold body?
- Thyroarytenoid muscle[3] (Fig. 7.2)

Vocal fold layers from medial to lateral
- Squamous epithelium
- Superficial layer of the lamina propria
- Vocal ligament

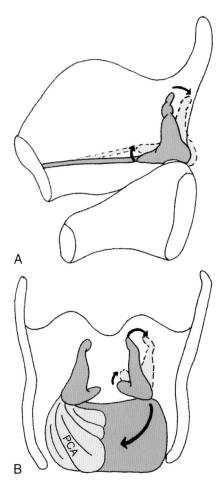

FIGURE 7.1 Three-Dimensional Effects of Posterior Cricoarytenoid Muscle Contraction. (**A**) Sagittal view. (**B**) Posterior view. (From Flint PW, Haughey BH, Lund VJ, et al. *Cummings Otolaryngology—Head and Neck Surgery.* 6th ed. Philadelphia, PA: Saunders; 2015, fig. 54-3.)

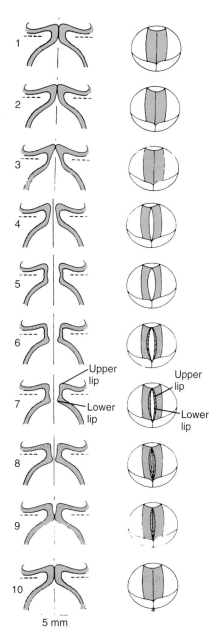

FIGURE 7.2 Movements of different portions of vocal folds during one cycle of vibration shown schematically in the coronal plane (*left*) and from above (*right*). Mucosal upheaval begins caudally (*1*) and then moves rostrally. The lower portion is closing as the upper margin is opening (*5*). (From Hirano M. *Clinical Examination of Voice.* New York, NY: Springer-Verlag; 1981; and Flint PW, Haughey BH, Lund VJ, et al. *Cummings Otolaryngology—Head and Neck Surgery.* 6th ed. Philadelphia, PA: Saunders; 2015, fig. 54-11.)

- Thyroarytenoid muscle
- Perichondrium and thyroid cartilage provides the lateral boundary of the vocal fold (Fig. 7.3)

VISUALIZATION OF THE LARYNX

Indirect Methods of Visualize the Larynx
1. Mirror laryngoscopy
2. Rigid indirect laryngoscopy
3. Flexible indirect laryngoscopy

Benefits of Rigid Indirect Laryngoscopy
1. Higher resolution
2. Brighter, clearer picture

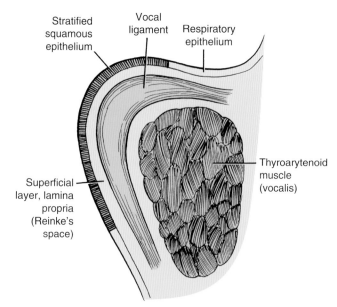

FIGURE 7.3 Cross Section of the Vocal Fold. (From Flint PW, Haughey BH, Lund VJ, et al. *Cummings Otolaryngology—Head and Neck Surgery.* 6th ed. Philadelphia, PA: Saunders; 2015, fig. 61-1.)

3. Image is more accurately magnified
4. Generally does not require topical anesthesia

Drawbacks of Rigid Indirect Laryngoscopy
1. Cannot visualize the larynx while patient performs complex speaking tasks
2. May be difficult to visualize arytenoid abduction/adduction in certain patients

Benefits of Flexible Indirect Laryngoscopy
1. Can visualize the larynx during speaking/singing tasks
2. The larynx is in a more natural configuration for neurological evaluation

Drawbacks of Flexible Indirect Laryngoscopy
1. Generally requires topical anesthesia
2. Distortion at the periphery of the image
3. Inferior light transport/magnification versus rigid

Key Structures and Finding to Be Evaluated with Laryngopharyngeal Endoscopy
1. Overall structure of vocal folds
   - Bowed (atrophy)
   - Scar/sulcus deformity
2. Masses or lesions
3. Abduction and adduction of true vocal folds
   - Vocal fold paresis/paralysis
   - Cricoarytenoid joint fixation
   - Posterior glottic stenosis
4. Supraglottic configuration
   - Relaxed: can see the whole vocal fold
   - Asymmetric: may imply paresis or be seen with paralysis
   - Symmetric: may be a normal variant or muscle tension dysphonia (MTD)
5. Pooling of secretions
   - Vallecula: consider tongue-base weakness
   - Piriform sinuses/postcricoid region
     - Pharyngeal weakness
     - Lack of sensation/neurologic deficit
     - Esophageal obstruction: see the dysphagia/esophageal section

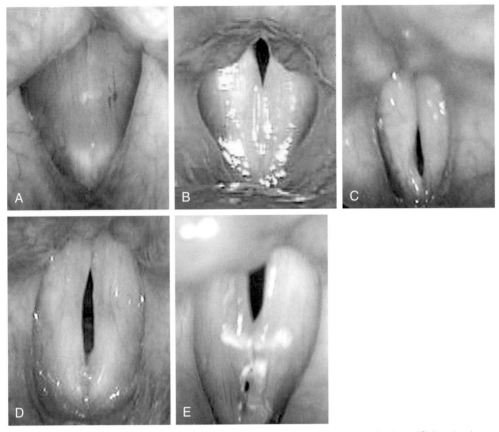

FIGURE 7.4 Glottal Closure and Gap Patterns. (**A**) Complete closure. (**B**) Posterior glottal gap. (**C**) Anterior glottal gap. (**D**) Spindle-shaped gap. (**E**) Hourglass-shaped gap. (From Flint PW, Haughey BH, Lund VJ, et al. *Cummings Otolaryngology—Head and Neck Surgery*. 6th ed. Philadelphia, PA: Saunders; 2015, fig. 55-3.)

Videostroboscopy Basics
- Used to assess vocal fold vibration
- Microphone uses pitch to calculate frequency of vocal fold vibration
- Strobe light set just off frequency to catch the vocal fold at various phases of vibration
- "Flip book" effect
- Requires a long enough phonatory segment to trigger the strobe light
- Cannot provide information about the phonation onset and offset, which are very short and irregular

Components of Stroboscopy Grading
1. Mucosal wave
   - Vertical upheaval of the vocal fold cover over the vocal fold body
   - Should cover approximately ½ of the superior surface of the true vocal fold
2. Amplitude of vibration
   - Lateral excursion of the vocal fold
   - Should be approximately ⅓ the width of the true vocal fold[4]
3. Vertical phase
   - Timing difference between the superior and inferior portions of the vocal fold
   - Inferior portion of the fold leads the superior portion in its movement away from and back to the midline
4. Phase symmetry
   - Symmetry of the motion of one vocal fold compared with the other vocal fold
5. Regularity/periodicity
   - Does one wave look the same as the next?

6. Adynamic segments
   - From scarring, sulcus, or cyst
   - May be seen better with high-speed digital imaging
7. Closure

Vocal Fold Closure Patterns (Fig. 7.4)
1. Complete
2. Anterior/posterior gap
   - May be a normal variant (females may have a posterior gap)
   - Postsurgical defect
   - Scar/sulcus
3. Spindle shaped
   - Bowed vocal folds from atrophy or presbylarynges
4. Hourglass
   - Seen with vocal fold nodules, prenodular edema, or a polyp/cyst with a reactive lesion

Voice Evaluation
History Evaluation for the Patient with Hoarseness
1. Onset and duration of symptoms (eg, upper-respiratory infection [URI] or screaming)
2. Perceived cause
3. Relapse/remit or constant
4. What makes it better and what makes it worse?
5. Does the patient have difficulty with swallowing, breathing, coughing, or throat clearing?
6. Pain
7. Occupation
8. Reflux
9. Talkativeness profile (intrinsic, personality-based tendency to use voice)

10. Vocal commitments or activities (extrinsic requirement, invitation, or opportunity to use voice), including voice type and training if the patient is a performer
11. Vocal abuse
12. Smoker/drinker
13. Hydration status
14. History of intubation
15. Psychological stressors
16. Neurologic history
17. Pulmonary history

Past Medical History Evaluation of a Patient with Hoarseness

1. Neurologic disorders
2. Head and neck/esophageal cancer history and risk factors
3. Reflux/treatment of such
4. Surgical history: especially spine surgery/head and neck surgery
5. Use of medications, including immunosuppressants

Voice Patient Physical Examination

1. Complete head and neck exam with special attention to cranial nerves and nasal exam
2. Palpate laryngeal framework: assess for tension (Fig. 7.5)
   a. There should be palpable space between the thyroid cartilage and hyoid bone
   b. There should be good lateral laryngeal mobility[5]
3. Assess voice quality with a perceptual assessment of vocal capabilities and limitations, particularly through elicitation of vocal tasks designed to detect mucosal disturbances
4. Laryngopharyngeal endoscopy
5. Stroboscopy

Objective Tools for Voice Assessment

1. Aerodynamic measurements
2. Acoustic measurements
3. Auditory perceptual assessment

Aerodynamic Measurements

1. Subglottal air pressure
   * Pressure required to sustain vocal fold vibration
   * Usually measured indirectly, transorally to avoid tracheal puncture
2. Phonation threshold pressure
   * Pressure required to initiate vocal fold vibration
   * Often corresponds to patient's sensation of vocal effort
   * Changes with viscoelastic changes in the vocal fold
3. Airflow
   * Mean flow of air (milliliter/second) during phonation

* May increase with vocal fold paralysis
* May decreased with maximum phonation time (MPT)
4. Laryngeal airway resistance
   * Ratio of translaryngeal air pressure to laryngeal airflow
5. MPT
   * Maximum time the patient can sustain phonation
   * Normal MPT: female 15-25 seconds and male 25-35 seconds[6]

Acoustic Measurements

1. Fundamental frequency (F_0)
   * Number of repeating cycles per second in the acoustic waveform
   * Pitch is a correlate of this
   * Voice disorders may manifest as altered or restricted pitch
2. Intensity
   * Loudness, measured in dB sound pressure level (SPL)
   * Conversational voice is generally approximately 70 dB SPL
3. Jitter
   * Cycle-to-cycle variation in *pitch/frequency*
   * Has not been shown to correspond to voice disorders
4. Shimmer
   * Cycle-to-cycle variation in *amplitude/loudness*
   * Has not been shown to correspond to voice disorders

Vocal Tasks to Be Performed for Assessment

* Average or anchor speech frequency
* Maximum frequency range
* Projected voice and yell
* Very-high-frequency, very-low-intensity tasks that detect mucosal disturbances
* Register use and phenomena
* MPT
* Instability and tremors
* Inconsistencies between spoken and sung capabilities

Auditory Perceptual Assessment

* Grading of voice by the trained listener
* Grade, Roughness, Breathiness, Asthenia, Strain (GRBAS) scale
* Consensus auditory-perceptual-evaluation-voice (CAPE-V)

GRBAS Scale, Graded from 0 to 3

1. Grade: overall severity
2. Roughness
3. Breathiness
4. Asthenia
5. Strain

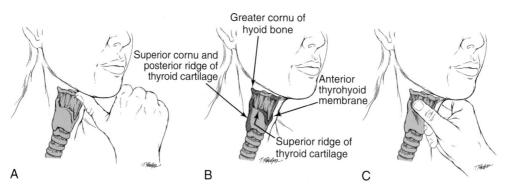

FIGURE 7.5 Manual Musculoskeletal Tension Evaluation. (**A**) Palpation of suprahyoid musculature. (**B**) Palpation of greater cornu of the hyoid bone, superior cornu of the thyroid cartilage, and lateral aspects of the thyroid cartilage. (**C**) Palpation of the thyrohyoid space. (From Flint PW, Haughey BH, Lund VJ, et al. *Cummings Otolaryngology—Head and Neck Surgery.* 6th ed. Philadelphia, PA: Saunders; 2015, fig. 56-4.)

CAPE-V, Rated by Marking Severity Along a 100-mm Line[7]

1. Overall severity
2. Roughness
3. Breathiness
4. Strain
5. Pitch
6. Loudness

NEUROLOGIC EVALUATION OF THE LARYNX

HISTORY ASSESSMENT FOR THE PATIENT WITH NEW-ONSET DYSARTHRIA

- History of neurologic defects (eg, cerebrovascular accident [CVA])
- History of neuromuscular disease (eg, amyotrophic lateral sclerosis [ALS]/Parkinson disease [PD])
- Presence of other areas of weakness
- Gait instability
- Dysphagia for solids and/or liquids

PHYSICAL EXAMINATION FOR THE PATIENT WITH NEW-ONSET DYSARTHRIA

1. Gross-motion clues of the oral cavity and oropharynx
   - Involuntary, slow, athetoid movements: tardive dyskinesia
   - Tongue with "bag of worms" appearance: ALS
   - Spasmodic motion of the tongue and jaw: oromandibular dystonia
   - Regular, repetitive jerking motions of the palate and/or pharynx: myoclonus
   - Soft voice that responds well to cuing: PD
2. Test lip motion: repeat "Pa"
3. Test tongue motion: repeat "Ta"
4. Test posterior tongue motion: repeat "Ga"
   - Decreased strength of action: lower motor neuron
   - Reduced rate with rhythm preserved: upper motor neuron
   - Erratic rhythm: cerebellar lesion
   - Fatigue: myasthenia gravis
5. Flexible laryngoscopy indications of poor swallow
   - Impaired pharyngeal squeeze
   - Pooling of secretions in the hypopharynx[8-10]

LARYNGEAL ELECTROMYOGRAPHY BASICS

- Assess integrity of RLN (paralysis vs. cricoarytenoid dislocation)
- May offer prognostic information in early paralysis
- Laryngeal electromyography (LEMG) will more often accurately predict poor prognosis in the setting of poor LEMG findings compared with predicting a good prognosis in the setting of positive LEMG findings[11]

COMMON LARYNGEAL ELECTROMYOGRAPHY FINDINGS

- Intact cricothyroid signal but absent thyroarytenoid signal: RLN injury but intact vagus nerve and SLN
- Fibrillation potentials with decreased activity: denervation
- Polyphasic action potentials: reinnervation
- Fatiguing: myasthenia gravis
- Decreased frequency: neuropathy
- Decreased amplitude: myopathy

NEUROLOGIC DISORDERS OF THE LARYNX

DIFFERENTIAL DIAGNOSIS FOR VOCAL INSTABILITY WITH NORMAL VOCAL STRUCTURE AND FULL ABDUCTION AND ADDUCTION OF THE TRUE VOCAL FOLDS

1. Spasmodic dysphonia (SD)
2. Vocal tremor (benign essential tremor)
3. MTD
4. Underlying neurologic disease

SPASMODIC DYSPHONIA DIAGNOSTIC FEATURES

- Unstable voice that improves with whispering, singing, or alcohol consumption
- May worsen with stress
- If voice is unstable through multiple sounds, with whisper and with singing, consider vocal tremor versus MTD
- 16% of SD patients will have another dystonia; 10% of SD cases are familial
- Consider Meige syndrome: dystonia of the eyelid, tongue, floor of mouth, and masseter, with 25% laryngeal involvement

ADDUCTOR SPASMODIC DYSPHONIA

- 87% of SD cases
- Choked, strangled-strained voice with abrupt initiation/ termination from thyroarytenoids (TA)/lateral cricoarytenoids (LCAs) dysfunction
- More with voiced vowels: "We eat eggs every Easter."
- Treatment: botulinum toxin to one or both TA muscles under electromyography (EMG) guidance
  - Demonstrated to improve speaking to mean 90% of normal function, with duration of effect between 3 and 4 months[12]

ABDUCTOR SPASMODIC DYSPHONIA

- 12% of SD cases
- Breathy, effortful voice with breaks; whispered segments of speech from PCA dysfunction
- Seen more in phrases with voiceless consonants: "Harry's happy hat"
- Treatment: botulinum toxin to one or both PCA muscles
- Return to mean maximal functional performance of 70% of normal[13]

BOTULINUM TOXIN BASICS

- Works by blocking presynaptic release of acetylcholine
- Recovery because of new nerve-terminal sprouting and increase in postjunctional receptors
- Potentiated by aminoglycosides
- Contraindicated in myasthenia gravis, Eaton-Lambert syndrome, and pregnancy

VOCAL TREMOR (BENIGN ESSENTIAL TREMOR)

- Tremoring persists with whisper, not sound specific, with vowel phonation
- Rhythmic at 6-8 Hz
- May have tremor elsewhere (eg, hands and head)

- 10-20% of patients with essential tremor will have vocal involvement[14]
- Treatment: B-blocker, primidone is considered first-line therapy
- Botulinum toxin injections to thyroarytenoid have also been shown to be effective[15]

OCULOPALATOPHARYNGEAL MYOCLONUS

- Rhythmic contractions of the palate, larynx, and pharynx at a rate of approximately 1-2/second
- Can involve the tensor veli palatine, causing repeating clicking noise
- Treated with botulinum toxin

PARKINSON'S DISEASE

- Systemic: resting tremor, rigidity, bradykinesia, and loss of postural reflexes
- Voice: soft, breathy, stimulable to loud voice
- May have bowed or adynamic vocal folds
- "Parkinson plus" (multisystem atrophy/progressive supranuclear palsy), may have unilateral vocal fold immobility

MUSCLE TENSION DYSPHONIA

- Strained, strangled voice with all sounds
- May cause a breathiness or a choppiness imitating a tremor or SD
- Treatment: voice therapy

HISTORY EVALUATION FOR THE VOCAL FOLD–MOTION-IMPAIRMENT PATIENT

1. Recent surgery, specifically thyroid, cardiothoracic, or cervical spine surgery
2. Breathing or swallowing complaints or other signs and symptoms of lung, thyroid, or esophageal malignancy
3. History of intubations
4. History of rheumatoid disease

POSSIBLE LARYNGEAL PATHOLOGIES CAUSED BY INTUBATION

1. Cricoarytenoid fixation
2. Posterior glottic stenosis
3. Vocal cord paralysis

VOCAL FOLD–MOTION-IMPAIRMENT PATIENT VOICE CHARACTERISTICS

1. Breathy quality
2. Phonatory dyspnea: patient runs out of air while talking
3. Decreased MPT (normal range: 20-25 seconds)

VOCAL FOLD–MOTION-IMPAIRMENT PATIENT WORKUP

1. Direct laryngoscopy and bronchoscopy in the operating room to assess for cricoarytenoid joint dislocation/fixation
2. Imaging: computed tomography with contrast of full course of RLNs, from the skull base to the aortic arch if no other temporal cause
3. Laboratory tests

PROFESSIONAL VOICE

Constituents in Professional Voice User Evaluation and Treatment Team

- Laryngologist
- Speech language pathologist
- Vocal pedagogue

Ways to Increase Subglottic Pressure and Sound Intensity

1. Increase airflow: more efficient
2. Increase force of vocal fold adduction: less efficient

Key Past Medical History Evaluation for a Professional Voice User

- Pulmonary status: pulmonary disease and medications, especially inhalers
- Hydration: diuretics and oral hydration
  - Singer should be taking at least 8 glasses (64 oz) of water per day
- Posture: musculoskeletal issues that may affect the vocal tract
- Personal habits
  - Caffeine and alcohol intake (diuretics)
  - High-fat, dairy diets will thicken mucus
- Thyroid function: may alter Reinke space

Key Physical Examination Components for a Professional Voice User

- Complete head and neck examination
- Nasal examination: obstruction may lead to mouth breathing and dry-air exposure to the larynx
- Anterior neck/strap muscle palpation: examine for excess tension
- Laryngeal endoscopy or stroboscopy

Vocal Misuse Basics

- Inefficient and/or excessive voice production when voice is produced with excess laryngeal tension or insufficient respiratory support
- Maladaptive patterns may begin with acute change, such as a URI

Treatment for the Singer with Laryngitis

- Voice rest: cancel performance if laryngitis is severe
- Hydration
- Antitussives for a prominent cough
- If patient chooses to perform, inform of the increased risk of hemorrhage and potential for permanent damage to the vocal folds

Indications to Cancel Singing Performance

1. Submucosal vocal fold hemorrhage
2. Enlarging varix
3. Vocal fold mucosal break
4. Severe laryngitis

Medications to Be Avoided by a Professional Singer

- Inhaled steroids
- Antihistamines
- Aspirin
- Decongestants
- Topical analgesics
- Mentholated products

Indications for Systemic Steroids for a Professional Singer

- Edema from episodic overuse

- Mild to moderate laryngitis
- Vocal fold hemorrhage

LASER SURGERY: BASIC PRINCIPLES AND SAFETY CONSIDERATIONS

Three Properties of Light Amplification by Stimulated Emission of Radiation Light (Fig. 7.6)

1. Monochromatic: single color, same wavelength
2. Collimated: emits organized light in the same direction
3. Coherent: in space and time

Light Amplification by Stimulated Emission of Radiation Basics

- Light amplification by stimulated emission of radiation (LASER) has an optical resonating chamber that contains medium (eg, argon or carbon dioxide [CO_2]) between two mirrors
- Medium is excited by a current
- Lens-focused beam to a small spot size
- Helium-neon visible aiming beam allows for visualization of wavelength in the nonvisible range

Three Variables in the Surgeon's Control

1. Power (watts)
2. Spot size (square millimeters or centimeters)
3. Exposure time (seconds)

Key LASER Formulas

- Irradiance (W/cm^2) = power/focal spot area
- Fluence (J/cm^2) = energy/target tissue = power density × time

LASER: Tissue Interactions

1. Reflection
2. Absorption (surgical interaction)
3. Transmission
4. Scattering

Argon Laser

- Blue-green light: 488 and 514 nm (tunable argon to 630 nm)
- Transmitted through clear aqueous tissues (eg, cornea, lens, and vitreous humor)
- Absorbed and reflected to varying degrees by tissues that are white in color (eg, skin, fat, and bone)
- Absorbed by hemoglobin and pigmented tissues
- Clinical use examples: stapedotomy, port wine stains, hemangiomas, telangiectasias, and photodynamic therapy
- Drawbacks: heat produced destroys the epidermis and upper dermis

Neodymium:Yttrium-Aluminum-Garnet LASER

- Near infrared: 1064 nm
- Transmitted through clear liquids
- Increased absorption in darkly pigmented tissues and charred debris
- Strong scattering leads to a zone of thermal coagulation and necrosis of approximately 4 mm
- Clinical use examples: ablation of tracheobronchial and esophageal lesions and photocoagulation of vascular and lymphatic malformations
- Benefit: control of hemorrhage is more secure because of the LASER beam's deep penetration in tissue
- Drawback: lacks precision

Carbon Dioxide

- 10,600 nm infrared, HeNe aiming beam
- Absorbed by water
- 60 and 65°C (140-149°F), protein denaturation occurs
  - Tissue effect: blanching
- > 100°C (212°F), vaporization of intracellular water occurs, craters, and tissue shrinkage
  - Tissue effect: carbonization, smoke, and gas generation
- Impact:
  - Zone of thermal necrosis about 100 µm wide
  - Adjacent zone of thermal conductivity and repair, which is usually 300-500 µm wide
  - Less postoperative edema, likely because heat seals vessels
- Minimize thermal damage by using a shorter pulse
- Can be used with micromanipulator, with pattern generator, or with flexible waveguide
- Clinical use examples: stapedotomy, cosmetic skin treatment, laryngology, and bronchoesophagology (cordotomy, medial arytenoidectomy, or total arytenoidectomy)
- Very precise, with increased hemostasis and decreased intraoperative edema

Potassium-Titanyl-Phosphate Laser

- 532 nm
- Absorbed by hemoglobin, specifically oxyhemoglobin
- Clinical use: otologic, rhinologic, and laryngologic surgery; tonsillectomy, pigmented dermal lesions, and stapes surgery
- Pulsed mode to decrease thermal damage
- Fiber based

Pulsed Dye Laser

- 585 nm
- Chromophore for the pulsed dye laser (PDL) is oxyhemoglobin (577 nm)

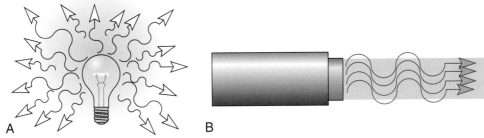

FIGURE 7.6 (A) Light emitted from a conventional lamp. The light travels in all directions, is composed of many wavelengths, and is not coherent. (**B**) Light emitted from a laser travels in the same direction and is a single wavelength, and all the waves are in phase; the light is coherent. (From Flint PW, Haughey BH, Lund VJ, et al. *Cummings Otolaryngology—Head and Neck Surgery*. 6th ed. Philadelphia, PA: Saunders; 2015, fig. 60-3.)

- Selectively absorbed by intraluminal blood of vascular lesions such as papillomas, vascular polyps, vocal fold ectasias, hemangiomas, and port wine stains
- Hemoglobin absorption is maximal with minimal scattering and absorption by melanin and other pigments

Laser Eye and Skin Safety Considerations

- Protect the eyes of the patient, surgeon, and other OR personnel
- Visible and near-infrared lasers can cause corneal or retinal burns
- CO_2 laser surgery: place double layer of saline-moistened eye pads over the eyes of the patient
- The patient's exposed skin and mucous membranes outside the surgical field should be protected by a double layer of saline-saturated surgical towels, surgical sponges, or lap pads

Laser Smoke Safety and Evacuation Considerations

- Have two separate suction setups
  - Smoke and steam evacuation
  - Blood and mucus from the operative wound
- Papillomavirus has been detected in the laser plume, but no cases of clinical transmission of diseases have been documented

Anesthetic Considerations for Laser Surgery

- Nonflammable general anesthetic should be used (eg, halothane and enflurane)
- Mixtures of helium, nitrogen, or air plus oxygen are commonly used
- Maintain the forced inspiratory oxygen <40%
- Nitrous oxide should not be used
- Protection should also be provided for the cuff of the endotracheal (ET) tube; saline-saturated cottonoids are then placed above the cuff
- Methylene blue–colored saline should be used to inflate the cuff
- In the event of tube ignition, the tube should be withdrawn simultaneously as saline is flushed down the ET tube and ventilation is stopped
- The airway must be reestablished immediately, and bronchoscopy should be performed to assess the degree of injury
- Intravenous steroids may be delivered, and the patient should remain intubated; repeat bronchoscopy should be performed daily until it is established that the airway is stable

BENIGN VOCAL FOLD MUCOSAL DISORDERS

RISK FACTORS FOR VOCAL INJURY

- High intrinsic tendency to use the voice (talkativeness and extroversion)
- High extrinsic opportunity or necessity to use the voice, driven by occupation, family needs, social activities, and avocations
- Visible vocal fold lesions may not cause an audible change in the speaking voice
- Visible vocal fold lesions that cause phonatory mismatch at the free margin or mucosal stiffness that are always detectable audibly in the singing voice, provided that the examiner knows how to elicit upper-range vocal tasks

SINGING-VOICE SYMPTOMS OF MUCOSAL INJURY

- Loss of the ability to sing softly at high pitches
- Increased day-to-day variability of singing-voice capabilities

- Phonatory onset delays
- Reduced vocal endurance
- Sense of increased effort

SINONASAL SYMPTOM MANAGEMENT IN THE VOICE

- Sinonasal conditions should be managed locally (topically) when possible
- Systemic drugs (eg, oral decongestants or antihistamine-decongestant combinations) dry not only nasal secretions but also secretions in the larynx and should be avoided
- Profuse rhinorrhea that accompanies the common cold can also be managed with ipratropium bromide inhalations

COMMON SYMPTOMS SUGGESTING REFLUX LARYNGITIS

- Exaggerated "morning mouth"
- Excessive phlegm
- Scratchy or dry throat irritation that is usually worse in the morning
- Habitual throat clearing
- Huskiness or lowered pitch of the voice in the morning

TREATMENT OF REFLUX LARYNGITIS

- Avoid caffeine, alcohol, and spicy foods
- Eat nothing <3 hours before bed
- Elevate the head of the bed
- Take antacid at bedtime, or H2 blocker 2-3 hours before bed
- Proton pump inhibitor (PPI) 30-60 minutes before dinner

TREATMENT OF ACUTE MUCOSAL SWELLING OF OVERUSE

- Relative vocal rest in context
- Pre-performance warm-up and solid vocal technique
- May consider short-term, high-dose tapering regimen of corticosteroids

SYSTEMIC MEDICATIONS THAT MAY AFFECT THE LARYNX

- Decongestants
- Antidepressants
- Antihypertensives
- Diuretics

VOICE THERAPY BASICS

- Success can be defined as a more consistent voice, without the exacerbations of hoarseness even if that now-more-reliable voice remains somewhat husky
- Success may require resolution of all upper-voice limitations in performers
- Some lesions are known at diagnosis to be irreversible except via surgery; aside from these exceptions, vocal fold microsurgery should follow an appropriate trial of voice therapy
- Nodules are expected to resolve, regress, or at least stabilize

SPECIFIC BENIGN VOCAL FOLD MUCOSAL DISORDERS

VOCAL FOLD NODULES BASICS

- Vocal nodules occur most commonly in boys and in women
- Almost always vocal "over-doers"

- Formation starts with localized vascular congestion with edema at the midportion of the membranous vocal folds, where shearing and collisional forces are greatest
- Maturation occurs with hyalinization of Reinke space and, in a subset of patients, to some thickening of the overlying epithelium
- Nodules do not occur unilaterally, although one may be larger than the other
- The larynx should be examined at high frequency to visualize subtle to small swellings, which can be poorly appreciated at lower frequencies
- Initial onset may be associated with a URI or acute laryngitis, after which the hoarseness never clears completely

COMMON VOCAL NODULE SYMPTOMS

- Loss of the ability to sing high notes softly
- Delayed phonatory onset, particularly with high, soft singing
- Increased breathiness (air escape), roughness, and harshness
- Reduced vocal endurance ("my voice gets husky easily")
- A sensation of increased effort for singing
- A need for longer warm-ups
- Day-to-day variability of vocal capabilities that is greater than expected for the singer's level of vocal training

VOCAL NODULE TREATMENT OPTIONS

- Voice therapy plays a primary role
- Good laryngeal lubrication should be ensured through general hydration
- Allergy and reflux, when present, should also be treated
- Surgical removal becomes an option when nodules of any size persist and when the voice remains unacceptably impaired after voice therapy for >3 months (Fig. 7.7)

CAPILLARY ECTASIA BASICS

- Capillary ectasia seems to happen most often in vocal over-doers

- Repeated vibratory microtrauma can lead to capillary angiogenesis
- Hoarse after relatively short periods of singing
- Additional symptoms reminiscent of nodules
- Treatment: voice therapy, consider stopping nonsteroidal antiinflammatory drugs/anticoagulants if medically appropriate

INDICATIONS FOR SURGICAL ABLATION OF CAPILLARY ECTASIAS

1. Persistent decreased vocal endurance
2. Intermittent bruising
3. Hemorrhagic polyp

VOCAL FOLD HEMORRHAGIC POLYP BASICS

- Capillary rupture causes accumulation of blood; similar to a blister
- May thicken overlying epithelium and stiffen vocal fold
- More common in men
- Intermittent severe voice abuse; working in noisy environments
- Abrupt onset of hoarseness during extreme vocal effort, such as at a party or sporting event

VOCAL FOLD HEMORRHAGIC POLYP APPEARANCE ON EXAMINATION (Fig. 7.8)

- Unilateral lesion in the "node position" with a possible small contralateral lesion
- May or may not have hemorrhagic or bruised appearance

TREATMENT OPTIONS FOR HEMORRHAGIC POLYPS AND VOCAL FOLD HEMORRHAGE

- Voice therapy
- For recent, large hemorrhage, evacuation of blood may be appropriate

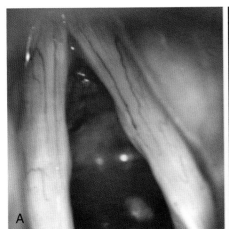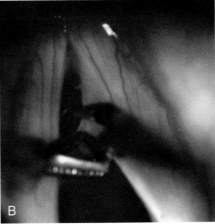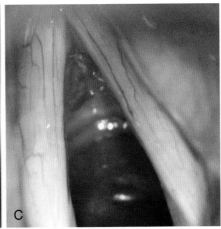

FIGURE 7.7 The operative sequence in a professional musical theater actor who had been experiencing vocal symptoms and limitations compatible with fusiform vocal nodules for more than 2 years. (**A**) The operative view after many months of conservative management. Not all fusiform swellings are reversible with conservative measures alone. (**B**) A polypoid nodule is grasped superficially and tented medially with Bouchayer forceps. Scissors that curve away from the vocal fold are used for removal. The nodule is thus removed in a very superficial plane, which minimizes the risk of scar between the remaining and regenerated mucosa and the underlying vocal ligament. (**C**) Vocal fold appearance after excision. The patient experienced dramatic normalization of vocal capabilities, and no evidence of scarring was found on postoperative stroboscopic examination. The dilated capillaries may predispose to recurrent nodule formation and can be spot coagulated with a microspot laser. (From Flint PW, Haughey BH, Lund VJ, et al. *Cummings Otolaryngology—Head and Neck Surgery*. 6th ed. Philadelphia, PA: Saunders; 2015, fig. 61-8.)

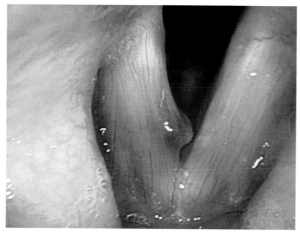

FIGURE 7.8 Hemorrhagic polyp, right fold. Note the blood-blister appearance. Recent further bleeding is evident from the yellowish discoloration of the upper surface of the fold because of breakdown products of a bruise, estimated to have occurred 2 weeks earlier. Hemorrhagic polyps sometimes rebruise intermittently. (From Flint PW, Haughey BH, Lund VJ, et al. *Cummings Otolaryngology—Head and Neck Surgery*. 6th ed. Philadelphia, PA: Saunders; 2015, fig. 61-11.)

- A long-standing polyp, whether hemorrhagic or end stage and pale, should be trimmed away superficially at the time the spot coagulations take place
- Prognosis for full return of vocal functioning after precision surgery is excellent

INTRACORDAL CYST BASICS

- Two types
  1. Mucus retention
  2. Epidermal inclusion
- Patients often demonstrate diplophonia in the upper vocal range
- May manifest an abrupt and irreducible transition to severe impairment at a relatively specific frequency
- Depth of lesion in Superficial layer of the lamina propria (SLP) changes the vibration of the affected vocal fold

INTRACORDAL CYST FINDINGS ON EXAMINATION

- Often originate just below the free margin of the fold with significant medial projection from the fold
- Reduction in mucosal wave over the lesion
- Open cyst: the sphere may be less discrete and may have a more mottled appearance on the superior surface of the vocal fold
- Opposite fold should be examined carefully because of the possibility of a more subtle cyst or sulcus

TREATMENT OPTIONS FOR INTRACORDAL CYST

- Voice therapy is considered
- Surgical excision should be performed with maximal mucosal preservation (Fig. 7.9)
- Surgical results are not as uniformly good as they are for nodules and polyps[16]

GLOTTIC SULCUS BASICS

- Epidermal cyst that has spontaneously emptied, leaving the collapsed pocket behind to form a sulcus
- Can be congenital and be seen in vocal over-doers

- Similar effect as scarring: stiffening of the mucosa inhibits oscillation and leads to dysphonia
- Not always visible during the office or voice laboratory examination: microlaryngoscopy is often required for definitive diagnosis

GLOTTIC SULCUS TREATMENT

- Trial of voice therapy
- Surgical excision: sulcus removal is technically demanding
  - Technique: hydrodissection via injection, circumcision of the lips of the sulcus and by dissection of the invaginated mucosal pocket from the underlying fold without injuring the vocal ligament (Fig. 7.10)
  - Voice outcomes less optimal than with polyp excision

BILATERAL DIFFUSE POLYPOSIS BASICS

- Middle-aged talkative women who have been long-term smokers
- Lower pitch than would be expected: a female being called "sir" on the telephone
- Exam: pale, watery bags of fluid attached to the superior surface and margins of the fold

TREATMENT OPTIONS FOR BILATERAL DIFFUSE POLYPOSIS

- Smoking cessation
- Consider thyroid function tests
- Polyp reduction with mucosal sparing
- May consider in-office laser ablation[17]

CONTACT ULCER OR GRANULOMA BASICS

- Contact granuloma or ulceration is seen primarily in men
- Chronic coughing or throat clearing traumatizes the posterior larynx
- Reflux of acid from the stomach into the posterior larynx during sleep
- Result: thin mucosa and perichondrium overlying the cartilaginous glottis become inflamed

PRESENTATION OF CONTACT ULCER OR GRANULOMA

- Unilateral discomfort over the midthyroid cartilage, occasionally with referred pain to the ipsilateral ear
- Hoarseness may develop when contact granulation tissue becomes large
- Exam: may appear as a depressed, ulcerated area with a whitish exudate clinging to it, or a bilobed, heaped-up lesion on the vocal process may be noted

TREATMENT OPTIONS FOR CONTACT ULCER OR GRANULOMA

- Antireflux regimen should be initiated
- Voice therapy
  - Abolish throat clearing
  - Raise average pitch for speech
- Injection of a depot corticosteroid directly into the lesion can be considered
- Botulinum injection into the thyroarytenoid muscle can be considered
- Due to high recurrence rate, removal should be limited, leaving the base or pedicle undisturbed[18]

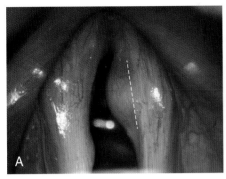
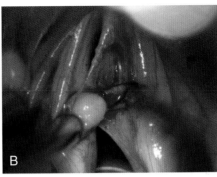
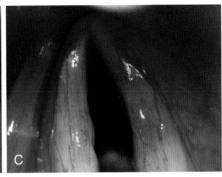

FIGURE 7.9 (**A**) Mucous retention cyst of right vocal fold. Yellowish spherical mass shines through overlying mucosa and was causing the patient severe hoarseness. Incision to enter the fold is made on the dotted line. (**B**) Near completion of dissection of the cyst from its final attachments using curved scissors. (**C**) After cyst removal. The patient's voice sounded virtually normal in the recovery room, although the upper voice was still abnormal. (From Flint PW, Haughey BH, Lund VJ, et al. *Cummings Otolaryngology—Head and Neck Surgery*. 6th ed. Philadelphia, PA: Saunders; 2015, fig. 61-17.)

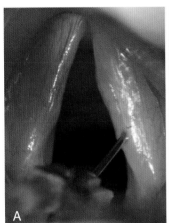
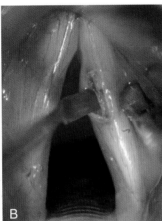
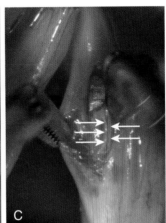
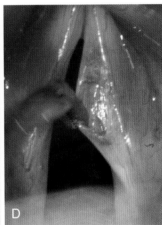

FIGURE 7.10 Glottic Sulcus. (**A**) At the beginning of surgery, the fold is infiltrated with lidocaine/epinephrine to provide hydrodissection and to expand the mucosa. The line of sulcus is seen proceeding anteriorly from the point of needle entry. (**B**) An elliptic incision has been made around the lips of the sulcus. (**C**) Right-curved alligator clip tents the medial mucosal flap. Arrows indicate the fine line that represents the opening into the sulcus. Curved scissors dissect the anterior aspect of the sulcus pocket from underlying vocal ligament. (**D**) After the sulcus pocket is removed, the gossamer mucosa is tented medially to show remaining flexibility. The voice is expected to improve, but normal upper-voice capabilities are only achieved sometimes. (From Flint PW, Haughey BH, Lund VJ, et al. *Cummings Otolaryngology—Head and Neck Surgery*. 6th ed. Philadelphia, PA: Saunders; 2015, fig. 61-19.)

INTUBATION GRANULOMA BASICS

- Patients who underwent acute or chronic intubation, rigid bronchoscopy, or other direct laryngeal manipulations
- Treatment: voice therapy, reflux regimen, and time

LARYNGOCELE AND SACCULAR CYST BASICS (Fig. 7.11)

- Air filled: laryngocele with patent saccular orifice
- Mucus filled: saccular cyst with blocked orifice
- Purulence filled: laryngopyocele with blocked orifice
- In infants, saccular disorders appear to be congenital
- Can be caused by transglottic pressure, such as that seen in trumpet players, glass blowers, and people using the voice in unusually forceful ways
- An uncommon cause of saccular cysts is laryngeal carcinoma, which causes obstruction of the saccular orifice

LARYNGOCELE AND SACCULAR CYST VARIANTS

- Anterior saccular cyst: tends to protrude from the anterior ventricle toward the laryngeal vestibule; when large, it may "push down" on the vocal fold and cause dysphonia

- Lateral saccular cyst or laryngocele, internal only: tends to dissect more superiorly and laterally up into the false and aryepiglottic folds, sometimes bulging not only those structures (medially) but also the medial wall of the piriform sinus (laterally), or even to fill the vallecula
- Lateral saccular cyst or laryngocele, internal/external: tends to dissect as described for the lateral cyst but also tends to penetrate through the thyrohyoid membrane and appear as a palpable swelling in the neck

TREATMENT CONSIDERATIONS FOR LARYNGOCELE AND SACCULAR CYSTS

- Researchers affirm complete endoscopic excision, instead of endoscopic marsupialization or transcervical removal, even for large recurrent lateral saccular cysts
- During endoscopic approach should note that even a large lateral cyst that bulges dramatically during awake endoscopy can virtually disappear under conditions of direct laryngoscopy with general anesthesia
- Can begin excising the false fold, during which maneuver the wall of the cyst is invariably encountered

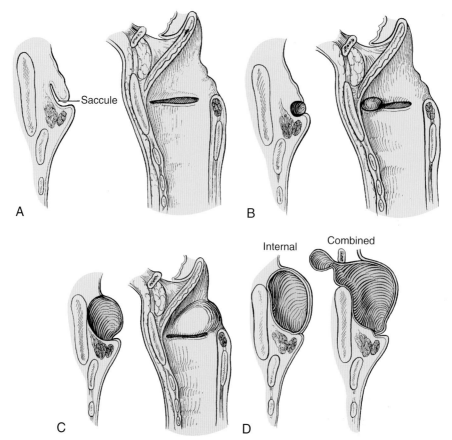

FIGURE 7.11 The Classification Scheme for a Laryngocele or Saccular Cyst. (**A**) Normal anatomy. (**B**) Anterior saccular cyst. (**C**) Lateral saccular cyst. (**D**) Laryngocele types. (From Flint PW, Haughey BH, Lund VJ, et al. *Cummings Otolaryngology—Head and Neck Surgery.* 6th ed. Philadelphia, PA: Saunders; 2015, fig. 61-29.)

RECURRENT RESPIRATORY PAPILLOMATOSIS BASICS

- Squamous papillomata caused by the human papillomavirus (HPV)
- Most common benign neoplasms seen by laryngologists
- Majority of infections are the result of subtypes 6 and 11; type 11 appears to predispose to more aggressive disease
- Juvenile form (HPV type 6 or 11) usually manifests in infancy or childhood as hoarseness and stridor and is usually aggressive and rapidly recurrent
- Adult-onset papillomata are occasionally solitary and more localized than juvenile-onset lesions are and are more likely to be of the so-called carpet variant (Fig. 7.12)

TREATMENT CONSIDERATIONS FOR RECURRENT RESPIRATORY PAPILLOMATOSIS

- Cold dissection, potassium-titanyl-phosphate, and 585-PDL, CO_2, and thulium lasers
    - CO_2 is the most widely accepted management for papilloma for depth control and hemostasis
    - Goal is to remove disease with preservation of vocal fold structures
    - Deep excision does not prevent recurrence
- Adjuvants
    - Intralesional cidofovir
    - Some consider bevacizumab
    - Investigational use of interferon and indole-3-carbinol

POLYPOID GRANULATION TISSUE BASICS

- Most common vascular tumor in the larynx
- Can be caused by laryngeal biopsy, intubation, direct external trauma to the larynx, and external penetrating wounds
- Treatment: conservative measures that include removal of the source of any ongoing irritation and intralesional corticosteroids
- For nonresponse and continuing symptoms, careful endoscopic removal may be considered

LARYNGEAL RHABDOMYOMA BASICS

- Most extracardiac rhabdomyomas are found in the head and neck region, in the pharynx and larynx
- Will not recur after local excision: approach should be as conservative

OTHER BENIGN NEOPLASMS OF THE LARYNX

- Benign mixed neoplasm (pleomorphic adenomas)
    - Extremely rare
    - Most commonly presents as a smooth, ovoid submucosal mass in the subglottis
    - Treatment is surgical excision with type of excision to be determined by location and size of the tumor
- Oncocytic tumor
    - Not a true neoplasm

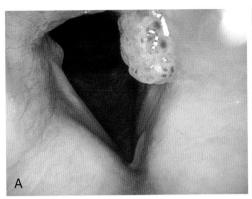 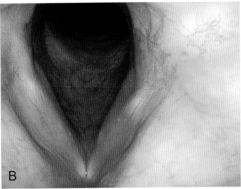

FIGURE 7.12 (**A**) Papillomata at posterior vocal folds; the left side is much larger than the right. (**B**) 2 weeks after microsurgical removal, cidofovir injection, and return of normal voice. (From Flint PW, Haughey BH, Lund VJ, et al. *Cummings Otolaryngology—Head and Neck Surgery.* 6th ed. Philadelphia, PA: Saunders; 2015, fig. 61-34.)

- Oncocytic metaplasia and hyperplasia of the ductal cell portion of glandular tissue
- Treated with simple excision
- Chondroma
  - Clinical behavior of chondromas and low-grade chondrosarcomas are so similar that histologic distinction has little practical significance
  - Slow growing and does not metastasize
  - Smooth, rounded mass in the subglottis: posterior aspect of the cricoid
  - Treatment with excision, most commonly with laryngofissure
- Granular cell neoplasm
  - The middle to posterior part of the true vocal fold is the most common site
  - Insufficiently deep biopsy of this lesion can lead to an incorrect diagnosis of squamous cell carcinoma from overlying pseudoepitheliomatous hyperplasia of the mucosa
  - Treatment: conservative but complete local excision
- Neurofibroma
  - Most commonly presents as lobulated nodules on the arytenoid or aryepiglottic fold
  - Recommend conservative, complete excision
- Neurilemmoma
  - Most commonly found on the aryepiglottic fold or false vocal fold
  - Treatment: conservative but complete local excision

POSTOPERATIVE DYSPHONIA

- Vocal fold surgery performed without extreme precision can lead to permanent dysphonia secondary to:
  - Scarring of the vocal fold cover with loss of pliability
  - Mismatch between the two vocal folds
- History must include voice-use patterns, which may explain previous lesion formation, as well as poor outcome from initial surgery
- Treatment: voice therapy with a voice-building strategy—gradual increase in voice use, which seems to soften the vocal scar and allow greater range
- >9-12 months should pass before reoperation is entertained
  - If glottic insufficiency is the main issue
    - May consider injection: collagen and fat
    - Thyroplasty

- If scarring is the main issue, may consider incision and elevation of mucosa with early postoperative phonation to prevent reformation of scar
- There is limited evidence to support any of these measures: proper preoperative patient education and careful surgical technique to prevent postoperative dysphonia are most important

ACUTE AND CHRONIC LARYNGITIS
ACUTE LARYNGITIS

Phonotrauma
- Vocal abuse, misuse, and overuse can contribute to phonotrauma
- Treatment: voice rest, steroids

Viral Laryngitis
- Most common types
  - Herpes zoster
  - Coronavirus
- Treatment options
  - Supportive care, rehydration, and vocal rest
  - In severe cases that result in airway embarrassment:
    - Steroids
    - Antibiotics for secondary infections
    - PPIs
    - Humidification

Acute Bacterial Laryngitis
- Presentation: drooling, febrile patient in respiratory distress
- Treatment options
  - Intubation in a controlled setting or awake tracheotomy may be appropriate
  - Most can be managed supportively with humidification, intravenous antibiotics, and close observation

Acute Fungal Laryngitis
- Typical history: patient on steroids (systemic or inhaled) or antibiotics
- Most common pathogen: *Candida*
- Presentation:
  - Hoarseness with or without accompanying throat discomfort

- Diffuse, whitish speckling of the vocal folds or supraglottis
- Differential diagnosis
  - Hyperkeratosis
  - Thick, dried mucus
  - Malignancy

Klebsiella Rhinoscleromatis
- Parts of the body are generally involved
  - Nose
  - Larynx
  - Trachea
- Pathology findings
  - Gram-negative coccobacillus, within macrophages (Mikulicz cells)
- Treatment
  - Fluoroquinolones
  - Tetracycline
  - Airway management

CHRONIC LARYNGITIS
Fungal Laryngitis
Blastomycosis
- Geographic region: southern United States
- Pathology findings
  - Broad-based budding yeast
  - Possible *pseudoepitheliomatous hyperplasia*, which may be mistaken for the advancing front of an epithelial malignancy
- Treatment: amphotericin B, ketoconazole, or itraconazole

Paracoccidioidomycosis
- Epidemiology: South American male farm workers
- Examination findings: ulcerative and exophytic lesions, which can resemble carcinoma
- Treatment: systemic antifungal therapy

Coccidioidomycosis
- Geographic region: "Valley fever" (San Joaquin Valley, CA) is a disease of the southwestern United States and northern Mexico
- Can present with airway obstruction
- Treatment: systemic antifungal therapy

Histoplasmosis
- Geographic region: Ohio and Mississippi River valleys
- Typical patient population: immunocompromised secondary to HIV infection, post transplant, or diabetes mellitus
- Presentation: localized pulmonary infection or systemic dissemination
- Treatment: amphotericin and fluconazole

Mycobacterial Laryngitis
- Geographic region: South America, Africa, and the Asian subcontinent
- Organisms: *Mycobacterium tuberculosis*, atypical mycobacteria
- Presentation: odynophagia and dysphonia
- Pathology findings: acid-fast bacilli and caseating granulomas
- True and false vocal folds were the most commonly affected sites
- Laryngeal manifestations of the disease are possible without systemic disease: generally, patient have either active pulmonary disease (47%) or inactive pulmonary tuberculosis (TB) (33%), whereas 15% had isolated laryngeal TB[19]

NONINFECTIOUS LARYNGITIS
Reflux Laryngitis
- Reflux irritation induces changes in the epithelium and stroma of laryngeal tissue that lead to organ dysfunction
- Bile has been implicated as a possible source of laryngeal injury
- Pepsin is active principally at acidic pH; however, pepsin was found to maintain its proteolytic activity at pH above 4 and was able to be "reactivated" after some time in a pH-neutral environment

LARYNGITIS ASSOCIATED WITH AUTOIMMUNE DISEASES
Pemphigoid and Pemphigus
- Presentation: 80% of the patients with pemphigus had otolaryngologic signs and symptoms, of which 40% were laryngeal in nature[20]
- Pathology: intraepithelial (pemphigus vulgaris) or subepithelial (pemphigoid) autoantibodies
- Treatment: high-dose corticosteroids combined with immunosuppressant therapy

Granulomatosis with Polyangiitis (Wegener Granulomatosis)
- Presentation: ~20% of all patients with granulomatosis with polyangiitis (GPA) will develop subglottic stenosis[21,22]
- Pathology: small- and medium-vessel vasculitis with *necrotizing granulomas*
- Laboratory studies
  - Autoantibodies against proteinase 3 (c-ANCA) and myeloperoxidase (p-ANCA)
  - Systemic disease, 95% are ANCA-positive
  - Head and neck, 75% are ANCA-positive[21]
- Treatment: immunosuppressant therapy and surgical intervention to maintain airway

Relapsing Polychondritis
- Presentation
  - 25-50% demonstrate symptoms of laryngeal dysfunction[23,24]
  - Most often affecting the cricoarytenoid joint, potentially causing immobility
  - Hoarseness, pain, cough, and airway obstruction
  - Most commonly manifests in the ears, nose, tracheobronchial cartilage, and joints
- Pathology
  - Inflammation in cartilages high in the glycosaminoglycans
  - Autoantibodies directed against type II collagen
- Diagnosis made clinically; no laboratory or pathology analysis
- Treatment: local or systemic steroids and immunomodulators

Sarcoidosis
- Presentation
  - Laryngeal manifestations occur in <1% of patients
  - Pulmonary, hepatic, cutaneous, cardiac, and lymphatic system involvement is common
  - Supraglottic and glottic larynx are most often involved in the form of diffuse edema
- Pathology
  - Noncaseating granulomas
  - Possible elevated serum calcium and angiotensin-converting enzyme levels

- Treatment
  - Work with a rheumatologist to treat the underlying condition
  - First-line treatment: systemic steroids
  - May require endoscopic resection if the mass is large enough to cause symptoms
  - Local steroid injection may also be of benefit

Amyloidosis
- Presentation
  - <1% of all benign laryngeal lesions
  - Nonulcerated, submucosal laryngeal mass or nodule often with a yellow or orange hue
  - Focal deposits can be secondary to extramedullary plasmacytomas and can occur in the mucosal-associated lymphoid tissue of the larynx
- Pathology
  - Extracellular deposition of abnormal proteinaceous debris
  - Can be associated with systemic lymphoproliferative or chronic inflammatory disorders such as multiple myeloma or rheumatoid arthritis
- Treatment
  - Consultation with pulmonary or rheumatology to assess for and treat systemic disease or underlying disorders causing the amyloidosis

Laryngeal Rhinoscleroma
- Organism: *Klebsiella rhinoscleromatis*
- Generally involves the nose and larynx and may involve the trachea
- Treatment: fluoroquinolones, tetracycline, and supportive airway management

VOCAL FOLD PARALYSIS
Laryngeal Electromyography and Palpation
- EMG provides data regarding prognosis, which may inform the timing of intervention, and choice of surgical procedures for the paralyzed larynx[25]
- Other causes of immobility such as joint ankylosis or cicatricle web formation can be discerned only by palpation of the vocal process, which must be done under general anesthesia

Vocal Cord Paralysis Prognostic Factors
- Favorable prognosis: blunt trauma, ET intubation, idiopathic vocal fold paralysis, and paralysis associated with viral pathogens (eg, Ramsay Hunt syndrome)
- Poor prognosis: injury after complete nerve section during surgical resection of tumor, cranial nerve involvement by tumor, paralysis associated with thoracic aneurysm, and paralysis from progressive neurologic disorders

High Vagal Injury Consequences
- Loss of abductor/adductor function
- Loss of cricothyroid muscle function and deafferentation of sensory fibers
- Greater difficulty with dysphonia, dysphagia, and aspiration

VOCAL FOLD MEDIALIZATION BY INJECTION
Indications for Vocal Fold Injection Medialization
- Early vocal fold paralysis (<12 months from insult)
- Patients who are not candidates for thyroplasty
- Patients with limited expected survival duration (eg, metastatic lung cancer) with severe dysphonia or aspiration symptoms

Materials Used for Vocal Fold–Injection Medialization
- Carboxymethylcellulose (Prolaryn Gel): lasts 3-6 months and with no foreign body reaction
- Autologous fat: requires overinjection; variable absorption; 62% overall success rate at 12 months[26]
- Micronized Alloderm (Cymetra): generally lasts 6-12 months[27] and requires some overinjection and reconstitution because it comes in powdered form
- Calcium hydroxyapatite (Prolaryn Plus): lasts 6-24 months and has a small potential for foreign body granulomatous reaction

Benefits and Drawbacks of In-Office Injection (Fig. 7.13)
- Safe and repeatable
- Lower cost
- Spares patient from general anesthesia
- Higher need for reinjection
- Higher rate of complication[28]

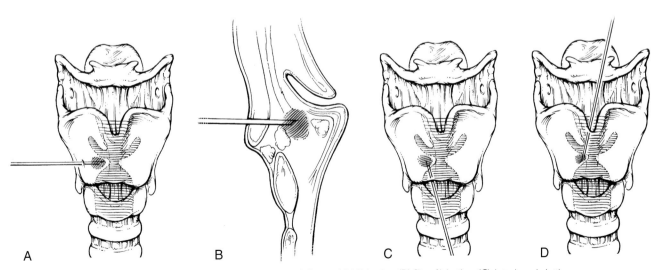

FIGURE 7.13 (**A**) Lateral percutaneous approach for vocal fold injection. (**B**) Site of injection. (**C**) Anterior subglottic percutaneous approach for vocal fold medialization. (**D**) Superior transthyrohyoid space approach. (Copyright 2008 by Johns Hopkins University, Art as Applied to Medicine.) (From Flint PW, Haughey BH, Lund VJ, et al. *Cummings Otolaryngology—Head and Neck Surgery*. 6th ed. Philadelphia, PA: Saunders; 2015, fig. 63-2.)

In-Office Vocal Fold–Injection Medialization Approaches

1. Transoral injection
   - Requires topical laryngeal and pharyngeal anesthesia
   - Easier to assess depth
2. Transcricothyroid
   - May be performed submucosally, so topical anesthesia is unnecessary
   - Must be careful to assess depth
3. Transthyrohyoid
   - Requires topical laryngeal and pharyngeal anesthesia
   - Easier to assess depth
4. Transthyroid cartilage
   - Performed submucosally, so topical anesthesia is unnecessary
   - Must be careful to assess depth
   - Cartilage can jam the needle

Vocal Fold–Injection Medialization Under General Anesthesia

- Good for patients who do not tolerate awake injection
- Needle is placed laterally in the vocal fold just anterior to the vocal process approximately at the depth of the lower margin of the true fold (Fig. 7.14)
- Advantages: lower need for reinjection and lower complication rate
- Disadvantages: cost, time, and cannot obtain vocal feedback from the patient during injection[28]

Complications of Vocal Fold–Injection Medialization

- Undeinjection
- Overinjection resulting in strained voice or potential airway compromise
- Improper placement with subglottal extension
- Laryngeal stenosis
- Migration into the superficial aspect of the vocal fold, which impairs vibratory capability
- Granuloma formation

MEDIALIZATION THYROPLASTY

Four Types of Laryngeal Framework Surgeries as Described by Isshiki

1. Type 1: medial displacement—corrects glottic insufficiency

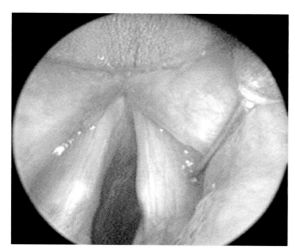

FIGURE 7.14 Vocal fold injection performed by direct laryngoscopy with a Brunings syringe. The injection needle is placed lateral to the vocal process and vocal ligament to prevent infiltration into the Reinke space. (From Flint PW, Haughey BH, Lund VJ, et al. *Cummings Otolaryngology—Head and Neck Surgery.* 6th ed. Philadelphia, PA: Saunders; 2015, fig. 63-3.)

2. Type 2: lateral displacement—used for SD
3. Type 3: shortening or relaxation—rarely used
4. Type 4: elongation—rarely used

Workup Before Considering Type I Thyroplasty

- Perceptual assessment: MPT and acoustic parameters
- Videostroboscopy: provides visual assessment of glottal closure and status of the mucosal wave

Advantages of Medialization Thyroplasty

- Performed with local anesthesia with minimal or no discomfort to the patient
- Long lasting
- Reversible

Disadvantages of Medialization Thyroplasty

- Open procedure
- Technically more difficult
- Closure of the posterior glottis may be limited

Indications for Medialization Thyroplasty

1. Permanent vocal fold paralysis (>12 months from insult, nerve sacrifice, and EMG findings)
2. Vocal fold bowing because of aging or cricothyroid joint fixation
3. Sulcus vocalis
4. Soft tissue defects from excision of pathologic tissue

Medialization Thyroplasty Implants

- Factors that affect outcome include size, shape, and position of the implant
- Silastic implants can be carved to any shape but take more time during surgery to produce
- Prefabricated implants with matched sizing templates may reduce operative time
- Gore-Tex strips have increased adaptability in some situations: better than prefabricated systems

Steps in Medialization Thyroplasty

1. Paramedian horizontal incision is outlined over the middle aspect of the thyroid lamina
2. Local anesthesia is administered subcutaneously and in four quadrants over the ipsilateral lamina
3. A 5-cm incision is made through the platysma
4. Elevate flaps
5. Strap muscles are split in the midline and are retracted laterally off the thyroid lamina, leaving the outer perichondrium intact
6. Single, large skin hook rotates the larynx
7. Cartilage window is outlined
8. Anterior aspect of the window is positioned 5-8 mm posterior to the ventral midline in women and 8-10 mm in men
9. Superior aspect of the window should be placed at the level of the true fold
10. A point half of the distance between the anterior-inferior border of the thyroid cartilage and the notch defines the level of the true fold
11. Outer perichondrium is incised and elevated
12. Window in cartilage is created
13. Size implant with flexible laryngoscopy guidance
14. Patient is asked to phonate while the template is moved through all four quadrants of the window
15. Place appropriate implant
16. Small suction drain is placed deeply to the strap muscles; the strap muscles and platysma are approximated with 4-0 absorbable suture, and the skin is closed with a running 5-0 subcuticular suture
17. Dexamethasone is given before surgery to minimize edema, and administration of prophylactic antibiotics is continued for 5 days

18. As a rule, regardless of the implant type used, it is preferable to use the largest prosthesis possible that maintains quality of voice (Fig. 7.15)

Limitations of Type I Thyroplasty
- Static change to the laryngeal framework but has no influence on dynamic function
- Average phonation time is increased from 4.6 to 15 seconds

Complications Associated with Type I Thyroplasty
- Penetration of the endolaryngeal mucosa
- Wound infection
- Chondritis
- Implant migration or extrusion
- Incomplete glottal closure: 10-15% of patients
- Airway obstruction
  - Potential for airway compromise requires overnight, inpatient observation
  - Combining medialization thyroplasty and arytenoid adduction increases risk of airway compromise

Arytenoid Abduction and Adduction Basics
- Variation in the position of the vocal fold and symptoms in vocal fold paralysis correlate with level of residual/regeneration of innervation of adductor vocal fold muscles[29,30]
  - More functional muscles: better function, smaller gap, and less likely to need arytenoid work
- Arytenoid abduction mimics the action of the PCA muscle: externally rotates the arytenoid to pull the vocal process superiorly and laterally
- Arytenoid adduction mimics the action of the LCA: pulls the vocal process medially and caudally
- Can also perform cricopharyngeal myotomy to reduce dysphagia[31,32]

Indications for Arytenoid Adduction
1. Large glottic gap/posterior gap
2. Insufficient voice improvement with thyroplasty alone
3. Vocal fold level (vertical height) mismatch

Steps for Arytenoid Adduction (Mimics Lateral Cricoarytenoid)
1. Create a thyroplasty window
2. Cricoid hook should then be placed on the superior cornu of the thyroid cartilage to rotate the larynx away from the field
3. Larynx is rotated to the opposite side by means of traction on the superior cornu of the thyroid cartilage

4. Inferior constrictor muscle is transected
5. Cricopharyngeal muscle comes into view, and this muscle can then be resected
6. Muscle can be defined by blunt dissection, just behind its attachment to the cricoid, and then a 1-2-cm segment of muscle is excised
7. Identification and displacement of the piriform sinus mucosa to expose the arytenoid cartilage and avoid entry into the hypopharynx
8. Piriform sinus is separated from the medial surface of the thyroid ala by blunt dissection
9. Sac is then reflected superiorly and anteriorly to expose the PCA
10. PCA fibers are followed to their convergence and insertion on the muscular process of the arytenoid
11. Muscular process of the arytenoid cartilage appears as a white prominence between the attachments of the anterior and posterior bellies of the PCA
12. Muscle tendon is grasped near its insertion, and the needle is passed from back to front through the cartilage process; care should be taken not to injure the piriform mucosa
13. Place suture in the muscular process of the arytenoid (origin of the LCA)
14. Pass the stitch anteriorly through the paraglottic space
15. Secure to the inferior thyroid ala

Indication for Arytenoid Abduction
- Bilateral vocal fold paralysis with good voice and airway obstruction symptoms

Steps in Arytenoid Abduction (Mimics Posterior Cricoarytenoid)
1. Same approach to arytenoid as arytenoid adduction
2. Place suture in the muscular process of the arytenoid
3. Pull posteriorly and inferiorly

LARYNGEAL REINNERVATION
Three Goals of Laryngeal Reinnervation
1. Restoration of vocal fold movement (nonselective laryngeal reinnervation does not result in *coordinated* movement)
2. Restoration of vocal fold position
3. Restoration of vocal fold bulk (tone)

Reinnervation Options for Unilateral Laryngeal Paralysis
1. The neuromuscular pedicle (NMP) procedure
2. Nerve transfer to the RLN, using the ansa cervicalis or hypoglossal

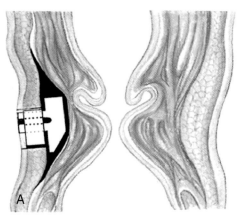
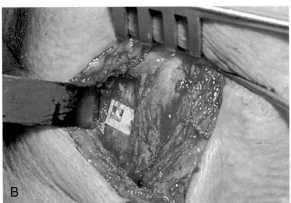

FIGURE 7.15 (A) Schematic rendition of an implant positioned within the fenestra and secured with a shim. **(B)** Intraoperative view of hydroxyapatite implant secured with a shim.

3. Direct implantation of a nerve (ansa hypoglossi) into the denervated muscle
4. Reanastomosis of the divided RLN

Reinnervation of the Posterior Cricoarytenoid Using the Phrenic Nerve
- Ideal in the setting of bilateral vocal fold paralysis
- Activates with inspiration
- Activity of the PCA muscle is synchronous with inspiration and precedes activation of the diaphragm by 40-100 ms

Only Internal Laryngeal Muscle with Bilateral Innervation
- Interarytenoid muscle

Actions Involving Cricothyroid Muscle Activation
1. Deep inspiration
2. Expiration
3. Phonation

Ansa Cervicalis for Laryngeal Reinnervation
- Most commonly used donor nerve
- Ansa provides motor supply to the infrahyoid muscles
- Reinnervation becomes less effective the longer a muscle is denervated
- Cricothyroid is innervated by the SLN, so muscle is not addressed by ansa-to-RLN reinnervation

Requirements for Restoration of Function in Laryngeal Reinnervation
1. A neuron that responds to the injury with the metabolic changes necessary to support axon regrowth
2. An environment around the injured axon that permits axon growth
3. Guidance clues for restoration of function

Neuromuscular Pedicle
- Transfer a nerve with a portion of its motor units intact to a denervated muscle
- Despite successful use in a few authors' experiences, widespread use of NMP has not materialized

Indications for Neuromuscular Pedicle in Bilateral Vocal Fold Paralysis
- Bilateral vocal fold paralysis that has persisted for 6 months to 1 year
- Ansa cervicalis nerve and its insertion into the appropriate strap muscle must be available and intact

Contraindications for Neuromuscular Pedicle in Bilateral Vocal Fold Paralysis
- Fixation or limitation of the cricoarytenoid joint; before planning reinnervation, must palpate the cricoarytenoid joints
- Central nervous system disease that results in bilateral vocal cord paralysis (relative contraindication)
- Only about 50% patients are suitable candidates[33]

Indications for Neuromuscular Pedicle in Unilateral Vocal Fold Paralysis
- Ansa cervicalis nerve intact
- Selected adductor muscle in suitable condition for reinnervation
- Mobile arytenoid on the paralyzed side
- Appropriate amount of time has passed that recovery of motion is unlikely (about 12 months)

Neuromuscular Pedicle Technique
1. NMP harvested from the omohyoid muscle
2. Branch of the ansa cervicalis nerve to the omohyoid is removed with a 2-3-mm attached block of muscle
3. Unilateral paralysis: NMP placed into the LCA via a window in the thyroid ala
4. Bilateral paralysis: NMP placed into the PCA after rotating the larynx and separating the fibers of the inferior constrictor

Ansa Cervicalis–to–Recurrent Laryngeal Nerve Transfer
- Procedure provides tone, position, and bulk to the denervated muscles
- Does not provide recovery of vocal fold function
- Voice outcomes versus thyroplasty
  - No significant difference in overall voice outcomes in randomized, controlled trial
  - Laryngeal reinnervation patients <52 years old had better voice outcomes compared with laryngeal framework surgery patients <52 years old
  - Laryngeal reinnervation patients <52 years old had better voice outcomes compared with laryngeal reinnervation patients >52 years old
  - Patients age >52 had significantly better voice outcomes with laryngoplasty/thyroplasty ± arytenoid adduction than with laryngeal reinnervation[34]

Contraindications for Ansa Cervicalis–to–Recurrent Laryngeal Nerve Transfer
1. Glottic airway compromise
2. Bilateral vocal fold paralysis
3. Absence of the distal RLN
4. Absence of the ansa cervicalis bilaterally
5. Poor general health
6. Limitations of time, voice, and surgery (relative contraindication)

Ansa Cervicalis–to–Recurrent Laryngeal Nerve Transfer Technique
1. RLN is identified in the tracheoesophageal groove to its entrance into the larynx
2. Ansa cervicalis can be identified along the lateral border of the sternothyroid muscle at the level of the omohyoid muscle or along the internal jugular vein
3. Ansa and RLN are transected; each nerve should be divided far enough inferiorly to permit a tension-free anastomosis
4. Anastomosis is completed
5. Absorbable material can be injected at the time of surgery

CHRONIC ASPIRATION

COMMON CAUSES OF CHRONIC ASPIRATION IN ADULTS
- Lower cranial nerve deficits secondary to CVA (most common)[35]
- Neuromuscular disorders
- Tumors (brainstem or laryngeal)
- Postoperative aspiration
- Postradiation swallowing dysfunction
- Traumatic or anoxic brain injury

COMMON CAUSES OF CHRONIC ASPIRATION IN THE PEDIATRIC POPULATION
- Cerebral palsy
- Anoxic encephalopathy

- Sequelae of neurologic trauma or surgery
- Tracheoesophageal fistula
- Other severe congenital or acquired neurologic disorders[36]

DYSPHAGIA HISTORY QUESTIONS

1. Onset
2. Pain: consider tumor, infection, and esophagitis
3. Solids (mass, lesion, immobility, and pouch) versus liquids (neurogenic)
4. Regurgitation
5. Weight loss
6. Aspiration/pneumonia (PNA)
7. Coughing while eating or drinking

DYSPHAGIA PAST MEDICAL HISTORY EVALUATION

1. Neurologic disorders
2. Head and neck or esophageal cancer risk factors
3. Reflux and current or past treatment
4. Previous spine or head and neck surgery
5. Immunosuppressant medications

DYSPHAGIA PHYSICAL EXAM

- Complete head and neck exam with special attention to cranial nerves and tongue strength
- Assess extremity motion and coordination: rule out underlying neurologic condition (eg, PD and ALS)
- Laryngoscopy (flexible scope vs. mirror) and assess for:
  - Pooling in the vallecula, piriform sinuses, and postcricoid region
  - Masses or lesions
  - Abduction and adduction of true vocal folds
  - Tongue-base retraction
  - Pharyngeal motion

OPTIONS FOR RADIOGRAPHIC EVALUATION OF THE SWALLOW

- Modified barium swallow study (MBSS)
  - Can show past the postcricoid region and upper-esophageal sphincter (UES)
  - Can have concurrent esophagogram
  - Will expose patient to radiation
  - Requires transport to radiology[37,38]
- Flexible endoscopic evaluation of swallowing
  - Allows indirect visualization of laryngeal and hypopharyngeal structures
  - Can perform at bedside
  - Can perform concurrent transnasal esophagoscopy
  - No radiation
  - Similar sensitivity/specificity for aspiration to MBSS[39]

SOLID DYSPHAGIA DIFFERENTIAL DIAGNOSES

1. Esophageal web
2. Achalasia
3. Zenker diverticulum
4. Cricopharyngeal achalasia
5. Esophageal dysmotility
6. Esophageal mass
7. Thyroid mass
8. Traction diverticulum
9. Scleroderma
10. Polymyositis/dermatomyositis
11. Diffuse esophageal spasm
12. Esophageal web
13. Esophageal ring

LIQUID OR MIXED DYSPHAGIA DIFFERENTIAL DIAGNOSES

1. CVA
2. Myopathies (muscular dystrophy and metabolic myopathy)
3. Status post head and neck cancer surgery
4. Status post radiation or chemoradiation of the head and neck
5. PD
6. ALS

GENERAL TREATMENT PRINCIPLES FOR DYSPHAGIA

- Assess risk using MBSS and ensure that patient is taking consistencies that are safe to avoid aspiration
- Swallowing therapy including swallowing exercises to strengthen the muscles of swallowing and techniques to avoid aspiration (eg, supraglottic swallow, chin tuck, and head turn)
- Referral to neurology if concern for underlying condition (eg, PD and ALS), for diagnosis and treatment

PATIENT NEWLY DIAGNOSED WITH CHRONIC ASPIRATION

- Stop oral feeding
- Aggressive pulmonary toilet (consider tracheostomy)
- Antibiotics if appropriate
- Alternative alimentation
  - Nasogastric feeding may increase aspiration risk[40]
  - If severe reflux, jejunostomy may be of more benefit compared with gastrostomy

LARYNGEAL AND ESOPHAGEAL TRAUMA

LARYNGEAL TRAUMA HISTORY QUESTIONS

1. Voice change
2. Breathing difficulty
3. Pain with coughing or swallowing
4. Hemoptysis

LARYNGEAL TRAUMA INITIAL ASSESSMENT

- First priority in managing a laryngeal trauma patient: establish a definitive, safe airway (consider awake tracheostomy)
- Second, follow advanced trauma life support (ATLS) protocol with trauma team
  - Keep neck immobile until cervical spine is cleared
  - 10% of laryngeal traumas will have concomitant cervical spine injuries[41]

LARYNGEAL TRAUMA PHYSICAL EXAMINATION

- Breathing: Is stridor or stertor detected?
- Voice: Can patient phonate?
- Visually inspect for signs of trauma
- Palpate the neck for:
  - Neck crepitus
  - Step-offs, deformities, and change in framework
  - Laryngeal tenderness

- Flexible laryngoscopy—if patient is stable
  - Vocal fold mobility
    - RLN trauma
    - Structural injury
  - Particular attention at vibratory edge of the vocal fold and anterior commissure

DEFINITIVE TREATMENT TIME FRAME FOR THE LARYNGEAL FRACTURE PATIENT

- 24 Hours (Fig. 7.16)

MOST COMMON CAUSES OF EXTERNAL LARYNGEAL TRAUMA

1. Motor vehicle accidents
2. Clothesline injuries (eg, sports)
3. Hanging (eg, attempted suicide)

MOST COMMON SYMPTOMS OF EXTERNAL LARYNGEAL TRAUMA

1. Hoarseness
2. Dysphagia
3. Pain

4. Dyspnea
5. Hemoptysis[42]

SCHAEFER CLASSIFICATION OF LARYNGEAL TRAUMA

1. Level I: minor hematoma/lacerations and no fractures
2. Level II: moderate edema, lacerations, mucosal disruptions without exposed cartilage, and nondisplaced fractures
3. Level III: massive edema, displaced fractures, and cord immobility
4. Level IV: massive edema, >2 displaced fractures, cord immobility, instability, and anterior commissure involvement

LARYNGEAL TRAUMA MANAGEMENT PRINCIPLES

- 24-Hour admission to an acute care unit
- Regular observations
- Serial flexible nasolaryngoscopy
- Humidified oxygen
- PPI therapy
- Systemic corticosteroids
- Prophylactic antibiotics

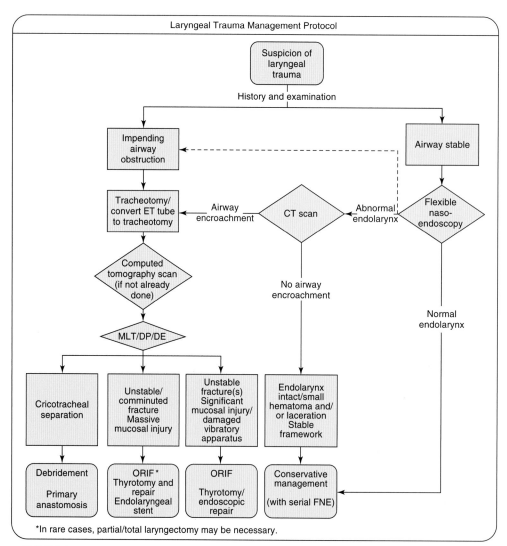

FIGURE 7.16 A Proposed Protocol for Managing Laryngeal Trauma. *CT*, Computed tomography; *DE*, direct esophagoscopy; *DP*, direct pharyngoscopy; *ET*, endotracheal; *FNE*, flexible nasoendoscopy; *MLT*, microlaryngoscopy; *ORIF*, open reduction with internal fixation. (From Flint PW, Haughey BH, Lund VJ, et al. *Cummings Otolaryngology—Head and Neck Surgery.* 6th ed. Philadelphia, PA: Saunders; 2015, fig. 63-8.)

- Head of the bed elevation
- Operative exploration typically not required for level I/II injuries, unless as needed for airway
- Levels III/IV require operative exploration
- Consider airway security with awake tracheostomy before sending the patient for imaging

INDICATIONS FOR SURGERY

1. Severe obstruction
2. Displaced fracture of laryngeal skeleton
3. Increasing subcutaneous emphysema
4. Hemorrhage
5. Lacerations involving the true vocal fold (TVC) or anterior commisure (AC)
6. Exposed cartilage
7. Dislocated arytenoids
8. Vocal cord immobility

PENETRATING NECK TRAUMA ZONES OF INJURY

1. Level I: clavicle/sternum to cricoid
2. Level II: cricoid to angle of mandible
3. Level III: angle of mandible to skull base

ALGORITHM FOR PENETRATING NECK TRAUMA

- Unstable: immediate exploration
- Stable
  - Symptomatic: angiography for zones I and III, then exploration or embolization
  - Asymptomatic: angiography for zones I and III; contrast esophagography and esophagoscopy for zone I
  - Zone II: directed by clinical exam; observe if no injury is identified

ASSESSMENTS TO BE PERFORMED IF SURGICAL INTERVENTION IS REQUIRED

- Direct Microlaryngoscopy
- Pharyngoscopy
- Tracheoscopy
- Esophagoscopy

ENDOLARYNGEAL PROCEDURES TO CONSIDER FOR LARYNGEAL TRAUMA

- Drainage of hematomas
- Repair of mucosal and selected vocal cord lacerations
- Reduction of dislocated cricoarytenoid joints
- Placement of stents or keels to prevent adhesions if injuries to opposing laryngeal mucosal surfaces are extensive

OPEN SURGICAL PROCEDURES TO CONSIDER FOR LARYNGEAL TRAUMA

- Open-reduction internal fixation of fractures
- Repair of lacerations with 5-0 or 6-0 absorbable sutures
- Rotation of mucosal flaps to replace denuded mucosa
- Deployment of a stent with significant framework comminution and to prevent anterior commissure webbing

POSTOPERATIVE CARE FOR LARYNGEAL TRAUMA PATIENTS

- Nasogastric tube until safe swallow is confirmed
- Antibiotics, especially if a stent was placed
- Antacid therapies, especially if there is a denuded epithelium
- Stent should be removed in 10-14 days
- Postoperative serial endoscopy

FACTORS INFLUENCING LARYNGEAL TRAUMA OUTCOMES

- Severity of initial injury
- Timing of surgery (early is better: should be <24 hours, Box 7.1)

CAUSTIC/THERMAL AIRWAY INJURY BASICS

- Inhalation burns occur in 30% of all burn patients
- 20% of patients with inhalation injury have extensive laryngeal injury[43]
- Alkali versus acid ingestion
  - Alkali injections is worse, resulting in liquefaction necrosis of muscle, collagen, and lipid, with injury worsening over time
  - Acid injection results in coagulative necrosis, which is generally superficial
- Tracheostomy versus ET intubation
  - In the setting of caustic injury, tracheostomy is favored over ET tube because of the high rate of laryngeal stenosis[44]

Box 7.1 FACTORS THAT DETERMINE THE NEED FOR AND THE NATURE OF SURGICAL INTERVENTION

Laryngeal Framework
Stable
  No fractures
  A single undisplaced fracture

Unstable
  A single displaced fracture
  More than one fracture line
  Cricoid fracture

Potentially Nonviable
  Framework comminution with devitalized cartilage fragments

Laryngeal Mucosa
Intact/Minimally Injured
  No mucosal injuries
  Small submucosal hematoma
  Linear laceration with no exposed cartilage

Injured
  Jagged/multiple linear lacerations
  Large hematoma(s)

Exposed Cartilage
Massively Injured
  Significant loss of mucosa
  Devitalized mucosal tissue

Vibratory Apparatus
Intact
Injured
  Anterior commissure
  Vibrating edge of the vocal cord(s)
  Arytenoid dislocation

Laryngotracheal Junction
Intact
Any degree of laryngotracheal separation

From Flint PW, Haughey BH, Lund VJ, et al. *Cummings Otolaryngology—Head and Neck Surgery.* 6th ed. Philadelphia, PA: Saunders; 2015, table 70-4.

MANAGEMENT OF CAUSTIC LARYNGEAL INJURY

- Establish safe airway
- Cardiovascular resuscitation per standard burn-care protocol
- If laryngeal and esophageal endoscopy is to be performed, should be within the first 24 hours to avoid more severe edema and ulceration later

GRADING OF ESOPHAGEAL INJURIES

- First degree: mucosal erythema
- Second degree: erythema with noncircumferential exudation
- Third degree: circumferential exudation
- Fourth degree: circumferential exudation with esophageal wall perforation[44]

CAUSTIC ESOPHAGEAL INJURY BASICS

- 30% of patients with caustic esophageal injuries do not have evidence of oropharyngeal damage[45]
- Adult injuries are generally more severe than pediatric because these are generally attempted suicide with ingestion of large volumes

MANAGEMENT OF CAUSTIC ESOPHAGEAL INJURY

- Irrigate upper-aerodigestive tract
- Insert large-bore nasogastric tube to maintain patency
- Broad-spectrum antibiotics
- Antacid therapy
- Steroids
- 10-35% of patients will develop esophageal strictures[44]
- One in seven patients who develop strictures will develop esophageal cancer; therefore, long-term follow-up is required[44]

SURGICAL MANAGEMENT OF UPPER-AIRWAY STENOSIS

DIFFERENTIAL DIAGNOSIS FOR ADULT LARYNGEAL AND UPPER TRACHEAL STENOSIS (Box 7.2)

- See box 7.2

MOST COMMON CAUSE AND MECHANISM OF ADULT LARYNGEAL AND UPPER TRACHEAL STENOSIS

- Prolonged intubation[46]
- Mucosal ulceration with possible bacterial infection can cause perichondritis/chondritis with cartilage resorption or granulation tissue, which results in submucosal fibrosis and scar contraction

MYER-COTTON CLASSIFICATION SYSTEM FOR GRADING CIRCUMFERENTIAL STENOSIS OF THE SUBGLOTTIS

1. Grade I: 0-50% of lumen obstructed
2. Grade II: 51-70% of lumen obstructed
3. Grade III: 71-99% of lumen obstructed
4. Grade IV: 100% of lumen obstructed[46]

Box 7.2 CAUSES OF ADULT LARYNGEAL AND UPPER-TRACHEAL STENOSIS

Trauma
Internal Laryngotracheal Injury
Prolonged ET intubation
Tracheotomy
Surgical procedure

External Laryngotracheal Injury
Blunt neck trauma
Penetrating injury of the larynx
Radiation therapy
ET burn
Thermal
Chemical

Idiopathic
Chronic Inflammatory Disease
Autoimmune
GPA
Sarcoidosis
Relapsing polychondritis
Granulomatous infection
TB

Neoplasms
Benign
Papillomas
Chondromas
Minor salivary gland neoplasms
Neural neoplasms

Malignant
Squamous cell carcinoma
Minor salivary gland neoplasms
Sarcomas
Lymphoma

From Flint PW, Haughey BH, Lund VJ, et al. *Cummings Otolaryngology—Head and Neck Surgery.* 6th ed. Philadelphia, PA: Saunders; 2015, box 68-1. Data from Herrington HC, Weber SM, Andersen PE: Modern management of laryngotracheal stenosis. *Laryngoscope.* 2006;116(9):1553-1557; Wester JL, Clayburgh DR, Stott WJ, et al. Airway reconstruction in Wegener's granulomatosis-associated laryngotracheal stenosis. *Laryngoscope.* 2011;121(12):2566-2571; and Parker NP, Bandyopadhyay D, Misono S, et al. Endoscopic cold incision, balloon dilation, mitomycin C application, and steroid injection for adult laryngotracheal stenosis. *Laryngoscope.* 2013;123(1):220-225.

MCCAFFREY CLASSIFICATION SYSTEM FOR GRADING SUBSITE-SPECIFIC LARYNGOTRACHEAL STENOSIS

1. Stage I: subglottic or tracheal lesion <1 cm
2. Stage II: subglottic lesion >1 cm long
3. Stage III: subglottic/tracheal lesions not involving glottis
4. Stage IV: glottis involved in stenosis with fixation of one or both vocal folds[47]

DESCRIBE THE DIFFERENCE IN FLOW-VOLUME LOOPS BETWEEN A PATIENT WITH A NORMAL AIRWAY, A FIXED OBSTRUCTION, AND A VARIABLE EXTRATHORACIC OBSTRUCTION (BILATERAL VOCAL FOLD PARALYSIS; Fig. 7.17)

DESCRIBE A NORMAL FLOW VOLUME LOOP

Normal result shows expiratory flow, indicated by positive deflection, and inspiratory flow, indicated by negative deflection Fig 7.17 (A).

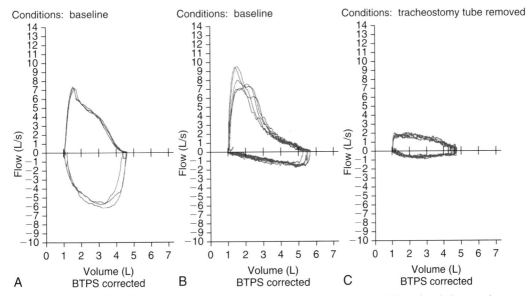

FIGURE 7.17 Flow-Volume Loop for Assessing Adequacy of the Upper Airway. (**A**) Normal result shows expiratory flow, indicated by positive deflection, and inspiratory flow, indicated by negative deflection. (**B**) Loop from a patient with bilateral vocal fold motion impairment shows variable extrathoracic obstruction with a mid-vital capacity inspiratory flow rate (Vi50) of < 1.5 L/sec. (**C**) Loop from a patient with an infiltrative tumor and a fixed obstruction. *BTPS*, body temperature and pressure saturation. (From Flint PW, Haughey BH, Lund VJ, et al. *Cummings Otolaryngology—Head and Neck Surgery*. 6th ed. Philadelphia, PA: Saunders; 2015, fig. 68-1.)

EXTRATHORACIC OBSTRUCTION

Fig 7.17 (**B**) Loop from a patient with bilateral vocal fold motion impairment shows variable extrathoracic obstruction with normal expiratory limb and limited mid-vital capacity inspiratory flow rate (Vi50) of <1.5 L/sec.

FIXED OBSTRUCTION

Fig 7.17 (**C**) Loop from a patient with a fixed obstruction with flattening of the inspiratory and expiratory limb.

FACTORS ASSOCIATED WITH POOR OUTCOME WITH ENDOSCOPIC REPAIR OF AIRWAY STENOSIS

1. Circumferential stenosis with scar contracture
2. Scarring wider than 1 cm in vertical dimension
3. Tracheomalacia with loss of cartilage
4. Previous history of severe bacterial infection–associated tracheostomy
5. Posterior laryngeal inlet scarring with arytenoid fixation

ENDOSCOPIC MANAGEMENT OF AIRWAY STENOSIS CONSIDERATIONS

- Indications: Myer-Cotton grade I and II stenosis
- Decannulation rate of approximately 85%
- Postoperatively, patients should be given 1-3 weeks of antibiotic therapies, reflux management, and wound reassessment in 6 weeks on endoscopy

AIRWAY SKELETAL FRAMEWORK/SCAFFOLD RECONSTRUCTION DONOR SITES

- Rib cartilage
- Thyroid cartilage
- Iliac crest
- Hyoid
- Auricular cartilage
- Septal cartilage

STENTING FOR AIRWAY STENOSIS CONSIDERATIONS

- May cause ischemic injury; capillary blood flow ceases with pressure 20-40 mm Hg[48]
- May help in keeping opposing raw surfaces apart, maintaining the lumen in a reconstructed area that lacks support, or allowing approximation of epidermal grafts

POSTERIOR GLOTTIC STENOSIS BASICS

- History: patient with prior prolonged intubation, followed by progressive dyspnea on exertion or stridor (inspiratory or biphasic)
- Nasolaryngoscopy reveals limitation of abduction of bilateral vocal folds on sniff maneuver and may see scar banding between arytenoids
- Must differentiate from bilateral vocal fold paralysis of neural origin, generally with intraoperative palpation of joints or laryngeal EMG

TREATMENT OPTIONS FOR POSTERIOR GLOTTIC STENOSIS

1. Divide scar band endoscopically in the operating room under jet ventilation and inject steroids (particularly helpful in early stenosis)[49-51]
2. Micro-trapdoor flap to move healthy mucosa into the region of the cut to prevent restenosis
3. Cordotomy/arytenoidectomy if cricoarytenoid joint has fused
4. Tracheotomy

DISEASES OF THE ESOPHAGUS

INDICATIONS FOR ESOPHAGOSCOPY

- Weight loss
- Upper gastrointestinal bleeding
- Dysphagia

- Odynophagia
- Chest pain
- Poor response to therapy
- Evaluation for Barrett esophagus

INDICATIONS FOR 24-HOUR PH MONITORING

1. Document excessive acid reflux in patients with suspected gastroesophageal reflux disease (GERD) without endoscopic findings
2. Assess the efficacy of medical or surgical therapy

INDICATIONS FOR MONITORING IN LIEU OF EMPIRIC TRIAL OF REFLUX THERAPY WITH MEDICATION AND LIFESTYLE CHANGES

- Dysphagia
- Odynophagia
- Weight loss
- Chest pain
- Choking/aspiration symptoms

MOST COMMON SYMPTOM OF INFECTIOUS ESOPHAGITIS

- Odynophagia (Fig. 7.18)

GLOBUS SENSATION

- Lump sensation in the throat that does not impede swallow
- May in fact be relieved with swallow

MANOMETRY BASICS (Table 7.1)

- Gold standard for diagnosis of motor disorders of the esophageal body and lower esophageal sphincter (LES)
- Upper sphincter pressures are highly variable, so manometry is less useful in UES assessment

AMBULATORY 24-HOUR PH PROBE BASICS

- Abnormal pH level: <4.0
- pH level at which pepsin is activated: <4.0
- Percent of time with pH <4.0 that is considered abnormal: ≥4.25%[52,53]

MULTICHANNEL INTRALUMINAL IMPEDANCE PROBE BASICS

- Measures both acid and nonacid refluxate
- Measures total resistance to current flow between adjacent electrodes

ESOPHAGEAL ACHALASIA BASICS

- Failure of LES to relax
- "Bird's beak" or "megaesophagus" on esophagogram
- Treatment: esophagoscopy with Botox or myotomy; referral to gastroenterology

ESOPHAGEAL DYSMOTILITY BASICS

- Normal contour on esophagogram
- Abnormal manometry
- Consider referral to gastroenterology

SCLERODERMA BASICS

- CREST Syndrome
  - Calcinosis
  - Raynaud phenomenon
  - Esophageal dysmotility
  - Sclerodactyly
  - Telangiectasia
- Esophogram: dilated *distal* esophagus
- Manometry: normal UES and LES

POLYMYOSITIS AND DERMATOMYOSITIS BASICS

- Striated muscle myopathy
  - Pharyngeal weakness with upper esophageal weakness

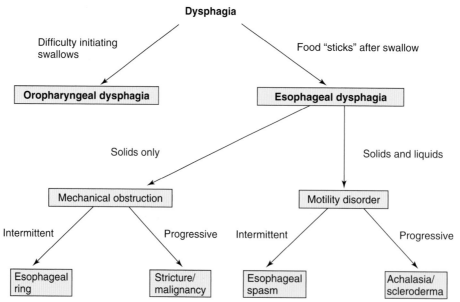

FIGURE 7.18 Algorithm for the Evaluation of Dysphagia. (From Flint PW, Haughey BH, Lund VJ, et al. *Cummings Otolaryngology—Head and Neck Surgery.* 6th ed. Philadelphia, PA: Saunders; 2015, fig. 69-1.)

Table 7.1   Esophageal Manometric Findings in Normal Patients and in Those with Motility Disorders

Finding	Normal	Achalasia	Diffuse Esophageal Spasm	Nutcracker Esophagus	Ineffective Esophageal Motility
Basal LES pressure	10-45 mm Hg	Normal or high	Normal	Normal	Low or normal
LES relaxation with swallow	Complete	Incomplete	Normal	Normal	Normal
Wave progression	Peristalsis	Aperistalsis	Peristalsis with at least 20% simultaneous contractions	Normal	30% or more failed nontransmitted contractions
Distal wave amplitude	30-180 mm Hg	Usually low (may be normal or high)	Normal	High	30% or more <30 mm Hg

LES, Lower esophageal sphincter.
From Flint PW, Haughey BH, Lund VJ, et al. *Cummings Otolaryngology—Head and Neck Surgery.* 6th ed. Philadelphia, PA: Saunders; 2015, table 69-1.

- • Skin rash
- • Proximal muscle weakness
- • Esophagogram: may see dilated *upper* esophagus

DIFFUSE ESOPHAGEAL SPASM BASICS

- • High-pressure nonperistaltic contractions
- • Esophagogram: "corkscrew" esophagus
- • Manometry: disorganized high-pressure contractions
- • Treatment: nitrates and calcium channel blockers

TRANSNASAL ESOPHAGOSCOPY BASICS

- • Lower cost
- • No need for sedation
- • High completion rate (83-99%); most common reason for failure is the inability to pass through the nasal vault
- • High degree of correlation between the endoscopic findings (sensitivity, 89%; specificity, 97%) of transnasal esophagoscopy and conventional esophagoscopy[54-56]
- • No significant difference in the rate of definitive histologic diagnosis[57]
- • In evaluating Barrett metaplasia, there is a 97% correlation between biopsy specimens obtained with transnasal esophagoscopy and conventional esophagoscopy[58]

ESOPHAGEAL INDICATIONS FOR TRANSNASAL ESOPHAGOSCOPY

- • Dysphagia
- • Esophageal symptoms that persist despite antireflux therapy
- • Screening for Barrett esophageal metaplasia
- • Visualization and biopsy of esophageal radiologic abnormalities
- • Long-standing (≥5 years) GERD

EXTRA-ESOPHAGEAL INDICATIONS FOR TRANSNASAL ESOPHAGOSCOPY

- • Chronic cough
- • Panendoscopy and biopsy for head and neck cancer
- • Moderate to severe laryngopharyngeal reflux
- • Globus pharyngeus[59]

EXTERNAL COMPRESSIONS OF THE ESOPHAGUS IN DESCENDING ORDER

1. Aortic compression: pulsating anterolateral prominence
2. Left mainstem bronchus: anterior compression 2 cm distal to aorta
3. Diaphragm: circumferential

TRANSNASAL ESOPHAGOSCOPY– COMPLICATION RATE

- • Epistaxis: most common, 0.5-2%
- • Vasovagal: 0.01-0.3%
- • Minor nasal discomfort: 1.3%[60-62]

CLASSIC ESOPHAGOSCOPY FINDINGS

- • Salmon-colored mucosa proximal to gastric rugae: Barrett esophagitis (Fig. 7.19)
- • Proximal extension of gastric rugae >2 cm from the diaphragm: hiatal hernia

ESOPHAGEAL DIVERTICULUM (Fig. 7.20) MOST COMMON HYPOPHARYNGEAL DIVERTICULUM

- • Zenker diverticulum

AREAS OF HYPOPHARYNGEAL WEAKNESS

1. Killian's triangle (site of Zenker diverticulum)
   - • Area of weakness between the inferior constrictor and the cricopharyngeus
2. Killian-Jameson dehiscence
   - • Area of weakness between the oblique and transverse cricopharyngeus fibers
3. Laimer triangle
   - • Area of weakness between the cricopharyngeus and the superior esophageal wall circular muscles

TRACTION AND PULSION DIVERTICULA

- • Pulsion: result from pressure from within the esophagus causing the esophageal mucosa and submucosa to be herniated through an area of weakness
- • Traction: result of pulling forces external to the esophagus; for example, inflammatory, neoplastic, or following cervical spine surgery

COMMON SYMPTOMS OF ZENKER DIVERTICULUM

- • Progressive dysphagia
- • Regurgitation of food, even hours after a meal
- • Unprovoked aspiration
- • Noisy deglutition (borborygmi)
- • Belching
- • Halitosis
- • Choking/coughing

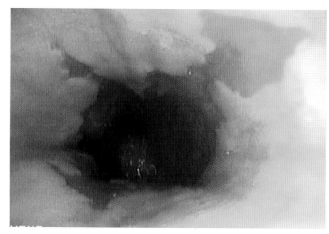

FIGURE 7.19 Evidence of Possible Barrett Metaplasia. Salmon-colored gastric mucosa extends into the distal esophagus. This area should be biopsied to evaluate for histologic changes consistent with Barrett metaplasia to make the diagnosis. (From Flint PW, Haughey BH, Lund VJ, et al. *Cummings Otolaryngology—Head and Neck Surgery.* 6th ed. Philadelphia, PA: Saunders; 2015, fig. 70-3.)

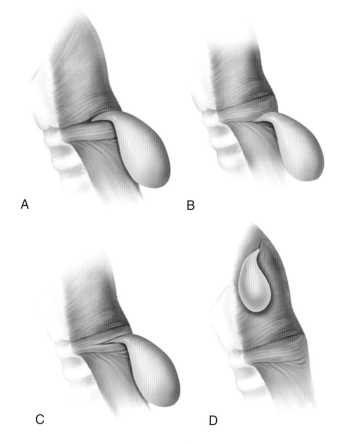

A   B

C   D

FIGURE 7.20 Types of Esophageal Diverticulae. (**A**) Killian triangle: region between the cricopharyngeal and inferior constrictor muscle. (**B**) Laimer triangle: region between the cricopharyngeal and most superior esophageal circular muscle. (**C**) Killian-Jamieson triangle: region between the oblique and transverse fibers of the cricopharyngeal muscle. (**D**) Lateral pharyngocele: variable location above and lateral to the cricopharyngeus. (From Flint PW, Haughey BH, Lund VJ, et al. *Cummings Otolaryngology—Head and Neck Surgery.* 6th ed. Philadelphia, PA: Saunders; 2015, fig. 71-1.)

- Globus pharyngeus
- Weight loss
- Recurrent respiratory infections

VAN OVERBEEK AND GROOTE STAGING SYSTEM FOR ZENKER DIVERTICULUM

1. Stage I: size of one vertebral body
2. Stage II: 1-3 vertebral bodies
3. Stage III: >3 vertebral bodies

TREATMENT OPTIONS FOR ZENKER DIVERTICULUM

1. Diet modification
2. Gastrostomy tube
3. Endoscopic diverticulotomy with cricopharyngeal myotomy
   - Endoscopic stapler (Fig. 7.21)
   - CO_2 laser
   - Harmonic scalpel
4. Open cricopharyngeal myotomy with or without diverticulectomy, diverticulopexy, or diverticular inversion

ADVANTAGES OF ENDOSCOPIC APPROACH TO ZENKER DIVERTICULUM[63,64]

1. Shorter operative time
2. Short hospital stay
3. Lower morbidity (2.6%) and mortality (0.3%)
4. Minimal risk of RLN injury
5. Shorter convalescence

DISADVANTAGES OF ENDOSCOPIC APPROACH TO ZENKER DIVERTICULUM[63]

1. Potential for persistent/recurrent symptoms
2. Risk of recurrent symptoms
3. May not be possible if cannot expose pouch
4. Bad option for larger pouches

ADVANTAGES OF OPEN APPROACH TO ZENKER DIVERTICULUM

1. Definitive procedure
2. No recurrence
3. May be the only possibility if the pouch cannot be exposed or if the pouch is >6 cm

DISADVANTAGES OF OPEN APPROACH TO ZENKER DIVERTICULUM[63]

1. Longer operative time
2. Increased morbidity (mediastinitis) and hospital stay
3. Complication rate 11.8%
4. Mortality 1.6%

TRACHEOBRONCHIAL ENDOSCOPY

Define Lobar and Segmental Bronchi

- Lobar bronchus: defines division of lung lobes
- Segmental bronchus: defines division of pulmonary lobules

Number of Lobes and Lobules of Each Lung

- Right lung: 3 lobes and 10 lobules
- Left lung: 2 lobes and 9 lobules

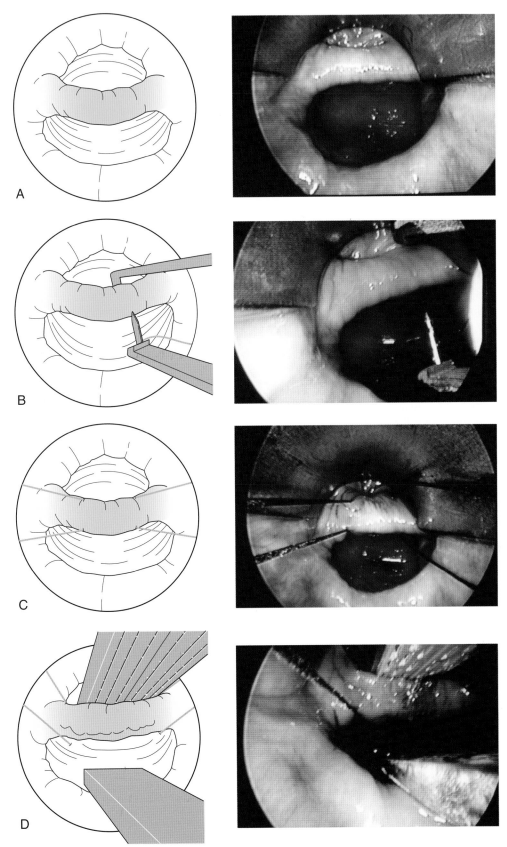

FIGURE 7.21 Technique of Endoscopic Staple Diverticulostomy as Seen with a Rigid Telescope. (**A**) Common wall visualized with a Weerda laryngoscope. (**B** and **C**) With an Endo Stitch suturing device (Covidien Autosuture), retraction sutures are placed on the lateral aspects of the common wall. (**D**) The common wall is positioned between the blades of the stapler.

Continued

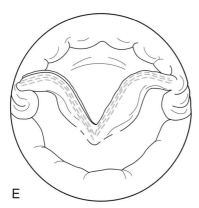
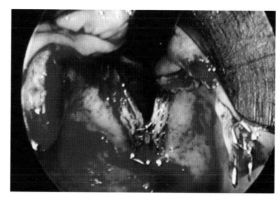

FIGURE 7.21, cont'd Technique of Endoscopic Staple Diverticulostomy as Seen with a Rigid Telescope. (**E**) The common wall is divided after the stapler is activated. The retraction sutures are cut and removed. (From Flint PW, Haughey BH, Lund VJ, et al. *Cummings Otolaryngology—Head and Neck Surgery*. 6th ed. Philadelphia, PA: Saunders; 2015, fig. 71-11.)

Services to Be Consulted Before Bronchoscopy for Massive Hemoptysis

- Thoracic surgery
- Interventional radiology

Topical Anesthesia

- Milligrams of lidocaine
  - 1 mL of 1% lidocaine has 10 mg lidocaine
  - 1 mL of 4% lidocaine has 40 mg lidocaine
- Maximum amount of lidocaine that can be administered at one time: 3-4 mg/kg

Advantages of Rigid Bronchoscopy

- Larger lumen for instrumentation/stenting
- Can ventilate through a side port using the Venturi jet ventilation system
- Can use the scope itself to tamponade bleeding or to core out the tumor

Disadvantages of Rigid Bronchoscopy

- Oral/dental trauma
- Laryngeal edema before surgery, especially with larger bronchoscope

What Is the Main Complication of Endobronchial Biopsy and How Is It Treated?

- Complication: bleeding
- Treatment: dispense small aliquots of oxymetazoline 0.05% or lidocaine 1% over the bleeding site (oxymetazoline is preferred because it causes less tachycardia)

REFERENCES

1. van den Berg J. Myoelastic-aerodynamic theory of voice production. *J Speech Hear Res*. 1958;1:227.
2. Sundberg J, Nordstrom PE. Raised and lowered larynx: the effect on vowel format frequencies. *J Res Sing*. 1983;6:7.
3. Hirano M. Morphological structure of the vocal cord as a vibrator and its variations. *Folia Phoniatr (Basel)*. 1974;26:89.
4. Hirano M, Bless DM. *Videostroboscopic Examination of the Larynx*. San Diego, CA: Singular Publishing Group; 1993.
5. Aronson AE, Bless DM. *Clinical Voice Disorders*. 4th ed. New York, NY: Thieme Medical Publishers; 2009.
6. Statham MM, Rosen C, Nandedkar S, et al. Quantitative laryngeal electromyography: turns and amplitude analysis. *Laryngoscope*. 2010;120:2036–2041.
7. Kempster GB, Gerratt BR, Verdolini Abbott K, et al. Consensus auditory-perceptual evaluation of voice: development of a standardized clinical protocol. *Am J Speech Lang Pathol*. 2009;18:124.
8. Woodson GE, Zwirner P, Murry T, et al. Use of flexible laryngoscopy to classify patients with spasmodic dysphonia. *J Voice*. 1991;5:85.
9. Smith ME, Yanagisawa E. Physical examination of the larynx and videolaryngoscopy. In: Blitzer A, Brin M, Ramig L, eds. *Neurologic Disorders of the Larynx*. New York, NY: Thieme; 2009: 54–58.
10. Bastian RW. Videoendoscopic evaluation of patients with dysphagia: an adjunct to the modified barium swallow. *Otolaryngol Head Neck Surg*. 1991;104(3):339–350.
11. Rickert SM, Childs LF, Carey BT, et al. Laryngeal electromyography for prognosis of vocal fold paralysis: a meta-analysis. *Laryngoscope*. 2012;122(1):158–161.
12. Black JD, Dolly JO. Interaction of 125I-labeled botulinum neurotoxins with nerve terminals I: ultrastructural autoradiographic localization and quantitation of distinct membrane acceptors for types A and B on motor nerves. *J Cell Biol*. 1986;103:521.
13. Blitzer A, Brin MF, Stewart CF. Botulinum toxin management of spasmodic dysphonia: a 12-year experience in more than 900 patients. *Laryngoscope*. 1998;108:1435.
14. Lebrun Y, Devreux F, Rousseau JJ, et al. Tremulous speech: a case report. *Folia Phoniatr*. 1982;34:134.
15. Adler CH, Bansberg SF, Hentz JG. Botulinum toxin type A for treating voice tremor. *Arch Neurol*. Sep. 2004;61(9):1416–1420.
16. Johns MM, Garrett CG, Hwang J, Ossoff RH, Courey MS. Quality of life outcomes following laryngeal endoscopic surgery for non-neoplastic vocal fold lesions. *Ann Otol Rhinol Laryngol*. 2004;113(8):597–601.
17. Koszewski IJ, Hoffman MR, Young WG, Lai Y-T, Dailey SH. Office-based photoangiolytic laser treatment of Reinke's edema: safety and voice outcomes. *Otolaryngol Head Neck Surg*. 2015;152(6): 1075–1081.
18. Lee SW, Hong HJ, Choi SH, et al. Comparison of treatment modalities for contact granuloma: a nation-wide multicenter study. *Laryngoscope*. 2013;124(5):1187–1191.
19. Lim JY, Kim KM, Choi EC, et al. Current clinical propensity of laryngeal tuberculosis: review of 60 cases. *Eur Arch Otorhinolaryngol*. 2006;263:838–842.
20. Hale EK, Bystryn JC. Laryngeal and nasal involvement in pemphigus vulgaris. *J Am Acad Dermatol*. 2001;44:609–611.
21. Taylor SC, Clayburgh DR, Rosenbaum JT, et al. Progression and management of Wegener's granulomatosis in the head and neck. *Laryngoscope*. 2012;122:1695–1700.
22. Lebovics RS, Hoffman GS, Leavitt RY, et al. The management of subglottic stenosis in patients with Wegener's granulomatosis. *Laryngoscope*. 1992;102:1341–1345.
23. Isaak BL, Liesegang TJ, Michet Jr CJ. Ocular and systemic findings in relapsing polychondritis. *Ophthalmology*. 1986;93:681–689.
24. Childs LF, Rickert S, Wengerman OC, et al. Laryngeal manifestations of relapsing polychondritis and a novel treatment option. *J Voice*. 2012;26:587–589.
25. Ingle JW, Young VN, Smith LJ, Munin MC, Rosen CA. Prospective evaluation of the clinical utility of laryngeal electromyography. *Laryngoscope*. 2014;124:2745–2749.

26. Laccourreye O, Papon JF, Kania R, et al. Intracordal injection of autologous fat in patients with unilateral laryngeal nerve paralysis: long-term results from the patient's perspective. *Laryngoscope.* 2003;113:541.

27. Milstein CF, Akst LM, Hicks MD, et al. Long-term effects of micronized alloderm injection for unilateral vocal fold paralysis. *Laryngoscope.* 2005;115:1691–1696.

28. Mathison CC, Villari CR, Klein AM, Johns III MM. Comparison of outcomes and complications between awake and asleep injection laryngoplasty: a case control study. *Laryngoscope.* 2009;119(7):1417–1423.

29. Hirano M, Nozoe I, Shin T, et al. Electromyography for laryngeal paralysis. In: Hirano M, Kirchner J, Bless D, eds. *Neurolaryngology: Recent Advances.* Boston, MA: College-Hill; 1987:232–248.

30. Woodson GE. Configuration of the glottis in laryngeal paralysis II: animal experiments. *Laryngoscope.* 1993;103:1235–1241.

31. Montgomery WM, Hilman RE, Varvares MA. Combined thyroplasty type I and inferior constrictor myotomy. *Ann Otol Rhinol Laryngol.* 1995;103:858–862.

32. Woodson GE. Cricopharyngeal myotomy and arytenoid adduction in the management of combined laryngeal and pharyngeal paralysis. *Otolaryngol Head Neck Surg.* 1997;117:339–343.

33. Tucker HM. Nerve-muscle pedicle reinnervation of the larynx: avoiding pitfalls and complications. *Ann Otol Rhinol Laryngol.* 1982;91:440–444.

34. Paniello RC, Edgar JD, Kallogjeri D, Piccirillo JF. Medialization versus reinnervation for unilateral vocal fold paralysis: a multicenter randomized clinical trial. *Laryngoscope.* 2011;121:2172–2179.

35. Horner J, Massey EW, Riski JE, et al. Aspiration following stroke: clinical correlates and outcome. *Neurology.* 1988;38:1359.

36. Lawless ST, Cook S, Luft J, et al. The use of a laryngotracheal separation procedure in pediatric patients. *Laryngoscope.* 1995;105:198.

37. Donner MW, Silbiger ML. Cinefluorographic analysis of pharyngeal swallowing in neuromuscular disorders. *Am J Med Sci.* 1966;251:600.

38. Splaingard ML, Hutchins B, Sulton LD, et al. Aspiration in rehabilitation patients: videofluoroscopy vs. bedside clinical assessment. *Arch Phys Med Rehabil.* 1988;69:637.

39. Wu CH, Hsiao TY, Chen JC, et al. Evaluation of swallowing safety with fiberoptic endoscope: comparison with videofluoroscopic technique. *Laryngoscope.* 1997;107(3):396.

40. Alessi DM, Berci G. Aspiration and nasogastric intubation. *Otolaryngol Head Neck Surg.* 1986;94:486.

41. Jewett BS, Shockley WW, Rutledge R. External laryngeal trauma analysis of 392 patients. *Arch Otolaryngol Head Neck Surg.* 1999;125:877–880.

42. Juutilainen M, Vintturi J, Robinson S, Bäck L, Lehtonen H, Mäkitie AA. Laryngeal fractures: clinical findings and considerations on suboptimal outcome. *Acta Otolaryngol.* 2008;128(2):213–218.

43. Nottet JB, Duruisseau O, Herve S, et al. Inhalation burns: apropos of 198 cases. Incidence of laryngotracheal involvement. *Ann Otolaryngol Chir Cervicofac.* 1997;114:220–225.

44. Arevalo-Silva C, Eliashar R, Wohlgelernter J, et al. Ingestion of caustic substances: a 15-year experience. *Laryngoscope.* 2006;116:1422–1426.

45. Ramasamy K, Gumaste VV. Corrosive ingestion in adults. *J Clin Gastroenterol.* 2003;37:119–124.

46. Herrington HC, Weber SM, Andersen PE. Modern management of laryngotracheal stenosis. *Laryngoscope.* 2006;116(9):1553–1557.

47. McCaffrey TV. Classification of laryngotracheal stenosis. *Laryngoscope.* 1992;102(12):1335–1340.

48. Nordin U, Lindholm CE, Wolgast M. Blood flow in rabbit tracheal mucosa and the influence of tracheal intubation. *Acta Anesthesiol Scand.* 1977;21:84.

49. Bogdasarian RS, Olson NR. Posterior glottic laryngeal stenosis. *Otolaryngol Head Neck Surg.* 1980;88:765.

50. Meyer TK, Wolf J. Lysis of interarytenoid synechia (Type I posterior glottic stenosis): vocal fold mobility and airway results. *Laryngoscope.* 2011;121(10):2165–2171.

51. Montgomery WW. Posterior and complete glottic stenosis. *Arch Otolaryngol Head Neck Surg.* 1973;98:170.

52. Johnson LF, Demeester TR. Twenty-four-hour pH monitoring of the distal esophagus. A quantitative measure of gastroesophageal reflux. *Am J Gastroenterol.* 1974;62(4):325–332.

53. Johnson LF. 24-hour pH monitoring in the study of gastroesophageal reflux. *J Clin Gastroenterol.* 1980;2(4):387–399.

54. Dean R, Dua K, Massey B, et al. A comparative study of unsedated transnasal esophagogastroduodenoscopy and conventional EGD. *Gastrointest Endosc.* 1996;44(4):422–424.

55. Ai ZL, Lan CH, Fan LL, et al. Unsedated transnasal upper gastrointestinal endoscopy has favorable diagnostic effectiveness, cardiopulmonary safety, and patient satisfaction compared with conventional or sedated endoscopy. *Surg Endosc.* 2012;26(12):3565–3572.

56. Thota PN, Zuccaro Jr G, Vargo 2nd JJ, et al. A randomized prospective trial comparing unsedated esophagoscopy via transnasal and transoral routes using a 4-mm video endoscope with conventional endoscopy with sedation. *Endoscopy.* 2005;37(6):559–565.

57. Walter T, Chesnay AL, Dumortier J, et al. Biopsy specimens obtained with small-caliber endoscopes have comparable diagnostic performances than those obtained with conventional endoscopes: a prospective study on 1335 specimens. *J Clin Gastroenterol.* 2010;44(1):12–17.

58. Saeian K, Staff DM, Vasilopoulos S, et al. Unsedated transnasal endoscopy accurately detects Barrett's metaplasia and dysplasia. *Gastrointest Endosc.* 2002;56(4):472–478.

59. Amin MR, Postma GN, Setzen M, et al. Transnasal esophagoscopy: a position statement from the American Bronchoesophagological Association (ABEA). *Otolaryngol Head Neck Surg.* 2008;138(4):411–414.

60. Dumortier J, Napoleon B, Hedelius F, et al. Unsedated transnasal EGD in daily practice: results with 1100 consecutive patients. *Gastrointest Endosc.* 2003;57(1):198–204.

61. Cho S, Arya N, Swan K, et al. Unsedated transnasal endoscopy: a Canadian experience in daily practice. *Canadian J Gastroenterol.* 2008;22(3):243–246.

62. Postma GN, Cohen JT, Belafsky PC, et al. Transnasal esophagoscopy: revisited (over 700 consecutive cases). *Laryngoscope.* 2005;115(2):321–323.

63. Chang C, Payyapilli R, Scher RL. Endoscopic staple diverticulostomy for Zenker's diverticulum: review of literature and experience in 159 consecutive patients. *Laryngoscope.* 2003;113:957–965.

64. Scher RL, Richtsmeier WJ. Endoscopic staple-assisted esophagodiverticulostomy for Zenker's diverticulum. *Laryngoscope.* 1996;106:951–956.

8 | Otolaryngic Allergy

INNATE AND ADAPTIVE IMMUNE SYSTEM

BASIC TYPES OF IMMUNITY

- Innate immune system (pattern-recognition receptors)
- Adaptive immune system (specific antigen recognition)
  - Humoral
  - Cellular

CELL LAYERS OF INNATE IMMUNE SYSTEM

- Epithelia cell layers
- Mucous cell layers

MUCOSAL IMMUNE SYSTEM

- Organized mucosal immune system
  - Tonsils
  - Peyer patches
  - Isolated lymphoid follicles
- Diffuse mucosal immune system
  - Intraepithelial lymphocytes
  - Lamina propria

CELLS OF INNATE IMMUNE SYSTEM

1. Neutrophils
2. Monocytes
3. Natural killer cells
4. Mast cells
5. Eosinophils
6. Basophils
7. Dendritic cells

ANTIMICROBIAL PEPTIDES OF INNATE IMMUNE SYSTEM

- Cathelicidins
- Defensins
  - Alpha defensins
  - Beta defensins
  - Theta defensins

RECEPTORS OF INNATE IMMUNE SYSTEM

- Pattern-recognition receptors
- Toll-like receptors

MECHANISMS OF INNATE IMMUNE SYSTEM

- Opsonize bacteria
- Activate coagulation
- Complement cascades

MEDIATORS OF ADAPTIVE IMMUNE SYSTEM (Fig. 8.1)

- B lymphocytes
- T lymphocytes
- Antibodies

T CELLS

- T helper 2 (TH2)—specialize in facilitating B-cell antibody response
- T helper 1 (TH1)—specialize in macrophage activation
- T helper 17 (TH17)—involved in autoimmunity
- Regulatory T cells—involved in autoimmunity

B CELLS

- Plasma
- Memory

IMMUNOGLOBULINS (Fig. 8.2)

- Immunoglobulin G (IgG) (75%, monomer): recall immune responses and can cross the placenta
- Immunoglobulin M (IgM) (10%, pentamer): antigen receptor of B cells
- Immunoglobulin A (IgA) (15%, dimer): found in external secretions, is the primary defense against local mucosal infections, and neutralizes foreign substances
- Immunoglobulin E (IgE) (<0.01%, monomer): binds mast cells and is involved in allergic and parasitic infections
- Immunoglobulin D (IgD) (0.2%, monomer): antigen receptor on B cells

LYMPHOID TISSUE OF ADAPTIVE IMMUNE SYSTEM

- Thymus
- Bone marrow
- Lymph nodes
- Spleen
- Epithelial immune system
- Mucosal immune system
  - Tonsils
  - Peyer patches and lymphoid follicles
  - Lymphoid follicles
  - Intraepithelial lymphocytes and lamina propria

HUMAN LEUKOCYTE ANTIGEN

- Class I: nucleated somatic cells
  - Human leukocyte antigen (HLA)-A
  - HLA-B
  - HLA-C

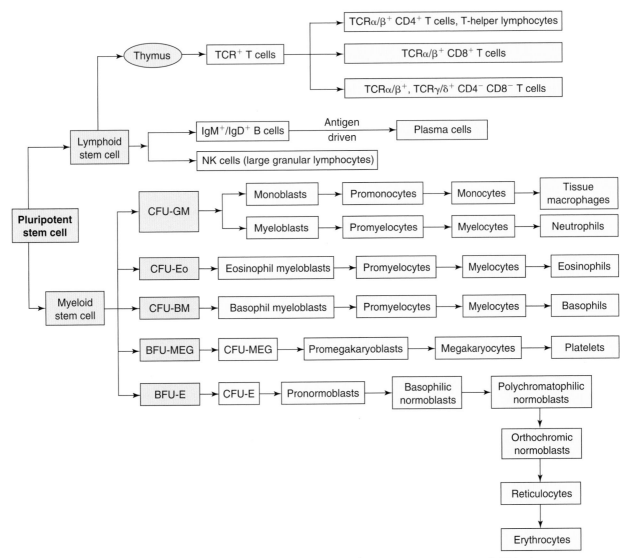

FIGURE 8.1 The Development of the Immune Cells. *BFU*, Burst-forming unit; *BM*, basophil mast cell; *CFU*, colony-forming unit; *E*, erythroid; *Eo*, eosinophil; *GM*, granulocyte-macrophage; *Ig*, immunoglobulin; *MEG*, megakaryocyte; *NK*, natural killer; *TCR*, T-cell receptor. (From Flint PW, Haughey BH, Lund VJ, et al. *Cummings Otolaryngology—Head and Neck Surgery*. 6th ed. Philadelphia, PA: Saunders; 2015, fig. 38-1.)

- Class II: immunocompetent antigen-presenting cells
  - HLA-DR
  - HLA-DQ
  - HLA-DP

MAJOR HISTOCOMPATIBILITY COMPLEX (Fig. 8.3)

- Class I: all nucleated cells
- Class II: antigen-presenting cells
  - Macrophage
  - Dendritic cells
  - B cells

COMPLEMENT SYSTEM (Fig. 8.4)

- Classic pathway
- Lectin pathway
- Alternative pathway

CYTOKINES (Table 8.1)

- Broad category of small proteins important in cell signaling

CHEMOKINES (Table 8.2)

- Small proteins important in signaling chemotaxis
- Four categories: CXC, CC, CX3C, and CX

CELL ADHESION (Fig. 8.5)

- Intercellular adhesion molecule (ICAM)-1
- ICAM-2
- E-selectin
- P-selectin
- Vascular cellular adhesion molecule (VCAM)

ALLERGIC TRIGGERS: CATEGORIES

1. Inhalants
2. Ingestions
3. Injectables
4. Contactants

STAGES OF DEVELOPMENT OF AN ALLERGY

- Early response: minutes after exposure antigen
  - Primary mediator is histamine

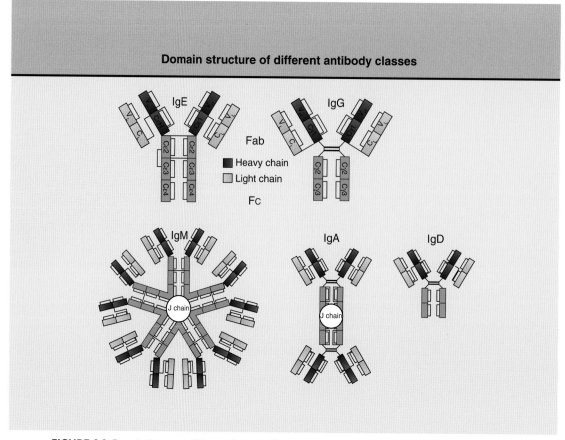

FIGURE 8.2 Domain Structure of Various Antibody Classes. (From Krouse JH. Introduction to allergy. In: Krouse JH, Derebery MJ, Chadwick SJ, eds. *Managing the Allergic Patient*. 1st ed. Philadelphia, PA: Saunders Elsevier; 2008. Originally reproduced from Holgate ST. *Allergy*. 2nd ed. London: Mosby/Elsevier; 2001:245, fig. 16.4.)

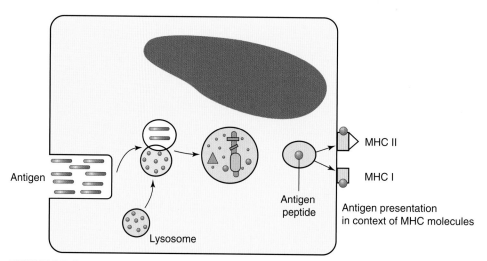

FIGURE 8.3 Antigen Processing and Presentation. The antigen undergoes hydrolytic cleavage within antigen-presenting cells, and the resultant oligopeptides are loaded on the antigen-binding grooves of major histocompatibility complex (MHC) molecules and are expressed at the cell surface. (From Flint PW, Haughey BH, Lund VJ, et al. *Cummings Otolaryngology—Head and Neck Surgery*. 6th ed. Philadelphia, PA: Saunders; 2015, fig. 38-2.)

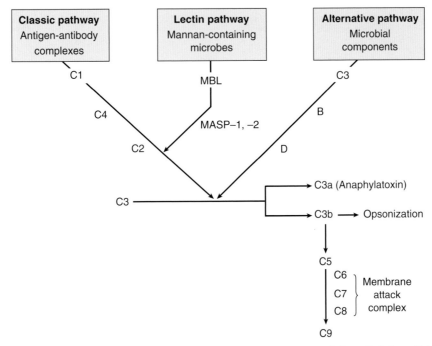

FIGURE 8.4 Complement Pathways. Three pathways of the complement system. *B*, Factor B; *D*, factor D; *MASP*, MBL-associated serine proteases; *MBL*, mannan-binding lectin. (From Flint PW, Haughey BH, Lund VJ, et al. *Cummings Otolaryngology—Head and Neck Surgery.* 6th ed. Philadelphia, PA: Saunders; 2015.)

Table 8.1 Cytokines

Cytokine	Cell Sources	Predominant Effects
Interleukins		
IL-1α, IL-1β functionally equivalent isoforms	Macrophages, neutrophils, epithelial and endothelial cells, monocytes, lymphocytes, and keratinocytes	Fever, local inflammation, T-cell and macrophage activation; principal mediator(s) of septic shock; differentiation of TH17 cells
IL-2	Activated T cells, DCs, and NK cells	Proliferation of effector T and B cells, development of Treg cells, and differentiation and proliferation of NK cells
IL-3	CD4+ T cells, thymic epithelial cells, mast cells, eosinophils, macrophages, and NK cells	Synergistic action in early hematopoiesis; activates and promotes recruitment of basophils and eosinophils in late allergic reactions
IL-4	TH2 cells, mast cells, basophils, NK T cells, eosinophils, and γ/δ–T cells	Differentiation and growth of TH2 subset, B-cell activation, survival factor for T and B cells, isotype switch to IgE and IgG1, suppression of TH1 cells, and growth factor for mast cells
IL-5	Activated TH2 cells and mast cells, NK cells, NK T cells, and eosinophils	Eosinophil survival, differentiation, and chemotaxis, differentiation and function of myeloid cells, and remodeling and wound healing
IL-6	T cells, mononuclear phagocytes, vascular endothelial cells, fibroblasts	T- and B-cell growth and differentiation; acute-phase protein production by the liver
IL-7	Stromal cells in bone marrow and thymus, B cells, monocytes, macrophages, epithelial cells, keratinocytes, and DCs	Growth of pre–B cells and pre–T cells; synthesis induction of inflammatory mediators in monocytes
IL-8, CXC chemokine	Activated mononuclear phagocytes, fibroblasts, and endothelial cells	Chemoattractant for neutrophils, NK cells, T cells, basophils, eosinophils; promotes neutrophil inflammatory responses, and mobilization of hematopoietic stem cells
IL-9	TH2 cells, TH9 cells, mast cells, and eosinophils	T-cell and mast-cell growth factor, inhibition of TH1 cytokines, proliferation of CD8+ T cells and mast cells, IgE production, and chemokine and mucus production in bronchial epithelial cells

Continued

Table 8.1	**Cytokines—cont'd**	
Cytokine	**Cell Sources**	**Predominant Effects**
IL-10	T cells, B cells, monocytes, macrophages, and DCs	Important in innate and adaptive immunity; immune suppression
IL-11	Stromal cells: fibroblasts, epithelial cells, endothelial cells, vascular smooth muscle cells, synoviocytes, and osteoblasts	Growth factor for myeloid, erythroid, and megakaryocyte progenitors; bone remodeling; protects epithelial cells and connective tissue; induction of acute-phase protein; inhibition of macrophage activity; promotion of neuronal development
IL-12	Macrophages, monocytes, neutrophils, DCs, B cells, and microglia	Induces TH1 differentiation and cytotoxicity
IL-13	T cells, NK T cells, mast cells, basophils, and eosinophils	Switching to IgG4 and IgE; upregulation of CD23; MHC-II on B cells; induction of CD11b, CD11c, CD18, CD29, CD23, and MHC-II on monocytes; activation of eosinophils and mast cells; recruitment and survival of eosinophils; defense against parasitic infections
IL-14	Activated T cells	Growth factor for B cells
IL-15	Monocytes, activated CD4+ T cells, keratinocytes, and skeletal muscle cells	Stimulates growth and development of NK cells; stimulates activation and proliferation of T and B cells
IL-16	T cells, mast cells, eosinophils, monocytes, DCs, fibroblasts, and airway epithelial cells	Chemotaxis and modulation of T-cell response
IL-17A	TH17 cells, CD8+ T cells, NK cells, NK T cells, γ/δ–T cells, and neutrophils	Induces proinflammatory cytokine and chemokine production by epithelial and endothelial cells and fibroblasts; recruitment of neutrophils
IL-17B	Neuronal cells and chondrocytes	Induces proinflammatory cytokine and chemokine production Chondrogenesis and osteogenesis
IL-17C	Immune cells under certain conditions	Induces proinflammatory cytokine and chemokine production
IL-17D	Resting B and T cells	Induces proinflammatory cytokine and chemokine production
IL-17F	TH17 cells, CD8+ T cells, NK cells, NK T cells, γ/δ–T cells, and neutrophils	Induces proinflammatory cytokine and chemokine production; recruitment of neutrophils
IL-18	Macrophages, Kupffer cells, keratinocytes, osteoblasts, astrocytes, and DCs	Induces IFN-γ production by T cells and NK cells; promotes TH1 or TH2 cell responses depending on cytokine milieu
IL-19	Monocytes, keratinocytes, airway epithelial cells, and B cells	Unknown
IL-20	Monocytes, keratinocytes, and epithelial and endothelial cells	Appears to have a role in skin development and is suspected of regulating inflammation in the skin
IL-21	T cells (predominantly TH17) and NK T cells	Regulates proliferation, differentiation, apoptosis, antibody isotype balance, and cytotoxic activity
IL-22	Activated T cells (predominantly TH17), NK T cells	Pathogen defense, wound healing, and tissue reorganization
IL-23	Macrophages and activated dendritic cells	Stimulates production of proinflammatory IL-17 and promotes memory
IL-24	Melanocytes, T cells, monocytes	Tumor suppression
IL-25	TH2 cells, mast cells, epithelial cells, eosinophils, and basophils from atopic individuals	Enhances allergic responses and promotes TH2 inflammation
IL-26	Activated T cells (predominantly TH17), NK T cells	Activates and regulates epithelial cells
IL-27	Activated DCs, macrophages, and epithelial cells	Promotes development along the TH1 phenotype, suppresses the TH2 phenotype, and inhibits TH17 response
IL-28 and IL-29	Monocyte-derived DCs	Induces an antiviral state in infected cells
IL-30 (p28 subunit of IL-27)	DCs and macrophages	Induces IL-12–mediated liver injury

Table 8.1	Cytokines—cont'd	
Cytokine	**Cell Sources**	**Predominant Effects**
IL-31	Activated CD4+ T cells (mainly TH2) and CD8+ T cells	Induces IL-6, IL-8, CXCL1, CXCL8, CC chemokine ligand 2, and CC chemokine ligand 8 production in eosinophils; upregulates chemokine mRNA expression in keratinocytes, expression of growth factors and chemokines in epithelial cells, and inhibits proliferation and apoptosis in epithelial cells
IL-32	Monocytes, macrophages, NK cells, T cells, and epithelial cells	Induces TNF-α, IL-8, and IL-6 apoptosis
IL-33	Necrotic cells	Induces TH2 inflammation
IL-34	Heart, brain, spleen, liver, kidney, thymus, testes, ovary, small intestine, prostate, and colon	Proliferation
IL-35	Treg cells	Proliferation of Treg cells and inhibition of TH17-cell function; suppression of inflammatory responses
IL-37	Monocytes, tonsil plasma cells, and breast carcinoma cells	Suppresses proinflammatory cytokines and inhibits DC activation
TSLP	Epithelial cells	Promotes T-cell proliferation and differentiation and activates DCs to prime for TH2 cell differentiation
Interferons		
IFN-γ	T cells, NK and NK T cells, macrophages, TH1 cells, and B cells	Macrophage activation, increased expression of MHC molecules and antigen-presenting components, Ig class switching, suppression of TH2 response, antiviral properties, and promotes cytotoxic activity
IFN-α	Leukocytes	Antiviral; increases MHC class I expression
IFN-β	Fibroblasts	Antiviral; increases MHC class I expression
Tumor Necrosis Factor and Related Molecules		
TNF	Activated monocytes/macrophages and T, B, and NK cells	Major inflammatory mediator induced by the presence of gram-negative bacteria and their components; potent immunoregulatory, cytotoxic, antiviral, and procoagulatory activities
LTα (previously called TNF-β)	Activated TH1, B, and NK cells	Promotes inflammation, has antiviral activity, and kills tumor cells by apoptosis
LTαβ	Activated TH1, B, and NK cells	Has a specialized role in secondary lymphoid organ development
OPGL	Osteoblasts, bone marrow stromal cells, and activated T cells	Stimulates osteoclasts and bone resorption
BAFF	Monocytes, macrophages, and dendritic cells	Survival factor required for the maturation of B cells
Transforming Growth Factor		
TGF-β	Chondrocytes, monocytes, and T cells	Antiinflammatory; inhibits cell growth; induces IgA secretion by B cells; plays a role in adhesion, proliferation, differentiation, transformation, chemotaxis, and immunoregulation
Hematopoietic Growth Factors		
SCF	Stromal cells in the fetal liver, bone marrow, and thymus; in the central nervous system; and in the gut mucosa	Supports the survival and growth of the earliest hematopoietic precursors in vivo
GM-CSF	Activated T cells, macrophages, stromal cells, and endothelial cells	Stimulates growth and differentiation of myelomonocytic lineage cells, particularly dendritic cells and inflammatory leukocytes
G-CSF	Activated T cells, endothelial cells, fibroblasts, and mononuclear phagocytes	Stimulates neutrophil development and differentiation
M-CSF	Endothelial cells, fibroblasts, and mononuclear phagocytes	Influences CFU-GM cells to differentiate into monocytes and macrophages in vitro

BAFF, B-lymphocyte–activating factor belonging to the TNF family; *CFU*, colony-forming unit; *CSF*, colony-stimulating factor; *DC*, dendritic cells; *G*, granulocyte; *GM*, granulocyte-macrophage; *IFN*, interferon; *Ig*, immunoglobulin; *IL*, interleukin; *LT*, lymphotoxin; *M*, macrophage; *MHC*, major histocompatibility complex; *mRNA*, messenger RNA; *NK*, natural killer; *OPGL*, osteoprotegerin ligand; *SCF*, stem cell factor; *TGF*, transforming growth factor; *TH*, helper T; *TNF*, tumor necrosis factor, *Treg*, regulatory T cells; *TSLP*, thymic stromal lymphopoietin.

From Flint PW, Haughey BH, Lund VJ, et al. *Cummings Otolaryngology—Head and Neck Surgery*. 6th ed. Philadelphia, PA: Saunders; 2015, table 38-1.

Table 8.2 **Chemokines**

Systematic Name	Common Name(s)/Ligand(s)	Target Cell(s)
CXC Chemokines		
CXCL1	GROα/MGSAα	Neutrophil
CXCL2	GROβ/MGSAβ	Neutrophil
CXCL3	GROδ/MGSAδ	Neutrophil
CXCL4	Platelet factor-4	Fibroblast
CXCL5	Epithelial neutrophil-activating peptide 78	Neutrophil
CXCL6	Granulocyte chemotactic protein 2	Neutrophil
CXCL7	Neutrophil-activating peptide 2	Neutrophil
CXCL8	IL-8	Neutrophil, basophil, and T cell
CXCL9	Monokine induced by IFN-γ	Activated T cell
CXCL10	IFN-γ–inducible protein 10	Activated T cell
CXCL11	IFN-inducible T-cell α–chemoattractant	Activated T cell
CXCL12	Stromal cell–derived factor 1a/b	CD34$^+$ bone marrow cell, T cell, dendritic cell, B cell, and activated CD4 cell
CXCL13	B-cell–attracting chemokine 1	Naïve B cell and activated CD4 cell
CXCL14	Breast and kidney–expressed chemokine	
CXCL15	Lungkine	
CXCL16	Small inducible cytokine B6	T cell and NK T cell
CC Chemokines		
CCL1	I-309 (a human chemokine)	Neutrophil, T cell
CCL2	MCP-1/monocyte chemotactic and activating factor/tumor-derived chemotactic factor	T cell, monocyte, and basophil
CCL3	MIP-1α	Monocyte, macrophage, T cell, NK cell, and basophil
CCL3L1	LD78β	
CCL4	MIP-1β	Monocyte, macrophage, T cell, NK cell, and basophil
CCL5	Regulated upon activation, normal T cell expressed and secreted (RANTES)	Monocyte, macrophage, T cell, NK cell, basophil, eosinophil, and dendritic cell
CCL6	None	
CCL7	MCP-3	T cell, monocyte, eosinophil, basophil, dendritic cell
CCL8	MCP-2	T cell, monocyte, eosinophil, and basophil
CCL9/10	MIP-1γ	
CCL11	Eotaxin	Eosinophil
CCL12	MCP-5	
CCL13	MCP-4	T cell, monocyte, eosinophil, basophil, and dendritic cell
CCL14	HCC-1	Monocyte
CCL15	HCC-2/leukotactin 1/MIP-1δ	T cell, monocyte, and dendritic cell
CCL16	HCC-4/liver-expressed chemokine	Monocyte
CCL17	Thymus- and activation-regulated chemokine	T cell, immature dendritic cell, T cell, and thymocyte
CCL18	MIP-4, dendritic cell–derived CC chemokine/pulmonary and activation-regulated chemokine/activation-induced, and chemokine-related molecule 1	Naïve T cell and T cell
CCL19	MIP-3β/exodus 3	Naïve T cell, mature dendritic cell, and B cell
CCL20	MIP-3α/liver- and activation-regulated chemokine/exodus 1	T cell, bone marrow, and dendritic cell
CCL21	6Ckine/secondary lymphoid tissue chemokine/exodus 2	Naïve T cell and B cell
CCL22	Macrophage-derived chemokine-stimulated T-cell chemoattractant protein 1	Immature dendritic cell and T cell

Table 8.2	Chemokines—cont'd	
Systematic Name	**Common Name(s)/Ligand(s)**	**Target Cell(s)**
CCL23	MPIF-1/CK 8/CK 8-1	Monocyte and T cell
CCL24	Eotaxin 2/MPIF-2	Eosinophil and basophil
CCL25	Thymus-expressed chemokine	Macrophage, thymocyte, and dendritic cell
CCL26	Eotaxin 3	
CCL27	Cutaneous T-cell–activating chemokine/IL-11 receptor α-locus chemokine	T cell
CCL28	Mucosa-associated epithelial chemokine	T cell and eosinophil
C Chemokines		
XCL1	Lymphotactin/SCM-1β/activation-induced, chemokine-related molecule	T cell and NK cell
XCL2	SCM-1β	
CXC3C Chemokine		
CXC3CL1	Fracktalkine	T cell and monocyte

CCL, CC ligand; *CK,* chemokine; *CXCL,* CXC ligand; *GRO,* growth-related oncogene; *HCC,* human CC chemokine; *IFN,* interferon; *IL,* interleukin; *MCP,* monocyte chemoattractant protein; *MGSA,* melanoma growth stimulatory activity; *MIP,* macrophage inflammatory protein; *MPIF,* myeloid progenitor inhibitory factor; *NK,* natural killer; *SCM,* single C motif.
From Flint PW, Haughey BH, Lund VJ, et al. *Cummings Otolaryngology—Head and Neck Surgery.* 6th ed. Philadelphia, PA: Saunders; 2015, table 38-2.

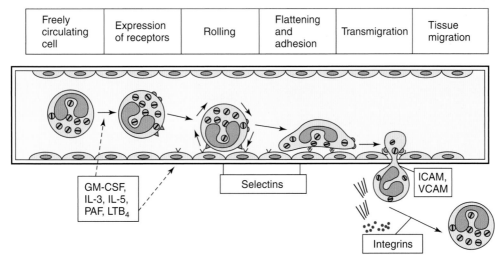

FIGURE 8.5 Cellular Adhesion and Recruitment. *GM-CSF,* Granulocyte-macrophage colony-stimulating factor; *ICAM,* intercellular adhesion molecule; *IL,* interleukin; *LTB₄,* leukotriene B₄; *PAF,* platelet-activating factor; *VCAM,* vascular cellular adhesion molecule. (From Flint PW, Haughey BH, Lund VJ, et al. *Cummings Otolaryngology—Head and Neck Surgery.* 6th ed. Philadelphia, PA: Saunders; 2015, fig. 38-4; and Mygind N, Dahl R, Pedersen S, Thestrup-Pedersen K, eds. *Essential Allergy.* 2nd ed. Oxford: Blackwell Scientific Publications; 1996.)

- Symptoms: largely nasal symptoms, including rhinorrhea, sneezing, itching, and congestion, as well as other symptoms, including tearing, wheezing, and, potentially, laryngospasm and bronchospasm
- Late response: hours after exposure to antigen
  - Mediators: leukotrienes and eosinophils
  - Symptoms: congestion, increased rhinorrhea, and wheezing

TYPES OF HYPERSENSITIVITIES (GELL AND COOMBS CLASSIFICATION)

1. Type I: immediate/anaphylaxis (IgE)
2. Type II: cytotoxic (IgG, IgM)
3. Type III: immune complex (IgG, IgM, IgA)
4. Type IV: cell mediated (T cells)

TYPE I: CAUSES OF ANAPHYLAXIS

- Inhalants
- Foods
- Drugs
- Insect stings

TYPE I: ANAPHYLAXIS SYMPTOMS

- Upper respiratory: sneezing, itching, rhinorrhea, and congestion
- Lower respiratory: cough, bronchospasm, and wheezing
- Skin: urticarial, angioedema, itching, and whealing
- Systemic: hypotension, tachycardia, and feelings of impending doom

TYPE I: ANAPHYLAXIS—MECHANISM

- Cross linking of IgE on mast cells
- Degranulation of mast cells
- Release of histamine

MAST CELL DEGRANULATION

- Vasodilation
- Increase capillary permeability
- Bronchoconstriction
- Tissue edema

TYPE II: CYTOTOXIC REACTION—MECHANISM

- IgG or IgM mediated
- Antibody reaction with antigens on the cell surface
- Activation of complement

TYPE II: CYTOTOXIC REACTION—EXAMPLES

- Hemolytic anemia
- Transfusion reaction
- Acute graft versus host disease
- Goodpasture syndrome
- Myasthenia gravis

TYPE III: IMMUNE COMPLEXES—MECHANISM

- Immune complexes form (binding of antibody to a soluble antigen)
- Complexes deposit in tissues

TYPE III: IMMUNE COMPLEXES—EXAMPLES

- Serum sickness
- Poststreptococcal glomerulonephritis
- Angioedema
- Gastrointestinal intolerance

TYPE IV: CELL MEDIATED—MECHANISM

- Direct T-cell activation
- Cell-mediated inflammation

TYPE IV: CELL MEDIATED—EXAMPLES

- Dermatitis
- Tuberculosis
- Sarcoidosis
- Candidiasis

ALLERGENS

PERENNIAL ALLERGENS

- Mites
- Cockroach
- Cotton particles
- Human skin scales
- Animal dander
- Molds

SEASONAL ALLERGIES

- Trees: winter and spring
- Grasses: spring, summer, and fall
- Weeds: summer and fall

POLLEN AS ALLERGEN

- Windborne
- Lightweight
- Large quantities
- Allergenic in sensitive individuals

HISTORY AND PHYSICAL EXAM OF PATIENT WITH ALLERGIES

HISTORY

- Particular emphasis on:
  - List of medications
  - Co-morbidities
  - Previous operations or treatments for allergy
  - Childhood history
  - Family history

PHYSICAL EXAM

- Eyes: allergic "shiners" and long eyelashes
- Ears: erythema, postauricular fissures, desquamation of external auditory canal, tympanosclerosis, tympanic membrane retraction and/or perforation, and serous effusion
- Nose: discharge, edema of turbinates, polyps, and "allergic salute"
- Neck: lymphadenopathy
- Chest: wheezing
- Pharyngeal: high, narrow arched palate; lymphoid hyperplasia; cobblestoning of the posterior pharyngeal wall; hypertrophy of the lateral nasopharyngeal bands; chronic cough, and edema of the uvula and glottis
- Systemic: eczema, heartburn, diarrhea, abdominal bloating, enuresis, and asthma

RHINITIS

DIFFERENTIAL DIAGNOSIS OF RHINORRHEA AND NASAL OBSTRUCTION (Box 8.1)

1. Allergic rhinitis
2. Nonallergic rhinitis
3. Nonallergic rhinitis eosinophilia syndrome
4. Infectious rhinitis
5. Granulomatous rhinitis
6. Drug-induced rhinitis
7. Rhinitis from mechanical obstruction
8. Neoplastic rhinitis
9. Chronic rhinitis and rhinosinusitis

ALLERGIC RHINITIS COMMON ALLERGENS: INFANTS/CHILDREN

- Milk
- Eggs
- Soy
- Wheat
- Dust mites
- Pet dander

ALLERGIC RHINITIS COMMON ALLERGENS: ADOLESCENTS/ADULTS

- Pollens
- Animal dander
- Insects
- Molds
- Foods

Box 8.1 DIFFERENTIAL DIAGNOSIS OF RHINORRHEA AND NASAL OBSTRUCTION

Allergic Rhinitis
Seasonal/perennial/episodic or intermittent/persistent

Local Allergic Rhinitis
Negative skin/radioallergosorbent testing but positive nasal allergen challenge

Nonallergic Rhinitis
Perennial (vasomotor): Constant symptoms of profuse, clear rhinorrhea and nasal congestion without correlation to specific allergen exposure or signs of atopy
  Cold air–induced: Nasal congestion and rhinorrhea upon exposure to cold, windy weather; occurs in both allergic and nonallergic individuals

Nonallergic Rhinitis with Eosinophilia Syndrome
Most often seen in adults; characterized by eosinophilia on nasal smears and with negative test results for specific allergens

Infectious Rhinitis
Bacterial, viral, and fungal

Granulomatous Rhinitis
Sarcoidosis and Wegener granulomatosis

Drug-Induced Rhinitis
Oral contraceptives, reserpine derivatives, hydralazine hydrochloride, topical decongestants (rhinitis medicamentosa), and beta-blockers (eyedrops)

Rhinitis from Mechanical Obstruction
Septal deviation: Common; might exacerbate nasal obstruction in allergic rhinitis
  Foreign body: Unilateral purulent nasal discharge is the usual manifestation of a foreign body; resolves after removal
  Choanal atresia or stenosis: Bilateral choanal atresia is usually diagnosed early in life, but unilateral choanal atresia or stenosis can go unnoticed for several years; it is easily diagnosed by nasal endoscopy and axial computed tomography of the midfacial skeleton
  Adenoid hypertrophy: Common cause of nasal obstruction in children
  Others: Encephaloceles, lacrimal duct cysts, and dermoids

Neoplastic Rhinitis
Benign: Polyps, juvenile angiofibroma, and inverted papilloma
  Malignant: Adenocarcinoma, squamous cell carcinoma, esthesioneuroblastoma, lymphoma, and rhabdomyosarcoma

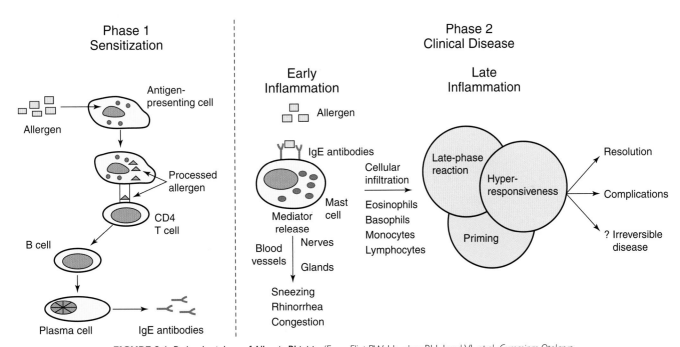

FIGURE 8.6 Pathophysiology of Allergic Rhinitis. (From Flint PW, Haughey BH, Lund VJ, et al. *Cummings Otolaryngology—Head and Neck Surgery.* 6th ed. Philadelphia, PA: Saunders; 2015, fig. 38-6; and Naclerio RM. Allergic rhinitis. *N Engl J Med* 1991;325:860.)

PATHOPHYSIOLOGY OF ALLERGIC RHINITIS (Fig. 8.6)

- Inflammation of nasal mucous membranes
- IgE mediated to allergens (type I)
- IgE attach to the surface receptors of mast cells

DEVELOPMENT OF ATOPY

- Genetics
- Environmental exposure
- Exposure to tobacco smoke
- Diesel exhaust

- "Hygiene hypothesis": lack of exposure to certain agents, such as infectious symbiotic microorganisms, during childhood increases susceptibility later in life

INFLAMMATORY MEDIATORS OF ALLERGIC RHINITIS

- Histamine
- Leukotrienes
- Cytokines
- Prostaglandins
- Platelet-activating factor

ALLERGIC RHINITIS EVALUATION

ALLERGIC RHINITIS DIAGNOSIS: HISTORY SPECIFIC QUESTIONS

- Nasal, ocular, otologic, oral, facial, and skin symptoms
- Time of year, relation to wind and weather patterns and geographic location
- Present environments—for example, home, school, work, and outdoors
- Family or childhood history of atopy (allergies, eczema, and asthma)
- History of anaphylaxis
- Quality of life
- Past and current allergy treatments

ALLERGIC RHINITIS DIAGNOSIS: PHYSICAL EXAM

- Periorbital puffiness
- Allergic shiners
- Long eyelashes
- Dennie lines
- Otitis media with effusion
- Clear rhinorrhea
- Gray/blue turbinates
- Allergic salute
- Adenoid facies
- Cobblestoning of pharyngeal lymphoid tissue

ALLERGIC RHINITIS–ASSOCIATED DISORDERS

1. Chronic rhinosinusitis
2. Nasal polyps
3. Asthma
4. Otitis media with effusion

ALLERGIC RHINITIS ADJUNCTIVE TESTING

1. Nasal endoscopy
2. Labs: IgE, eosinophilia
3. Nasal smear
4. Nasal allergen challenge
5. Skin allergy testing
6. In vitro allergy testing
7. Pulmonary function tests if asthma is suspected

DIFFERENTIAL DIAGNOSIS OF ALLERGIC RHINITIS

1. Infectious rhinitis
2. Perennial nonallergic rhinitis
3. Pollutants and irritants
4. Hormonal rhinitis
5. Medication-induced topical rhinitis
6. Anatomic deformity
7. Tumor
8. Foreign body

SKIN TESTING

ALLERGIC RHINITIS IN VIVO ALLERGY TESTING

- Scratch test
- Prick test
- Intradermal test
- Skin endpoint titration/intradermal dilutional testing

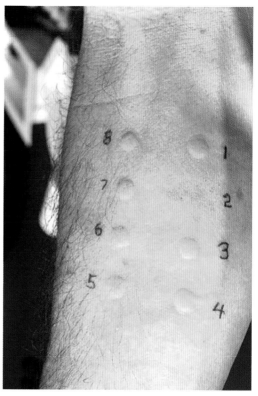

FIGURE 8.7 Prick Test. (From Chadwick SJ. Principles of allergy management. In: Krouse JH, Derebery MJ, Chadwick SJ, eds. *Managing the Allergic Patient*. 1st ed. Philadelphia, PA: Saunders; 2008.)

SCRATCH TEST

- 2-mm superficial laceration made in the patient skin (usually on the patient's back)
- Drop of antigen is applied to the scratch
- Observation in change of the laceration
- Advantages: safe, systemic, reactions are unlikely, and a large surface area for testing
- Disadvantages: false positives, painful, and poor reproducibility

PRICK TEST (Fig. 8.7)

- Drop of antigen is placed on the skin, and a small-gauge needle is used to penetrate into the epidermis and deliver the antigen
- Alternate: use of an automated prick device
- Measurement after 10-20 minutes
- Quantitative (size of wheal) and qualitative scoring of wheal (eg, 0-4+)
- Advantages: rapid test, easy to perform, strong reproducibility, and rare systemic reactions
- Disadvantages: mostly qualitative assessment and false negatives

INTRADERMAL TEST (Fig. 8.8)

- Small-gauge needle (eg, #26) used to inject a small amount of antigen (0.01-0.05 mL intradermally)
- Concentrations of antigens: 1:500 to 1:1000 weight/volume
- 10-20 minutes to allow for skin reaction
- Quantitative (size of wheal) and qualitative scoring of wheal (eg, 0-4+)
- Advantages: highly sensitive, moderately reproducible
- Disadvantages: poor specificity and false positives

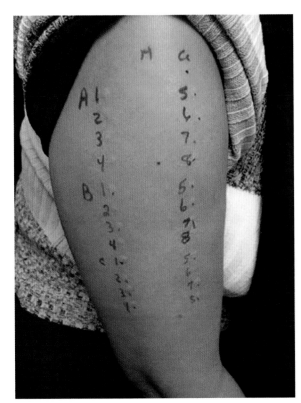

FIGURE 8.8 Intradermal Testing. (From Chadwick SJ. Principles of allergy management. In: Krouse JH, Derebery MJ, Chadwick SJ, eds. *Managing the Allergic Patient.* 1st ed. Philadelphia, PA: Saunders; 2008.)

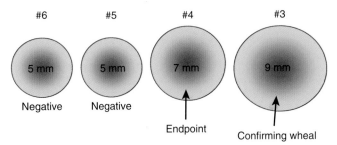

FIGURE 8.9 Example of Intradermal Dilutional Testing. Circles represent the wheal sizes 10 minutes after placing a 4-mm wheal of fivefold dilutions. The increase from 4 to 5 mm is independent of hypersensitivity and is expected. The #6 dilution on the left would be placed first, and if negative, then a #5 dilution would be placed. In this example, the #4 dilution increases to 7 mm, which suggests a positive response (the endpoint), and the #3 dilution increases greater than or equal to 2 mm more than the #4, "confirming" the reaction. (Adapted from Haydon RC. Allergic rhinitis—current approaches to skin and in vitro testing. *Otolaryngol Clin North Am.* 2008 Apr;41(2):331-46, vii.)

PRICK VERSUS INTRADERMAL TESTING

- Prick: more specific
- Intradermal: more sensitive

SKIN ENDPOINT TITRATION/INTRADERMAL DILUTIONAL TESTING

- Fivefold dilution of each antigen made and placed in vials labeled 1-6
  - 1 cc of antigenic concentrate (1:20 weight/volume) mixed with 4 cc of inert diluent
  - First diluted preparation is referred to as the #1 dilution
  - Each dilution is subsequently diluted fivefold; for example, vial #1 is 1:100; vial #2 is 1:500; and vial 3 is 1:2,500 v/w
- Vial #6 or stronger dilution is injected intradermally (Fig. 8.9) with the goal of creating a precise 4-mm-diameter wheal in the skin
- Measurement after 10 minutes
- Wheal of 7 mm or greater in diameter is considered a "positive whealing response"
  - Note: 4-mm → 5-mm wheal in 10 minutes via diffusion
  - If no response, the next stronger dilution (#5) is injected
  - Absence of allergy: no positive whealing response with any concentration
- After demonstration of a first positive wheal ("endpoint"), the next stronger concentration is applied as a 4-mm-diameter wheal
  - Positive second wheal is called the "confirming wheal," and it must be ≥2 mm larger in diameter than the first positive wheal
- Advantages
  - Quantitative and qualitative
  - Reproducible, sensitive
  - Safe, low risk of systemic response

- Disadvantages
  - Decreased specificity with high concentrations of antigen
  - Time consuming
  - Tester dependent
  - Increased costs
  - Possible false positive
  - Current allergic medications—for example, antihistamines or steroids, may suppress wheal and flare response

ALLERGIC RHINITIS IN VITRO ALLERGY TESTING

- Indications
  - Patients with suspected or documented severe allergic reaction: for example, anaphylaxis
  - Patients on certain medications: for example, antihistamines, beta-blockers, and angiotensin-converting enzyme inhibitors
  - Children and infants
  - Patients with existing skin conditions: for example, dermatographism or dermatitis
  - IgE-mediated food or venom sensitivities
  - Convenience: testing can be performed during a single visit
  - Suspect false-negative skin response
- Radioallergosorbent test (RAST)
  - First in vitro test for allergy
  - Highly specific
  - Based on detection of radiolabeled IgE that is added to a patient's serum and suspected allergen
  - Original RAST testing for the quantification of IgE and diagnosis of allergy has largely been abandoned in favor of the modified RAST test (MRT), which is both specific and sensitive; examples of MRT are radioisotope or enzyme linked
  - Classic technique:
    - Disc is placed in a test tube with the patient's serum
    - The patient's IgE binds to the disc and excess serum is washed away
    - Radiolabeled anti-IgE binds to the patient's IgE
    - Measure radioactivity
- Enzyme-linked immunosorbent assay
  - Commonly used form of immunoassay, which may be solid or liquid phase
  - Advantages: specific, safe, and useful in children or persons with skin conditions

- Disadvantages: lower sensitivity, fewer antigens available, and can be more costly
- Technique: an allergen is bound to a matrix, and the patient's serum, including associated antibodies, is added; the patient's antibodies bind to the allergen, and any unbound are washed away; secondary antibodies, such as to the patient's IgE, may be added and detected by a variety of methods

ALLERGIC RHINITIS TREATMENT

1. Avoidance
2. Symptomatic relief
3. Management of severe symptoms
4. Immunotherapy
5. Management of complications

ALLERGIC RHINITIS TREATMENT: AVOIDANCE

- Allergen avoidance
- HEPA filters
- Barriers: mattress and pillow covers and pollen-rated masks

HOW TO DECREASE ALLERGENS

- Reduce household humidity to 40-50%
- Wash bed linens in hot water weekly
- Encase bedding in hypoallergenic covers
- Eliminate cockroaches
- Close windows during pollination

ALLERGIC RHINITIS TREATMENT: SYMPTOMATIC RELIEF

1. Intranasal corticosteroids (Table 8.3)
2. Intranasal antihistamines
3. Intranasal decongestants
4. Intranasal anticholinergics

5. Intranasal mast cell stabilizers
6. Intranasal cromolyn sodium
7. Second-generation oral antihistamines
8. Oral antileukotrienes
9. Systemic steroids

MECHANISM OF ACTION OF ALLERGIC RHINITIS MEDICATIONS

- Antihistamines: block binding on the H_1 receptor
- Decongestants: act on alpha-adrenergic receptors of mucosa
- Steroids: wide range of cell types and mediators
- Mast cell stabilizers: decrease release of mediators from degranulated mast cells
- Anticholinergic agents: antagonize acetylcholine (Ach) at the muscarinic receptors
- Leukotriene modifiers: antagonize the action of leukotriene receptors or inhibit 5-lipoxygenase and the formation of leukotrienes

IMMUNOTHERAPY

ALLERGIC RHINITIS TREATMENT: IMMUNOTHERAPY

1. Subcutaneous immunotherapy (SCIT)
2. Sublingual immunotherapy (SLIT)
3. Specific nasal immunotherapy
4. Monoclonal antibodies

SUBCUTANEOUS IMMUNOTHERAPY MECHANISMS

- Rise in serum-specific IgG
- Increase levels of IgG and IgA antibodies in nasal secretions
- Reduction of the reactivity of peripheral basophils
- Reduced in vitro lymphocyte responsiveness to allergens

Table 8.3	**Commonly Used Intranasal Steroid Preparations**				
Chemical Name	**Trade Name**	**Formulation**	**Dose/ Actuation**	**Recommended Dosage**
Triamcinolone acetonide	Nasacort	Propellant, aqueous	55 µg	*2-5 years:* 1 spray/nostril qd (110 µg/day) *6-11 years:* 2 sprays/nostril qd (220 µg/day) *≥12 years:* 2 sprays/nostril qd (220 µg/day)
Budesonide	Rhinocort	Propellant	32 µg	*≥6 years:* 2 sprays/nostril qd (128 µg/day) *>12 years:* 2 sprays/nostril qd up to 4 sprays/nostril qd (128-256 µg/day)
Flunisolide	Nasalide Nasarel	0.025% Solution	25 µg	*6-14 years:* 1 spray/nostril tid (150 µg/day); 2 sprays/nostril bid (200 µg/day) *≥14 years:* 2 sprays/nostril bid-tid (200-300 µg/day)
Fluticasone propionate	Flonase	0.05% Nasal spray (aqueous)	50 µg	*4 years to adolescence:* 1 spray/nostril qd (100 µg/day) *Adults:* 2 sprays/nostril qd (200 µg/day)
Mometasone furoate	Nasonex	Aqueous	50 µg	*2-11 years:* 1 spray/nostril qd (100 µg/day) *≥12 years:* 2 sprays/nostril qd (200 µg daily)
Ciclesonide	Omnaris	Suspension	50 µg	*>6 years:* 2 sprays/nostril qd (200 µg/day)
Fluticasone furoate	Veramyst	Suspension	27.5 µg	*2-11 years:* 1 spray/nostril qd, can increase to 2 sprays/nostril qd (55-110 µg/day) *>11 years:* 2 sprays/nostril qd (110 µg/day)
Beclomethasone dipropionate	Qnasl	Nonaqueous aerosol	80 µg	*≥12 years:* 2 sprays/nostril qd (320 µg/day)
Ciclesonide	Zetonna	HFA-propelled aerosol	37 µg	*≥12 years:* 1 spray/nostril qd (74 µg/day)

HFA, Hydrofluoroalkane.

From Flint PW, Haughey BH, Lund VJ, et al. *Cummings Otolaryngology—Head and Neck Surgery.* 6th ed. Philadelphia, PA: Saunders; 2015, table 38-3.

- Reduction in inflammatory cells in nasal mucosa and nasal secretions and a shift from the TH2 to the TH1 cytokine profile
- Suppression of the seasonal elevation of IgE antibodies

ADVANTAGES OF SUBLINGUAL IMMUNOTHERAPY

- Ease of administration
- Avoidance of clinic visit
- Strong safety profile

DISADVANTAGES OF SUBLINGUAL IMMUNOTHERAPY

- Lesser immune response than occurs with SCIT
- Longer time for clinical response
- Long-term benefit is unknown
- Currently variable insurance coverage

MEDICAL TREATMENT VERSUS SUBCUTANEOUS IMMUNOTHERAPY VERSUS SUBLINGUAL IMMUNOTHERAPY

- Medical treatment: seasonal or episodic rhinitis
- SCIT/SLIT: perennial and seasonal allergens

IMMUNOTHERAPY INDICATIONS

1. Moderately severe and severe symptoms
2. Allergy to allergens that cannot be treated or avoided
3. Failed maximal medical therapy
4. Avoid need for chronic medications
5. Co-existing asthma

IMMUNOTHERAPY CONTRAINDICATIONS

1. Initiating immunotherapy during pregnancy; therapy can be continued during pregnancy; retesting should not be performed
2. Immunocompromised
3. Unstable asthma
4. Medications (beta-blockers)
5. Noncompliant patients

DOSING IMMUNOTHERAPY

- Starting dose
  - General principles: high enough to initiate response, low enough to prevent systemic and/or local reaction

- Intradermal dilutional testing: 0.05 cc of endpoint
- RAST: 0.05 cc of endpoint minus 1 or 2 for safety in patients at high risk
  - Dose escalation/maintenance dose
- Initially weekly and then every 2-3 weeks
  - Increase 0.05-0.20 cc depending on the patient and the season
  - Stop titration when evidence of clinical improvement appears

SUGGESTED READINGS

1. Naseri I, Sobol SE. Management of Acute Sinusitis and Its Complications. In: Wetmore RF, ed. *The Requisites in Pediatrics: Pediatric Otolaryngology.* Philadelphia, PA: Mosby/Elsevier; 2007.
2. Tom WC. Diagnosis and Management of Chronic Sinusitis. In: Wetmore RF, ed. *The Requisites in Pediatrics: Pediatric Otolaryngology.* Philadelphia, PA: Mosby/Elsevier; 2007.
3. Khoury P, Naclerio RM. Immunology and Allergy. In: Bailey BJ, Johnson JT, eds. *Head & Neck Surgery –Otolaryngology.* Philadelphia, PA: Lippincott; 2006.
4. Krouse JH. Allergic and Nonallergic Rhinitis. In: Bailey BJ, Johnson JT, eds. *Head & Neck Surgery –Otolaryngology.* Philadelphia, PA: Lippincott; 2006.
5. Golub JS, Marks SC, Pasha R. Rhinology and Paranasal Sinuses. In: Pasha R, Golub JS, eds. *Otolaryngology –Head and Neck Surgery: Clinical Reference Guide.* Plural Publishing; 2014.
6. Salamone FN, Tami TA. Acute & Chronic Sinusitis. In: Lawani AK, ed. *Current Diagnosis & Treatment: Otolaryngology Head and Neck Surgery.* New York, NY: McGraw-Hill Medical; 2008. Lange Series.
7. Shah SB, Emanuel IA. Nonallergic & Allergic Rhinitis. In: Lawani AK, ed. *Current Diagnosis & Treatment: Otolaryngology Head and Neck Surgery.* New York, NY: McGraw-Hill Medical; 2008. Lange Series.
8. Houck J. Immunology and Allergy. In: Lee KJ, ed. *Essential Otolaryngology: Head & Neck Surgery.* New York, NY: McGraw-Hill; 2008.
9. Goldenberg D, Goldstein BJ. *Rhinology. Handbook of Otolaryngology: Head and Neck Surgery.* New York, NY: Thieme; 2011.
10. Baroody FM, Naclerio RM. Allergy and immunology of the upper airway. *Cummings Otolaryngology.* 2014.
11. Derebery MJ, Berliner KI. Allergy and the contemporary otologist. *Otolaryngol Clin North Am.* 2003.
12. Derebery MJ, Berliner KI. Allergy for the otologist. External canal to inner ear. *Otolaryngol Clin North Am.* 1998;31(1):157–173.
13. Nolte H, Kowal J, Dubuske L. Overview of in vitro allergy tests. In: Bochner BS, Feldweg AM (eds.) UpToDate. Waltham, MA: *UpToDate.* Accessed on June 1, 2015. http://www.uptodate.com/contents/overview-of-in-vitro-allergy-tests
14. Mims JW. Allergy testing. In: Johnson JT, Rosen CA, eds. *Bailey's Head and Neck Surgery: Otolaryngology.* 5th ed. Philadelphia, PA: Lippincott Williams & Wilkins; 2014.
15. Krouse JH. Introduction to allergy. In: Krouse JH, Derebery MJ, Chadwick SJ, eds. *Managing the Allergic Patient.* 1st ed. Philadelphia, PA: Saunders Elsevier; 2008.
16. Chadwick SJ. Principles of allergy management. In: Krouse JH, Derebery MJ, Chadwick SJ, eds. *Managing the Allergic Patient.* 1st ed. Philadelphia, PA: Saunders Elsevier; 2008.

9 | Sleep Medicine

NORMAL SLEEP PHYSIOLOGY

IDEAL LENGTH OF SLEEP

- Infants: 14-16 hours
- Children: 9 hours
- Adults: 7-8 hours

FACTORS THAT DETERMINE SLEEP LENGTH

- Genetic
- Circadian rhythm
- Voluntary control: for example, an alarm clock

STAGES OF SLEEP

- Nonrapid eye movement sleep (NREM)
- Rapid eye movement (REM) sleep

NONRAPID EYE MOVEMENT SLEEP STAGES OF SLEEP

- N1: transition to sleep (2-5%)
- N2: sleep (45-55%)
- N3: deep sleep (15-20%)

RAPID EYE MOVEMENT SLEEP STAGES

- Tonic: parasympathetically driven and no eye movements
- Phasic: sympathetically driven, REMs, irregular cardiac and respiratory patterns, and loss of peripheral muscle tone

AGING AND SLEEP STAGES

- Young infants and children: increased REM and stage N3 NREM
- Elderly: decreased stage N3 NREM

SLEEP WAVES AND RHYTHMS

- Beta: 13-30 Hz (wakefulness)
- Alpha: 8-12 Hz (relaxed wakefulness)
- Theta: 4-8 Hz (N1 and REM)
- Delta: 1-4 Hz (N3)
- K complex (N2)
- Vertex sharp waves (N1)
- Sleep spindle (N2)
- Sawtooth waves (REM)

SLEEP-WAKE CYCLES

- Homeostatic drive (Process S; increasing sleep propensity with wakefulness)
- Circadian rhythm (Process C; internal sleep/wake cycle)

SLEEP CENTERS OF THE BRAIN

- Reticular activating system
- Hypothalamus
- Basal forebrain
- Thalamus

SLEEP-RELATED BRAIN NUCLEI

- Locus coeruleus
- Substantia nigra
- Ventral tegmental region
- Laterodorsal tegmental nuclei
- Pedunculopontine nuclei
- Dorsal raphe nucleus

HORMONES RELATED TO SLEEP FUNCTION

- Cortisol
- Thyroid-stimulating hormone
- Growth hormone
- Prolactin
- Glucose/insulin
- Hypocretins/orexins
- Melatonin
- Leptin
- Ghrelin

MUSCLES THAT MAINTAIN AIRWAY PATENCY

1. Tensor veli palatini
2. Pterygoid
3. Genioglossus
4. Geniohyoid
5. Sternohyoid

SLEEP DISORDER CLASSIFICATION AND DEFINITIONS (Table 9.1)

FOUR MAJOR CATEGORIES OF INTERNATIONAL CLASSIFICATION OF SLEEP DISORDERS

1. Dysomnias: for example, obstructive sleep apnea (OSA)
2. Parasomnias: for example, sleep walking
3. Medical-psychiatric sleep disorders
4. Proposed sleep disorders: for example, subwakefulness syndrome, which is a category of sleep disorders for which there is insufficient information available to confirm the disorder

APNEA

- >90% reduction of air flow by the nose or mouth AND
- 10 seconds or longer

Table 9.1	**Respiratory Event Definitions and Types**
Respiratory Event	**Definition**
Apnea	A cessation of airflow for at least 10 s
Hypopnea	A reduction in airflow (≥30%) for at least 10 s with ≤4% oxyhemoglobin desaturation
	OR a reduction in airflow (≥50%) at least 10 s with ≥3% oxyhemoglobin desaturation or an electroencephalogram arousal
Respiratory effort–related arousal	Sequence of breaths for at least 10 s with increasing respiratory effort or flattening of the nasal pressure waveform, leading to an arousal from sleep, when the sequence of breaths does not meet the criteria for an apnea or a hypopnea
Obstructive	Continued thoracoabdominal effort in the setting of partial or complete airflow cessation
Central	Lack of thoracoabdominal effort in the setting of partial or complete airflow cessation
Mixed	Respiratory event with both obstructive and central features, with mixed events generally beginning as central events and ending with thoracoabdominal effort without airflow

From Flint PW, Haughey BH, Lund VJ, et al. *Cummings Otolaryngology—Head and Neck Surgery.* 6th ed. Philadelphia, PA: Saunders; 2015, table 18-1. Originally from Kushida CA, Littner MR, Morgenthaler T, et al. Practice parameters for the indications for polysomnography and related procedures: an update for 2005. *Sleep* 2005;28:499-521.

HYPOPNEA (VARIES BASED ON LABORATORY)

- Decrease in airflow to ≥30% baseline AND
- Period of 10 seconds AND
- ≥4% oxygen desaturation

RESPIRATORY EFFORT-RELATED AROUSAL

- Absence of apnea/hypopnea AND
- 10 seconds or more duration of progressive negative esophageal pressure or flattening of the nasal pressure waveform AND
- Electroencephalogram (EEG) arousal

INDICES OF APNEA (Table 9.2)

- Apnea index (apneas/per hour of sleep)
- Apnea-hypopnea index (apneas and hypopneas/per hour of sleep)
- Respiratory disturbance index (apneas, hypopneas, and respiratory effort-related arousals (RERAs)/per hour of sleep)

TYPES OF APNEAS

- Obstructive
- Central
- Mixed

OBSTRUCTIVE SLEEP APNEA

OBSTRUCTIVE SLEEP APNEA SPECTRUM

- Primary snoring
- Upper-airway resistance syndrome
- OAS syndrome (OSAS)

Table 9.2	**Indexes of Sleep-Disordered Breathing**
Index	**Definition**
Apnea index	Number of apneas per hour of total sleep time
Hypopnea index	Number of hypopneas per hour of total sleep time
Apnea-hypopnea index	Number of apneas and hypopneas per hour of total sleep time
RERA index	Number of RERAs per hour of total sleep time
Respiratory disturbance index	Number of apneas, hypopneas, and RERAs per hour of total sleep time
Central apnea index	Number of central apneas per hour of total sleep time
Mixed apnea index	Number of mixed apneas per hour of total sleep time

RERA, Respiratory effort–related arousal.
From Flint PW, Haughey BH, Lund VJ, et al. *Cummings Otolaryngology—Head and Neck Surgery.* 6th ed. Philadelphia, PA: Saunders; 2015, table 18-2.

- Overlap syndrome (OSAS and chronic obstructive pulmonary disease [COPD])
- Obesity-hypoventilation syndrome

LEVELS OF AIRWAY OBSTRUCTION

1. Nasal cavity/nasopharynx
   - Septal deviation, turbinate hypertrophy, nasal valve collapse, nasal polyps, and adenoid hypertrophy
2. Oral cavity/oropharynx
   - Elongation of the soft palate and uvula, palatine and lingual tonsil hypertrophy, macroglossia, retrognathia, and poor upper-airway muscle tone
3. Hypopharynx/larynx
   - Omega-shaped epiglottis, laryngotracheal malacia, or stenosis

CATEGORIES OF OBSTRUCTIVE SLEEP APNEA BASED ON APNEA-HYPOPNEA INDEX

1. Mild (5-15 events/hour)
2. Moderate (15-30 events/hour)
3. Severe (>30 events/hour)

SNORING

ANATOMIC SITES OF ORIGIN OF SNORING

- Soft palate
- Tonsillar pillars
- Base of tongue
- Epiglottis/supraglottis

NONSURGICAL MANAGEMENT OF SNORING

- Weight loss
- Eliminate alcohol, tobacco, caffeine, and sedative use
- Positioning while asleep
- Medically treat reflux, sinusitis, and nasal polyps
- Nasal breathing strips
- Oral appliance (Fig. 9.1)

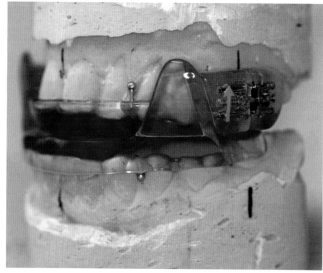

FIGURE 9.1 Oral Appliance. Mandibular advancement appliance for mild to moderate sleep apnea. (From Flint PW, Haughey BH, Lund VJ, et al. *Cummings Otolaryngology—Head and Neck Surgery.* 6th ed. Philadelphia, PA: Saunders; 2015, fig. 18-11.)

SURGICAL MANAGEMENT OF SNORING

- Septoplasty/turbinate reduction
- Radiofrequency palatoplasty/somnoplasty (ablation of upper-airway tissue, including the palate, turbinates, and tongue base)
- Palatal implants (Fig. 9.2)

UPPER-AIRWAY RESISTANCE SYNDROME

UPPER-AIRWAY RESISTANCE SYNDROME DIAGNOSIS

- 15 or more RERAs per hour

RISK FACTOR FOR UPPER-AIRWAY RESISTANCE SYNDROME

- Female gender
- Nonobese
- Younger age
- Nasal obstruction

OBSTRUCTIVE SLEEP APNEA SYNDROME

OBSTRUCTIVE SLEEP APNEA SYNDROME DIAGNOSIS

- ≥5 respiratory events/hour AND respiratory effort with symptoms OR
- ≥15/hour respiratory events with respiratory effort without symptoms

OBSTRUCTIVE SLEEP APNEA SYNDROME PATHOPHYSIOLOGY

- Upper-airway collapse
- Inability for airway dilators to respond
- Decreased sensitivity of chemoreceptors

- Decreased central respiratory drive
- Defective ventilator receptors

OBSTRUCTIVE SLEEP APNEA SYNDROME RISK FACTORS: BASIC

- Obesity
- Family history
- Anatomy (maxillary hypoplasia; retrognathia)
- Increased age
- Allergies
- Postmenopausal status
- Sedatives and alcohol
- Smoking

OBSTRUCTIVE SLEEP APNEA SYNDROME: SYSTEMIC

- Down syndrome
- Marfan syndrome
- Neuromuscular disorders
- Muscular dystrophy
- Kyphoscoliosis
- Amyloidosis
- Endocrine abnormalities

OBSTRUCTIVE APNEA SYNDROME RISK FACTORS: MISCELLANEOUS

- South Asian ancestry
- ApoE4 allele

CLINICAL CONSEQUENCES OF OBSTRUCTIVE SLEEP APNEA

- Sleep-related
  - Daytime somnolence and fatigue, morning headache, motor vehicle accidents, poor job performance, depression, and familial stress
- Cardiovascular consequences
  - Hypertension, coronary artery disease, cardiac arrhythmia, and cerebrovascular accidents
- Pulmonary consequences
  - Pulmonary hypertension
  - Cor pulmonale
- Shorter life expectancy

WORKUP OF OBSTRUCTIVE SLEEP APNEA

- Loud nightly snoring
- Daytime sleepiness/fatigue (Box 9.1)
- Unrefreshing sleep
- History from bed partner (witnessed breathing pauses and gasps)
- Physical exam
  - Vital signs
  - Body mass index (BMI)
  - Head and neck exam
  - Awake supine flexible laryngoscopy with Mueller maneuver
- Laboratory studies
  - Polysomnography
  - Cephalometric films
  - Oximetry
  - Thyroid and cardiac studies

BASIC SLEEP HISTORY

- Bedtimes
- Arousal times

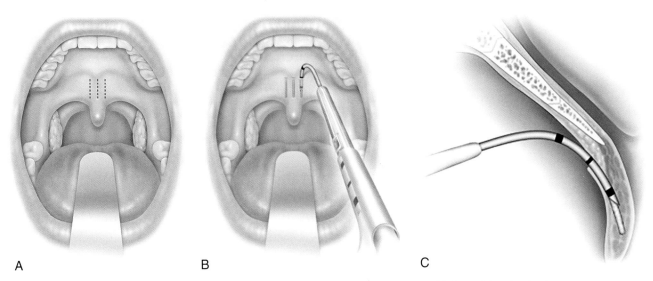

A   B   C

FIGURE 9.2 Placement of Palatal Implants. (**A**) Approximate location of implant. (**B**) Coronal view showing placement of implant. (**C**) Sagittal view showing placement of implant. Pillar® implant technique may be conducted in the office or operating room. (Modified from Maurer JT. Palatal implants for primary snoring: Short- and long-term results of a new minimally invasive surgical technique. In: Friedman M, ed. *Sleep Apnea and Snoring.* Philadelphia, Elsevier, 2009.)

Box 9.1   MEDICAL CONDITIONS THAT CAUSE FATIGUE

- Severe anemia
- Endocrine dysfunction, including hypothyroidism and Addison disease
- Chronic fatigue syndrome
- Pulmonary disease, including asthma, emphysema, and Pickwickian syndrome
- Cardiovascular disease, including congestive and left heart failure
- Neoplasms, including disseminated and central nervous system lesions
- Anticancer chemotherapy
- Collagen vascular diseases
- Chronic infections, including mononucleosis, hepatitis, and influenza
- Depression and other psychiatric disorders
- Malnutrition
- Neurologic disorders, including Parkinson disease and multiple sclerosis
- Medication side effects

From Flint PW, Haughey BH, Lund VJ, et al. *Cummings Otolaryngology—Head and Neck Surgery.* 6th ed. Philadelphia, PA: Saunders; 2015, box 18-2.

- Awake times
- Body position during sleep
- Restless sleep
- Leg movements/kicking
- Alcohol or sedative use
- Caffeine intake
- Mouth breathing at night
- Menopause status

PHYSICAL EXAM FINDINGS OF OBSTRUCTIVE SLEEP APNEA (Table 9.3)

- Neck circumference (≥17 inches males; ≥15.5 inches females)
- Waste/hip ratio (≥0.9 male; ≥0.85 female)
- Cricomental distance (≥15 mm excludes OSA)
- Kyphosis
- Micro/retrognathia (class II occlusion)
- Enlarged tonsils
- High arched palate
- Maxillary retrusion (class III occlusion)

Table 9.3	**Physical Exam Findings of Obstructive Sleep Apnea**
Nasal obstruction	• Septal deviation • Turbinate hypertrophy • Nasal valve collapse • Adenoid hypertrophy nasal tumors or polyps
Oropharyngeal obstruction	• Large soft palate • Palatine tonsillar hypertrophy • Posterior pharyngeal wall banding • Macroglossia • Large mandibular tori • Narrow skeletal arch
Hypopharyngeal obstruction	• Lateral pharyngeal wall collapse • Omega-shaped epiglottis • Hypopharyngeal tumor • Lingual tonsillar hypertrophy • Macroglossia • Retrognathia and micrognathia
Laryngeal obstruction	• True vocal cord paralysis • Laryngeal tumor
General neck obstruction	• Increased neck circumference • Redundant cervical adipose tissue
General body habitus	• Obesity • Achondroplasia • Chest wall deformity • Marfan syndrome
Cardiovascular signs	• Arterial hypertension, especially morning hypertension • Peripheral edema

From Flint PW, Haughey BH, Lund VJ, et al. *Cummings Otolaryngology—Head and Neck Surgery.* 6th ed. Philadelphia, PA: Saunders; 2015, box 18-3.

- Tracheo/laryngomalacia
- Enlarged tongue (modified Mallampati III or IV)

EVALUATION OF MAXILLARY RETRUSION

- Frankfurt plane
- Line dropped from the nasion to the subnasale should be perpendicular to the Frankfurt plane

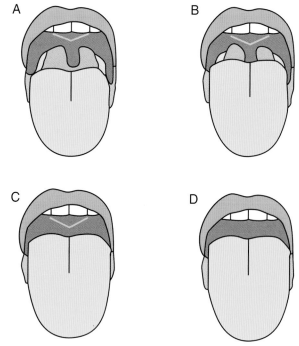

FIGURE 9.3 Modified Mallampati Palate Position. (**A**) The entire uvula can be seen with the tongue at rest. (**B**) A partial view of the uvula is seen. (**C**) Only the soft and hard palate can be seen. (**D**) Only the hard palate can be seen. (From Flint PW, Haughey BH, Lund VJ, et al. *Cummings Otolaryngology—Head and Neck Surgery*. 6th ed. Philadelphia, PA: Saunders; 2015, fig.18-12.)

TONSIL EVALUATION

- 1: 0-25% lateral narrowing of oropharynx (in tonsillar fossa)
- 2: 25-50% lateral narrowing of oropharynx (fills fossa)
- 3: 50-75% lateral narrowing of oropharynx (extends beyond fossa)
- 4+: >75% lateral narrowing of oropharynx (touching tonsils)

EVALUATION OF RETROGNATHIA

- Frankfurt plane
- Line bisecting vermilion border of the lower lip with the pogonion should be perpendicular to the Frankfurt plane

MALLAMPATI SCORE (Fig. 9.3)

- Class I: full view of the uvula and tonsils
- Class II: partial view of tonsils
- Class III: soft palate edge but the uvula is not visible
- Class IV: soft palate is not visible

OBSTRUCTIVE SLEEP APNEA SYNDROME TESTS

- Drug-induced sleep endoscopy
- Polysomnography
- Lateral cephalometric analysis
- Subjective sleep questionnaires

POLYSOMNOGRAPHY PARAMETERS

- EEG
- Electrooculum (EOG)
- Electromyogram (EMG)
- Electrocardiogram (ECG)
- Oronasal airflow
- Respiratory effort

- Oximetry
- Vital signs
- Snoring volume

ELECTROENCEPHALOGRAM: ALLOWS SLEEP STAGING; GIGANTIC PYRAMIDAL CELLS FROM BRAIN REGIONS

- Frontal
- Central
- Occipital

MEASURES OF RESPIRATORY EFFORT BY THE FOLLOWING

- Esophageal manometry
- Respiratory inductance plethysmography
- Thoracoabdominal strain gauge

POLYSOMNOGRAPHY REPORT (Fig. 9.4)

- Sleep latency
- Sleep efficiency
- Sleep architecture
- Types of respiratory disturbances/quantification
- Volume/presence of snoring
- Effect of position on respiratory airflow
- Effect of sleep stage on respiratory airflow
- Number/severity of the oxygen desaturation events ≥4%
- Percentage sleep time with O_2 saturation <90%
- Lowest O_2 saturation level

CATEGORIES OF PORTABLE SLEEP-MONITORING DEVICES

- Type 1: in-laboratory sleep study with sleep technologist
- Type 2 (home sleep test): in-home polysomnogram with a minimum of seven channels, including EEG with sleep technologist
- Type 3 (home sleep test): minimum of four channels including respiratory airflow, respiratory effort, electrocardiogram, and oxygen saturation
- Type 4 (home sleep test): minimum of three channels including airflow or actigraphy, peripheral arterial tone, and oxygen saturation

RADIOLOGIC EVALUATION OF OBSTRUCTIVE SLEEP APNEA

- Lateral cephalometry and plain x-rays
- Computed tomography/magnetic resonance imaging: not used routinely

FINDINGS OF OBSTRUCTIVE SLEEP APNEA SYNDROME ON CEPHALOMETRIC ROENTGENOGRAMS

- Retrognathia
- Narrowed posterior airway space (retropalatal; retroglossal)
- Increased mandibular plane to the hyoid bone (low hyoid)
- Shortening of the anterior cranial base
- Elongated/thickened soft palate

SUBJECTIVE SLEEP QUESTIONNAIRES

- Epworth Sleepiness Scale
- Stanford Sleepiness Scale
- Functional Outcome of Sleep Questionnaire

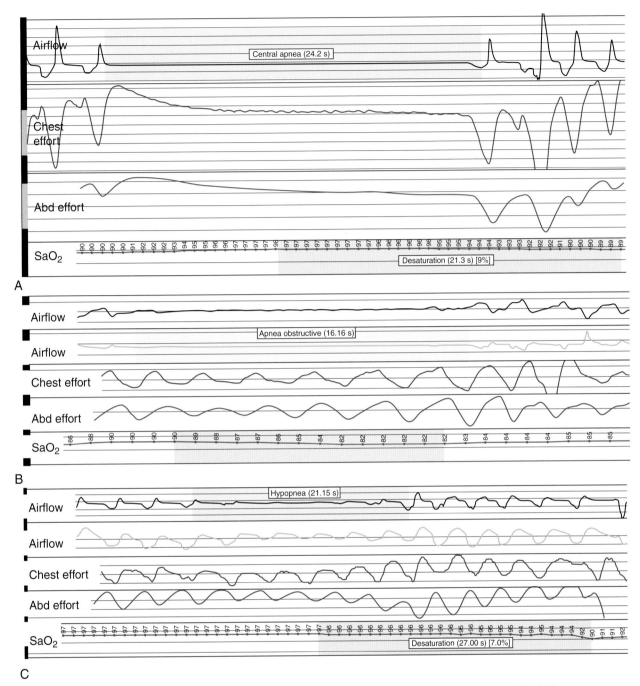

FIGURE 9.4 Polysomnographic tracing of a central apnea (**A**), obstructive apnea (**B**), and hypopnea (**C**). *Abd,* Abdominal. (From Flint PW, Haughey BH, Lund VJ, et al. *Cummings Otolaryngology—Head and Neck Surgery.* 6th ed. Philadelphia, PA: Saunders; 2015, figs. 18-10, 18-8, and 18-9.)

MANAGEMENT SEQUENCE OF OBSTRUCTIVE SLEEP APNEA

1. Behavioral (weight loss and limit alcohol, tobacco, caffeine, and sedatives)
2. Medical management (nasal blockage; reflux)
3. Continuous positive airway pressure (CPAP)/bilevel positive airway pressure (BiPAP)
4. Oral or nasal appliances
5. Mandibular repositioning
6. Surgery

INCREASE CPAP PATIENT COMPLIANCE

- Add humidity
- Treat nasal congestion/obstruction
- Desensitization
- Reassess mask
- Chin-strap for mouth leak
- Pressure reduction
- Brief trial of hypnotic medication while adjusting to the device

BIPAP INDICATIONS

- Pressure support for obesity-hypoventilatory patients
- COPD
- Hypoxemic patients
- Respiratory muscle weakness
- Neurologic dysfunction
- Poor CPAP compliance because of high PAP pressure (≥16 cm H_2O)

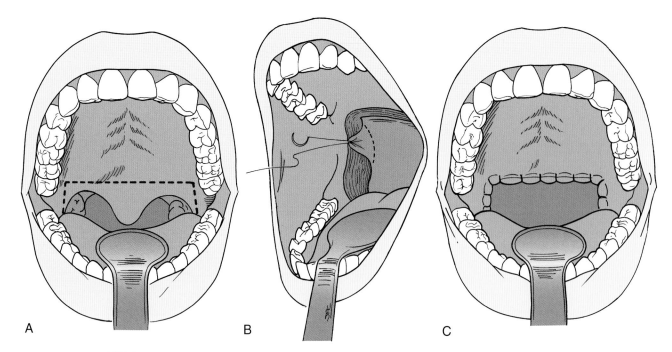

A   B   C

FIGURE 9.5 Uvulopalatopharyngoplasty. (**A**) The incision along the anterior pillar meets the horizontal incision through the palate at approximately a 90-degree angle. (**B**) The mucosa of the posterior tonsillar pillar is advanced and sutured to the anterior pillar employing long-lasting absorbable sutures. The free edge of the soft palate is closed on itself, employing long-lasting absorbable sutures. (**C**) The result is a wide opening into the oropharynx. (From Flint PW, Haughey BH, Lund VJ, et al. *Cummings Otolaryngology—Head and Neck Surgery.* 6th ed. Philadelphia, PA: Saunders; 2015, figs. 21-5, 21-7, and 21-9.)

CPAP/BIPAP CONTRAINDICATIONS

- No respiratory drive
- Risk of aspiration
- Hypotension
- Cerebrospinal fluid leak
- Bullous lung disease
- Pneumocephalus
- Pneumothorax
- History of transasal skull-base surgery

INDICATIONS FOR OBSTRUCTIVE SLEEP APNEA SURGERY

- Loud snoring
- Poor sleep quality
- Daytime sleepiness
- Failed CPAP after 3-6 months' trial
- Identifiable anatomic site amendable to surgical therapy

RELATIVE CONTRAINDICATIONS FOR OBSTRUCTIVE SLEEP APNEA SURGERY

- Severe obesity (BMI ≥ 40)
- Cardiopulmonary disease
- Substance abuse
- Bleeding disorder

ANATOMIC LOCATIONS OF SURGERY FOR OBSTRUCTIVE SLEEP APNEA

- Nasal
- Oropharyngeal
- Hypopharyngeal
- Mandibular and midface advancement
- Tracheostomy

NASAL SURGERY

- Septopalsty
- Turbinate reduction
- Polypectomy
- Nasal valve reconstruction
- Functional rhinoplasty

OROPHARYNGEAL SURGERY

- Adenotonsillectomy
- Uvulopalatopharyngoplasty
- Palatal stiffening

STEPS OF UVULOPALATOPHARYNGOPLASTY (Fig. 9.5)

1. Remove tonsils if present
2. Incision made through anterior pillar to the square edge of the soft palate
3. Uvula removed and debulked at its base
4. Posterior tonsillar pillar as a flap is rotated anteriorly and sutured to the anterior pillar
5. Dorsal soft palate mucosa is advanced and sutured to the ventral mucosa closing the uvula/soft palate incision

HYPOPHARYNGEAL SURGERY

- Lingual tonsillectomy
- Tongue-base reduction (radiofrequency; coblation; robotic)
- Genioglossal advancement (Fig. 9.6)
- Genioglossal suspension
- Hyoid myotomy and suspension (Fig. 9.7)
- Epiglottoplasty

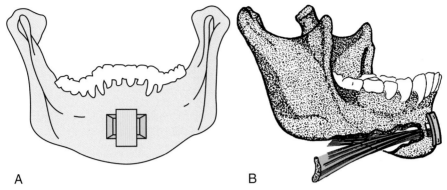

A   B

FIGURE 9.6 Genioglossal Advancement Procedure: Rectangular Geniotubercle Osteotomy Modification. (**A**) Anterior view. The rectangular geniotubercle osteotomy modification provides tension on the genioglossus muscle with a minimal fracture risk. The geniotubercle fragment is rotated enough to allow bony overlap. A single inferiorly placed miniscrew is used to fix the fragment. (**B**) Lateral view. (From Flint PW, Haughey BH, Lund VJ, et al. *Cummings Otolaryngology—Head and Neck Surgery*. 6th ed. Philadelphia, PA: Saunders; 2015, fig. 18-16. Originally from Troell RJ, Riley RW, Powell NB, Li K. Surgical management of the hypopharyngeal airway in sleep disordered breathing. *Otolaryngol Clin North Am.* 1998;13:983.)

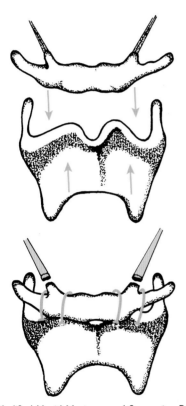

FIGURE 9.7 Modified Hyoid Myotomy and Suspension Procedure. (From Flint PW, Haughey BH, Lund VJ, et al. *Cummings Otolaryngology—Head and Neck Surgery*. 6th ed. Philadelphia, PA: Saunders; 2015, fig. 18-17. Originally from Riley R, Powell N, Guilleminault C. Obstructive sleep apnea and the hyoid: a revised surgical procedure. *Otolaryngol Head Neck Surg.* 1994;111:717.)

MANDIBULAR AND MIDFACE ADVANCEMENT (Fig. 9.8)

- Increases the retropalatal and retrolingual airway
- Maxilla and mandible are advanced by Le Fort I maxillary and sagittal-split mandibular osteotomies

HYPOGLOSSAL NERVE STIMULATION

- Early reports demonstrate potential to increase the muscular tone of the pharynx and improve inspiratory airflow

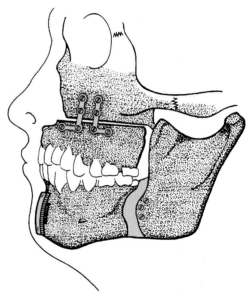

FIGURE 9.8 Maxillomandibular Advancement Procedure. Le Fort I maxillary osteotomy with rigid plate fixation and a bilateral sagittal-split mandibular osteotomy with bicortical screw fixation. The advancement is at least 10 mm. A previous genioglossal advancement is shown. (From Flint PW, Haughey BH, Lund VJ, et al. *Cummings Otolaryngology—Head and Neck Surgery*. 6th ed. Philadelphia, PA: Saunders; 2015, fig. 18-18; and Powell NB, Riley RW, Guilleminault C. The hypopharynx: upper airway reconstruction in obstructive sleep apnea syndrome. In: Fairbanks DNF, Fujita A, eds. *Snoring and Obstructive Sleep Apnea*. 2nd ed. New York, NY: Raven Press; 1994:205.)

- Stimulation electrode is placed on the hypoglossal nerve to stimulate tongue protrusion
- Sensing lead placed between the internal and external intercostal muscles to detect respiratory effort
- Neurostimulation device implanted in the right ipsilateral mid-infraclavicular region
- Stimulation timed with inspiratory phase of respiration to prevent patient awakening

EMERGENCIES OF SURGICAL TREATMENT OF SLEEP APNEA

- Intraoperative
  - Preoperative sedation resulting in airway obstruction

- Inability to intubate with airway obstruction (consider awake fiberoptic)
- Premature extubation with airway obstruction (prevent with patient sitting up following commands)
- Postoperative
  - Airway obstruction as a result of oversedation
  - Postoperative pulmonary edema
  - Postoperative bleeding
  - Postoperative subcutaneous emphysema, pneumomediastinum, and pneumothorax

COMPLICATIONS OF SURGICAL PROCEDURES FOR SLEEP APNEA

- Uvulopalatopharyngoplasty
  - Bleeding
  - Foreign-body sensation
  - Velopharyngeal insufficiency
  - Nasopharyngeal stenosis
- Septoplasty/turbinate reduction
  - Septal perforation
  - Upper incisor anesthesia (lesser palatine nerve)
- Radiofrequency tissue ablation of the tongue (infection, hematoma, and nerve paralysis)
- Tongue-base suspension (dysphagia, extrusion, and infection)
- Genioglossal advancement with hyoid myotomy (mandibular fracture, anesthesia of incisors/lower lip, and dysphagia)

SLEEP APNEA IN CHILDREN: PATHOGENESIS

- Adenotonsillar hypertrophy
- Poor muscle tone
- Upper-airway narrowing

SLEEP APNEA IN CHILDREN: SIGNS AND SYMPTOMS

- Snoring
- Choking and gasping
- Restless sleep
- Witnessed apneas
- Enuresis
- Nonspecific findings: chronic mouth breathing, hyponasality, dysphagia, halitosis, aggression, hyperactivity, and learning disabilities

SLEEP APNEA IN CHILDREN: EVALUATION

- Physical exam
  - Nasal cavity: masses, choanal stenosis/atresia
  - Nasopharynx: adenoids
  - Oral cavity: macroglossia
  - Oropharynx: obstructing tonsils
  - Palpation of soft and hard palate
- Polysomnography indicated when clinical assessment suggests sleep apnea
- Other: sleep questionnaires, nighttime recordings, and sleep somnograpy (no strong data)

SLEEP APNEA IN CHILDREN: COMPLICATIONS

- Cardiopulmonary complications
- Failure to thrive
- Poor growth
- Learning disabilities

SLEEP APNEA IN CHILDREN: NONSURGICAL TREATMENT

- CPAP, in patients with contraindications to surgery
- Weight loss
- Treatment of other medical conditions: nasal obstruction, asthma, and reflux

SLEEP APNEA IN CHILDREN: SURGICAL TREATMENT

- Adenotonsillectomy
- Less common: uvulopalatopharyngoplasty (UPPP), upper-airway radiofrequency ablation, tongue reduction, osteotomies and advancements, and tracheostomy

CENTRAL SLEEP APNEA

TYPES OF CENTRAL SLEEP APNEAS

- Primary central sleep apnea (CSA)
- Cheyne-Stokes breathing
- High-altitude CSA

CHEYNE-STOKES BREATHING

- Three cycles of crescendo and decrescendo breathing amplitude AND
- Lasting 10 minutes OR
- Associated with five or more central apneas or hypopneas
- Associated with heart failure (prolonged circulatory time)

TREATMENT OF CENTRAL SLEEP APNEA

- Treat underlying disorder
- CPAP
- Servo ventilator
- Triazolam
- Respiratory stimulants
- Nasal oxygen

CAUSES OF HYPOVENTILATION SYNDROME

- Obesity
- Interstitial lung disease
- Pulmonary hypertension
- Sickle cell anemia
- Myxedema

DIAGNOSIS OF HYPOVENTILATION SYNDROME

- Pulmonary function tests (PFTs)
- Pulmonary artery catheterization
- Echocardiogram

TREATMENT OF HYPOVENTILATION SYNDROME

- Treat underlying cause
- BiPAP
- Tracheotomy with nocturnal ventilation
- Weight loss

SLEEP-RELATED MOVEMENT DISORDERS

- Restless leg syndrome
- Periodic limb movement disorder

- Rhythmic movement disorder
- Nocturnal leg cramps
- Excessive fragmentary myoclonus
- Bruxism

RESTLESS LEG RISK FACTORS

- Female
- Family history
- BTBD9 gene

RESTLESS LEG DIAGNOSIS

- Clinical diagnosis (URGE): *U*rge to move legs; *R*est makes worse; *G*ets better with activity; *E*vening and nighttime symptoms
- Labs (serum ferritin, renal function, glucose, anemia, thyroid, B_{12}, Mg, antinuclear antibody (ANA), and rheumatoid factor (RF)
- Cerebrospinal fluid (CSF) transferrin levels

TYPES OF RESTLESS LEGS

- Primary: onset in youth; is familial
- Secondary: iron deficiency (central iron deficiency causing dopamine depletion), renal failure, pregnancy, peripheral neuropathy (diabetes), and medications
- Idiopathic

MEDICATIONS CAUSING RESTLESS LEG SYNDROME

- Selective serotonin reuptake inhibitor (SSRI)
- Serotonin–norepinephrine reuptake inhibitor (SNRI)
- Tricyclic antidepressant (TCAs)
- Lithium
- Antihistamines
- Antipsychotics
- Antiemetics
- Dopamine antagonists

DIFFERENTIAL DIAGNOSIS OF RESTLESS LEG

- Nocturnal leg cramps
- Frontal lobe seizures
- Neuropathies
- Pain syndrome
- Myoclonus
- Vascular disease
- Hypnic jerks

TREATMENT OF RESTLESS LEG

- Address secondary causes
- Behavior modification
- Dopamine agonists (ropinirole; pramipexole)

SLEEP-RELATED BRUXISM

- Sustained or phasic
- Elevation of chin EMG for >2 seconds
- Measured in masseter muscle

OTHER PEDIATRIC SLEEP DISORDERS

NONOBSTRUCTIVE PEDIATRIC SLEEP DISORDERS: DYSSOMNIAS

- Primary idiopathic insomnia
- Narcolepsy
- Primary idiopathic hypersomnia
- Limb movement disorders
- Limit-setting sleep disorder
- Insufficient sleep disorder
- Circadian rhythm sleep disorder

NONOBSTRUCTIVE PEDIATRIC SLEEP DISORDERS: PARASOMNIAS

- Sleep terrors
- Somnambulism
- Confusional arousal
- Nightmares
- Sleep paralysis
- REM sleep behavior disorder
- Bruxism
- Somniloquy
- Nocturnal enuresis
- Rhythmic movement disorders

SUGGESTED READINGS

1. Wetmore RF. Sleep-Disordered Breathing. In: Wetmore RF, ed. *The Requisites in Pediatrics: Pediatric Otolaryngology.* Philadelphia, PA: Mosby Elsevier; 2007.
2. Johnson LD. Pediatric Sleep-Disordered Breathing. In: Bailey BJ, Johnson JT, Newlands SD, eds. *Head & Neck Surgery–Otolaryngology.* Philadelphia, PA: Lippincott; 2006.
3. Walker RP. Snoring and Obstructive Sleep Apnea. In: Bailey BJ, Johnson JT, Newlands SD, eds. *Head & Neck Surgery–Otolaryngology.* Philadelphia, PA: Lippincott; 2006.
4. Pasha R, Takashima M, Golub JS. In: Pasha R, Golub JS, eds. *Otolaryngology –Head and Neck Surgery: Clinical Reference Guide.* San Diego: Plural Publishing; 2011.
5. Cote V, Prager JD, Ou H, Kelley PE, Pasha R, Golub JS. Pediatric Otolaryngology. In: Pasha R, Golub JS, eds. *Otolaryngology–Head and Neck Surgery: Clinical Reference Guide.* San Diego: Plural Publishing; 2011.
6. Welch KC, Goldberg AN. Sleep Disorders. In: Lalwani AKm, ed. *Current Diagnosis & Treatment: Otolaryngology Head and Neck Surgery.* New York, NY: McGraw-Hill Medical; 2008. Lange Series.
7. Bruch JM, Busaba NY. Obstructive Sleep Apnea. In: Lee KJ, ed. *Essential Otolaryngology: Head & Neck Surgery.* New York, NY: McGraw-Hill; 2008.
8. Westerman DE. *The Concise Sleep Medicine Handbook.* Atlanta, GA: GSSD Publishers; 2011.
9. Wakefield TL, Lam DJ, Ishman SL. Sleep apnea and sleep disorders. In: Flint PW, Haughey BH, Lund VJ, et al., eds. *Cummings Otolaryngology—Head and Neck Surgery.* Philadelphia, PA: Mosby Elsevier; 2014.
10. Kepchar J, Brietzke S. Non-obstructive pediatric sleep disorders. In: Flint PW, Haughey BH, Lund VJ, et al., eds. *Cummings Otolaryngology—Head and Neck Surgery.* Philadelphia, PA: Mosby Elsevier; 2014.
11. Strollo PJ, Soose RJ, Maurer JT, et al. Upper-airway stimulation for obstructive sleep apnea. *N Engl J Med.* 2014;370(2):139–149.

10 Oral Surgery

DENTAL TERMINOLOGY[1]

- Incisal: refers to the biting surface of an anterior tooth (incisor and canine)
- Occlusal: refers to the biting surface of a posterior tooth (premolar and molar)
- Apical: toward the root tip
- Mesial: toward the midline
- Distal: away from the midline
- Lingual: toward the tongue (mandibular teeth)
- Palatal: toward the palate (maxillary teeth)
- Buccal: toward the cheek
- Labial: toward the lip
- Crown: portion of the tooth covered by enamel (anatomic) or visible within the oral cavity (clinical)
- Root: portion of the tooth covered by cementum

PEDIATRIC DENTITION

- Primary dentition (baby teeth)
- 2 incisors, 1 canine, and 2 molars in each quadrant (20 teeth total)
- No premolars
- Teeth are referenced by letter (A-T)
- Right maxillary second molar (A) → left maxillary second molar (J)
- Left mandibular second molar (K) → right mandibular second molar (T)
- Primary teeth begin to erupt around 8 months of age, with completion of the primary eruption sequence by 24 months of age

ADULT DENTITION

- Succedaneous (permanent) dentition
- Two incisors, 1 canine, 2 premolars, and 3 molars in each quadrant (32 teeth total)
- Teeth are referenced by number (1-32)
- Right maxillary third molar (1) → left maxillary third molar (16)
- Left mandibular third molar (17) → right mandibular third molar (32)
- General ages for eruption:
  - Incisors, 6-9 years
  - Canines, 9-11 years
  - Premolars, 10-12 years (first) and 11-12 years (second)
  - Molars, 6-7 years (first), 11-13 years (second), and 17-20 years (third)

OCCLUSION

- Overbite: vertical overlap between incisors (normal, ~2 mm)
- Overjet: horizontal overlap between incisors (normal, ~2 mm)

- Crossbite: malpositioning of teeth in the horizontal plane, such that the mandibular anterior teeth are anterior to the maxillary anteriors (ie, negative overjet) or the mandibular posterior teeth are buccal to the maxillary posterior teeth
- Open bite: malpositioning of the teeth in the vertical plane, most commonly manifests as a gap between the incisal edges of the maxillary anterior teeth and the mandibular anterior teeth (negative overbite)
- Retrognathia: retruded jaw position (most commonly used in reference to mandibular position)
- Prognathia: protruded jaw position (most commonly used in reference to the mandible)
- Centric relation: position of the mandible when the condyles are seated within the glenoid fossa in the most anterior-superior position
- Centric occlusion: occlusion achieved with the mandibular condyles in centric relation
- Maximal intercuspal position: best fit of teeth, independent of condylar position. May or may not coincide with centric occlusion
- Based upon the relationship between the mesiobuccal cusp of the maxillary first molar to the buccal groove of the mandibular first molar
  - Normal occlusion: mesiobuccal cusp occludes with the groove, and there is a smooth arc of curvature along the dental arch, without malpositioned or rotated teeth
- Considered a malocclusion when teeth are malpositioned or rotated

MALOCCLUSION CLASSES

- Class I: the mesiobuccal cusp occludes with the mesiobuccal groove
- Class II: the mesiobuccal cusp is mesial (anterior) to the mesiobuccal groove
  - Division I: normal incisal angulation (usually has an excessive overjet)
  - Division II: incisors retroclined ("deep bite": usually has a less excessive overjet and an excessive overbite)
- Class III: the mesiobuccal cusp is distal (posterior) to the mesiobuccal groove

DENTOFACIAL DEFORMITIES

- An integrated orthodontic-surgical approach is required
- Communication (patient-orthodontist-surgeon) is critical
- Characterized by the skeletal relationship between the maxilla and mandible
- Orthodontics cannot correct facial disharmony related to skeletal discrepancies but can camouflage the effects of skeletal disharmony on occlusion

- Skeletal malocclusions require skeletal correction
- Dental compensations occur naturally, may mask skeletal discrepancies, and should be addressed before surgical correction (ie, the teeth should be decompensated before surgical correction)

SURGICAL EVALUATION OF DENTOFACIAL DEFORMITIES

- Assess pathologic/etiologic factors (obstructive sleep apnea, craniofacial anomalies, clefts, and maxillofacial trauma)
- Growth: surgical correction is typically delayed until completion of skeletal growth (girls, 2-3 years after menarche; boys, ages 16-18). Completion of growth may be assessed by serial radiographic examination (eg, hand-wrist radiographs)
- Identify the sagittal relationship between the maxilla and mandible (excessive or negative overjet, class I, class II, or class III skeletal profile)
- Identify vertical discrepancies (eg, excessive overbite, open bite, deep bite, and gummy smile)
- Identify transverse discrepancies (crossbite and occlusal cant)

CEPHALOMETRIC EVALUATION OF DENTOFACIAL DEFORMITIES

- Allows for standardized assessment of the relationship between the skull base, maxilla, and mandible
- Establishes the anatomic basis for deformity
- For diagnostic purposes—does not dictate the type or magnitude of surgical movement (ie, do not treat the numbers, treat the patient)

AESTHETIC EVALUATION OF DENTOFACIAL DEFORMITIES

- Surgical decisions based on aesthetics (eg, it may be better to correct a skeletal class III deformity in a male with a Le Fort I osteotomy rather than a mandibular setback to preserve a strong chin, whereas the opposite may be true in a female)
- Clinical evaluation of frontal repose and profile
- Evaluate the upper, middle, and lower facial thirds in both the horizontal and vertical planes
- Balance of proportions is the key
- Consider adjunctive treatments to obtain ideal balance, either in conjunction with orthognathic surgery or following correction of skeletal malocclusion (eg, malar alloplastic augmentation and rhinoplasty)

COMMON DENTOFACIAL DEFORMITY DIAGNOSES

- Maxillary hypoplasia
- Maxillary hyperplasia
- Mandibular hypoplasia
- Mandibular hyperplasia
- Combination

MAXILLARY HYPOPLASIA

- May occur in the sagittal, vertical, or transverse planes
- Seen as a secondary deformity in patients with cleft lip/cleft palate
- Manifests as a concave facial profile, deficient infraorbital/perinasal regions, poor tooth show at rest/smiling, short lower facial third, deficient upper lip, and anterior or posterior crossbite

- Primary treatment is Le Fort I osteotomy
- Segmental (eg, two- or three-piece) Le Fort I osteotomies may be performed for complex deformities
- Bone grafting may be required, depending on the magnitude and direction of movement

MAXILLARY EXCESS

- Most commonly occurs in the vertical plane
- Vertical maxillary excess characterized by elongated lower facial third, narrow alar base, excessive tooth/gingival show, lip incompetence, and often with a convex facial profile
- May be associated with anterior open bite (apertognathia)
- Surgical treatment is Le Fort I osteotomy, with segmental osteotomies and bone grafting as needed

MANDIBULAR HYPOPLASIA

- Class II molar/canine relationship with excessive overjet
- Manifest as a convex facial profile, retruded chin, acute labiomental fold, abnormal lip posturing, and short thyromental distance
- May be associated with syndromes/other pathology (Marfan, Pierre Robin, craniofacial microsomia, Treacher Collins, Nager, and obstructive sleep apnea)
- Primary treatment is bilateral sagittal split osteotomy (BSSO)

MANDIBULAR HYPERPLASIA

- Class III molar/canine relationship with negative overjet
- Prominent lower facial third, protrusive chin, and a concave facial profile
- Surgical correction can include either Le Fort I osteotomy for advancement, BSSO for mandibular setback, or a combination of both
- Intraoral vertical ramus osteotomies of the mandible may also be used for mandibular setback, but require maxillomandibular fixation

STABILITY OF ORTHOGNATHIC CORRECTION

- Relapse may occur, and patients should be counseled about this
- Most important contributing factors: jaw being moved (maxilla vs. mandible), magnitude of movement, and direction of movement
- Orthodontic factors: inadequate decompensation, inadequate alignment of dental arches, and presurgical correction of surgical problem (eg, transverse discrepancy)
- Surgical factors: inaccurate condylar positioning, inadequate fixation, and condylar resorption

INNERVATION OF TEETH/GINGIVA

- Maxillary anterior teeth: anterior-superior alveolar nerve (labial gingiva and pulp) and nasopalatine nerve (palatal gingiva)
- Maxillary premolars: middle superior alveolar nerve (buccal gingiva and pulp) and greater palatine nerve (palatal gingiva)
- Maxillary molars: posterior superior alveolar nerve (buccal gingiva and pulp) and greater palatine nerve (palatal gingiva)
- Mandibular anterior teeth: incisive nerve (labial gingiva and pulp) and lingual nerve (lingual gingiva)
- Mandibular premolars: inferior alveolar nerve (buccal gingiva and pulp) and lingual nerve (lingual gingiva)

- Mandibular molars: inferior alveolar nerve (pulp +/− buccal gingiva), long buccal nerve (buccal gingiva), and lingual nerve (lingual gingiva)

DENTAL ANESTHESIA

- Nerve blocks are very effective for anesthetizing individual teeth or portions of the oral cavity for procedures (eg, biopsies, tooth extraction, and arch bar placement)
- Infraorbital block: local anesthetic deposited at the infraorbital foramen (located 5-7 mm below the inferior orbital rim, in line with the medial limbus)
- Nasopalatine block: local anesthetic deposited at the foramen (5-7 mm posterior to the maxillary dental midline)
- Greater palatine block: local anesthetic deposited halfway between the maxillary second molar and palatal midline (Fig. 10.1)
- Posterior superior alveolar block: local anesthetic deposited into the alveolar mucosa immediately above maxillary second molar, with needle oriented at a 45-degree angle to bone
- Inferior alveolar block: local anesthetic deposited adjacent to the medial aspect of the mandibular ramus; enters the mucosa medial to the ramus, ~1 cm superior to the mandibular occlusal plane, with the needle at 45 degrees relative to the ramus
- Long buccal block: the needle is inserted into the retromolar buccal mucosa along the ascending ramus, at the level of the mandibular occlusal plane
- Maxillary anterior teeth: infraorbital and nasopalatine blocks
- Maxillary premolars: infraorbital and greater palatine blocks
- Maxillary molars: posterior superior alveolar and greater palatine blocks
- Mandibular anterior teeth: inferior alveolar block
- Mandibular premolars: inferior alveolar block
- Mandibular molars: inferior alveolar block and long buccal block

ODONTOGENIC INFECTIONS[2]

- May be localized or may involve one or more fascial spaces
- Mortality is most often related to airway compromise: airway, breathing, and circulation (ABCs) first
- Polymicrobial infections (aerobic/anaerobic gram-positive cocci and anaerobic gram-negative rods [GNRs])
- Greater than 50% of infections are mixed aerobic/anaerobic
- Important pathogens: *Streptococcus*, *Peptostreptococcus*, *Fusobacterium*, *Prevotella*, and *Porphyromonas*

- Empiric treatment should include anaerobic coverage
- Pathogenesis: occurs either from uncontrolled dental caries → pulpal necrosis → periapical infection that spreads into the alveolar bone or a deep periodontal pocket → periodontal infection
- Periapical infections are the most common sources
- Clinical manifestation of infection is dependent upon muscle attachments (eg, buccinator and mylohyoid)
  - Maxillary alveolar infections that erode the bone below the buccinator attachment will present with intraoral mucosal swelling (maxillary vestibular infection). Those that erode above the buccinator attachment will present as infraorbital swelling
  - Mandibular alveolar infections involving the molars will often present with submandibular swelling because the roots of the molars are below the insertion of the mylohyoid. Alveolar infections of the premolars and anteriors may present with sublingual swelling because the roots are above the mylohyoid

TREATMENT OF ODONTOGENIC INFECTIONS

1. ABCs first (always), be prepared to secure emergency surgical airway as often as needed
2. Determine severity of infection
   - Fever, tachycardia, tachypnea, and hypotension
   - Trismus, dysphonia, dysphagia, inability to control secretions, and respiratory distress
   - Identify potential high-risk space involvement
3. Assess host defenses
   - Immunocompromised (steroids/chemotherapy, human immunodeficiency virus infection, diabetes, substance abuse, and malnutrition)
4. Provide surgical drainage and source control
   - Incision and drainage of all affected spaces
   - The source of the infection must be treated (ie, tooth extraction)
5. Antibiotic treatment
   - Drainage and source control are the primary treatment
   - All infections should be cultured
   - Antibiotic treatment begins empirically with penicillin or clindamycin (if penicillin allergic)
   - Severe infections may necessitate additional antibiotics (eg, piperacillin/tazobactam and metronidazole) for broader gram-negative or anaerobic coverage
   - Antibiotic therapy tailored to culture results

TEMPOROMANDIBULAR JOINT DISORDERS

1. Myofascial pain
2. Internal derangement of temporomandibular joint (TMJ)
3. Osteoarthritis
4. Rheumatoid arthritis
5. Infectious arthritis
6. Traumatic arthritis
7. TMJ ankylosis
8. Condylar hyperplasia
9. Condylar hypoplasia
10. Mandibular dislocation
11. Idiopathic condylar resorption

MYOFASCIAL PAIN

- History/exam: intermittent pain that is dull, aching, and usually unilateral; limited mouth opening, associated with headaches/earaches; tenderness to muscles of mastication; and pain that increases with function or stress

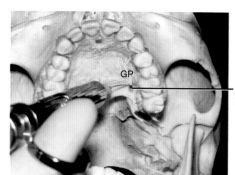

FIGURE 10.1 Placement of the Needle in Greater Palatine Foramen for a Greater Palatine Nerve Lock. *GP,* Greater palatine. (The Anatomical Basis of Dentistry; 2011. Applied Anatomy, fig. 11.7, pii: B978-0-323-06807-9.00011-9.)

- Diagnosis: clinical exam, panoramic radiograph to rule out condylar/mandibular pathology
- Treatment:
  - Phase 1, soft diet, intermittent moist heat, nonsteroidal antiinflammatory drugs (NSAIDs), and muscle relaxation; symptoms should improve within 1 month of treatment
  - Phase 2, if not better after 1 month of phase 1, bite appliance and occlusal equilibration; should improve within 1 month of treatment
  - Phase 3, physical and relaxation therapy
  - Phase 4, stress reduction and psychotherapy ± pain management (about 10% of patients will not respond to escalation of therapy through phase III)

INTERNAL DERANGEMENT OF THE TEMPOROMANDIBULAR JOINT

- History/exam: traumatic injury, parafunctional habits (tooth grinding and clenching), joint pain, joint clicking/popping/locking, and limited mouth opening
- Diagnosis: clinical exam, panoramic radiograph or maxillofacial computed tomography (CT) to rule out condylar/mandibular pathology, magnetic resonance imaging (MRI) of the TMJ to assess articular disc positioning (static and dynamic), and arthroscopy
  - Wilkes classification[3]:
    - I Painless clicking, slightly forward disc that reduces on opening, and the joint contour appears normal on radiograph
    - II Occasional painful clicking/headache, early disc deformity, and forward position
    - III Frequent pain, joint tenderness, headache, locking, restricted motion, anterior disc, early reducing disc progresses to nonreducing, disc thickened, fibrillations, and no bone changes
    - IV Chronic pain, headache, restricted motion, nonreducing disc, and bony changes including degeneration, osteophyte, and adhesions, but no disc perforation
    - V Variable pain, joint crepitus, painful function, anterior disc displacement, perforated disc, adhesions, and multiple degenerative changes
- Treatment
  - Clicking or popping: NSAIDs, soft diet, jaw rest, and bite appliance; consider surgical intervention (arthrocentesis, discplasty, or discectomy) if conservative measures fail
  - Locking: anterior disc displacement without reduction (arthrocentesis, arthroscopic surgery, or discplasty); disc adhesion to articular eminence → arthrocentesis

OSTEOARTHRITIS OF THE TEMPOROMANDIBULAR JOINT

- History/exam: jaw trauma, constant aching pain that increases with function, parafunctional habits, decreased mouth opening, TMJ tenderness, and joint crepitus
- Diagnosis: clinical exam, panoramic radiograph or maxillofacial CT to assess for condylar changes (subcondylar sclerosis, condylar flattening, condylar erosion, and osteophyte formation); consider bone scan to assess for active disease process within condyles; rule out rheumatoid arthritis
- Treatment:
  - Primary: NSAIDs, soft diet, limit jaw function, bite appliance, and establish a stable occlusion
  - If not improvement after 6 months of primary treatment → TMJ arthroplasty

RHEUMATOID ARTHRITIS OF THE TEMPOROMANDIBULAR JOINT

- History/exam: bilateral TMJ swelling/tenderness, dull/aching pain, TMJ stiffness—worse in the morning, limited mouth opening, history of rheumatoid disease, and anterior open bite/condylar, or retrognathia in severe cases
- Diagnosis: panoramic radiograph, CT scan, MRI, rheumatoid factor, antinuclear antibody, and erythrocyte sedimentation rate (ESR)
- Treatment:
  - Active disease: medical management (NSAIDs, soft diet, moist heat, range of motion exercises, and short-term steroids). If no improvement → disease-modifying therapy, coordinated with rheumatologist; if no improvement with disease-modifying therapy → surgical intervention (arthrocentesis and synovectomy)
  - Inactive disease: surgical correction of ankylosis, open bite, or retrognathia as needed

INFECTIOUS ARTHRITIS OF THE TEMPOROMANDIBULAR JOINT

- History/exam: history of tuberculosis/syphilis/gonorrhea, associated infection in the ear/mandible/parotid gland/pharynx, fever or malaise, TMJ pain, swelling, redness, and tenderness
- Diagnosis: clinical exam, panoramic radiograph, MRI, joint aspiration for culture and Gram stain, complete blood count (CBC) with differential, and ESR
- Treatment:
  - Empiric antibiotics (penicillin for simple infections and third-generation cephalosporin for GNRs)
  - Joint aspiration or incision and drainage
  - If improvement → 2 weeks of antibiotics and TMJ physical therapy once active issues are resolved
  - If no improvement → change antibiotics based on cultures, consider intravenous (IV) antibiotic therapy and surgical debridement

TRAUMATIC ARTHRITIS OF THE TEMPOROMANDIBULAR JOINT

- History/exam: trauma to mandible/TMJ, TMJ pain and tenderness, and limited motion
- Diagnosis: panoramic radiograph ± CT scan
- Treatment: NSAIDs, intermittent moist heat, soft diet, steroid injection, and jaw rest
- If improvement → jaw physical therapy to prevent ankylosis
- If no improvement → arthrocentesis

TEMPOROMANDIBULAR JOINT ANKYLOSIS

- History/exam: history of trauma or infection to the TMJ, facial asymmetry, and trismus
- Diagnosis: panoramic radiograph, maxillofacial CT with three-dimensional reconstructions—consider angiography if a large ankylotic mass is present with possible intimate association with internal maxillary artery or pterygoid plexus
- Treatment:
  - Pseudoankylosis (postsurgical scar, radiation fibrosis, coronoid hyperplasia, osteochondroma, untreated zygomatic arch fracture, paramandibular neoplasia, myositis ossificans, and psychogenic) → site-specific treatment
  - Ankylosis: mechanical dilation of jaws with physical therapy or appliance (eg, Therabite) if onset is recent. If unsuccessful or for long-standing ankylosis → surgical correction with resection of the ankylotic mass and

reconstruction of the ramus-condyle unit (bone graft, distraction osteogenesis, and alloplastic reconstruction), followed by orthognathic surgery or facial aesthetic surgery to achieve facial balance

CONDYLAR HYPERPLASIA

- History/exam: facial asymmetry (usually starting in puberty), deviation of chin point away from the affected side, crossbite or open bite malocclusion, prognathic appearance, and asymmetric mandibular projection
- Diagnosis: panoramic radiograph, anterior-posterior and lateral cephalograms, review of historical photographs to document time course and evolution of deformity, CT scan, and technetium-99 (Tc99) bone scan to assess activity and growth
- Treatment: based on Tc99 bone scan
  - Positive bone scan: partial condylectomy on the affected side with compensatory contralateral mandibular osteotomy, inferior-border contour correction, and possible genioplasty
  - Negative bone scan: orthodontic treatment to address the dental component of malocclusion with subsequent orthognathic surgery and contour correction

CONDYLAR HYPOPLASIA

- History/exam: history of mandibular trauma, inflammation, or radiation. Facial deformity with chin point deviation toward the affected side, micrognathia, mandibular contour asymmetry, and exaggerated antigonial notching
- Diagnosis: clinical exam, panoramic radiograph, anterior-posterior and lateral cephalograms, and CT scan
- Treatment: based on growth
  - Still growing: costochondral graft or distraction osteogenesis
  - Done growing: orthodontics → orthognathic surgery or genioplasty/contour correction

MANDIBULAR DISLOCATION

- History/exam: external trauma, wide mouth opening (sudden or prolonged), joint subluxation, muscular disease, and open lock
- Diagnosis: clinical exam and panoramic radiograph or CT scan
- Treatment: based on time course
  - Acute: manual reduction and immobilization (Intermaxillary Fixation or head wrap for 5-7 days)
  - Chronic: manual reduction under general anesthesia; if unsuccessful → manual reduction with angle traction wires; if unsuccessful → temporalis myotomy, if unsuccessful → subcondylar osteotomy or condylectomy

IDIOPATHIC CONDYLAR RESORPTION

- History/exam: history of orthodontic treatment or orthognathic surgery, female predilection (age 15-35 years, "Cheerleader" syndrome), class II skeletal profile, class II malocclusion, high mandibular plane angle, and anterior open bite
- Diagnosis: clinical exam, panoramic radiograph, CT scan, and rule out rheumatoid arthritis, scleroderma, and other autoimmune processes
- Treatment: based on Tc-99 bone scan (Fig. 10.2)
  - Positive scan: delay treatment until scan is negative
  - Negative scan: orthognathic surgery ± condylectomy with TMJ reconstruction

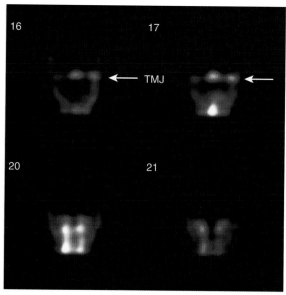

FIGURE 10.2 Technetium-99m Bone Scan. A nuclear medicine bone scan evaluates metabolic activity in the condyles. The bone scan is sensitive to increased activity, and it serves as a guide for determining the stability of the asymmetry. (Farrell BB, Tucker MR. Mandibular asymmetry: diagnosis and treatment considerations. In: Bagheri SC, Bell RB, Khan HA, eds. *Current Therapy in Oral and Maxillofacial Surgery.* Philadelphia, PA: Saunders; 2012:671-684, fig. 80.8.)

COMMON ODONTOGENIC CYSTS AND TUMORS[4,5]

1. Radicular (periapical) cyst
2. Dentigerous cyst
3. Residual cyst
4. Lateral periodontal cyst
5. Eruption cyst
6. Traumatic bone cyst
7. Odontogenic keratocyst (OKC)
8. Calcifying epithelial odontogenic tumor (CEOT, Pindborg tumor)
9. Clear cell odontogenic carcinoma (clear cell odontogenic tumor)
10. Adenomatoid odontogenic tumor
11. Odontogenic myxoma
12. Calcifying odontogenic cyst (Gorlin cyst)
13. Ameloblastoma
14. Ameloblastic carcinoma
15. Ameloblastic fibroma
16. Ameloblastic fibro-odontoma
17. Odontoma

RADICULAR (PERIAPICAL) CYST

- Round or oval lesion that arises from residual odontogenic epithelium and nonvital pulp
- Treatment: enucleation of cyst, endodontic treatment, or extraction of tooth

DENTIGEROUS CYST (Fig. 10.3)

- Develops in relationship to the crown of the erupting tooth
- Uni- or multilocular
- Most common in the third molar and maxillary canine regions
- Treatment: removal of the impacted tooth and enucleation or decompression of the cyst

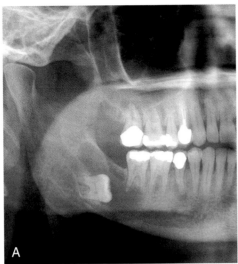
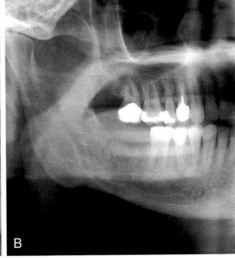

FIGURE 10.3 Dentigerous Cyst Radiograph. Note that the lesion surrounds a tooth, and radiographic margins begin at the cement-enamel junction. (**A**) Dentigerous cyst. (**B**) Bone regeneration after removal of the dentigerous cyst. (Marx RE. Jaw cysts, benign odontogenic tumors of the jaws, and fibro-osseous diseases. In: Bagheri SC, Bell RB, Khan HA, eds. *Current Therapy in Oral and Maxillofacial Surgery.* Philadelphia, PA: Saunders; 2012:390-410, fig. 50.2.)

RESIDUAL CYST

- Persistent cyst after the tooth is removed
- Treatment: enucleation

LATERAL PERIODONTAL CYST

- Interradicular lesion that develops from epithelial rests in periodontal ligament
- Commonly located in the mandibular canine and premolar regions and maxillary lateral incisor regions
- Treatment: enucleation

ERUPTION CYST

- Dentigerous cyst that is associated with an erupting tooth
- Treatment: excision of overlying soft tissue and exposure of tooth

TRAUMATIC BONE CYST

- Mandibular lesion of unknown etiology
- Usually found in asymptomatic patients <25 years of age
- Not a true cyst because the bony cavity is typically not epithelium lined
- Aspiration is necessary to rule out other possible diagnoses (hemorrhagic bone cyst and arteriovenous malformation [AVM])
- The area can be explored surgically to confirm the diagnosis
- Serial radiographs are used for follow-up

ODONTOGENIC KERATOCYST (ALSO KNOWN AS KERATOCYSTIC ODONTOGENIC TUMOR) (Fig. 10.4)

- Differentiated from other odontogenic cysts because it has an orthokeratinized lining
- Mandible > maxilla
- Up to 40% recurrence rate with simple enucleation

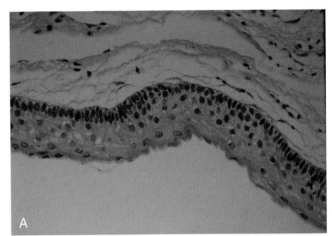
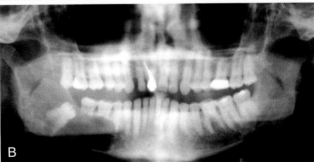

FIGURE 10.4 Keratocystic Odontogenic Tumor Radiograph and Histology. (**A**) Histologic appearance of a typical keratocystic odontogenic tumor showing a tumor lining five to six cells in thickness, with parakeratinization and polarization of the basal layer. (H & E; original magnification ×40. (**B**) Panoramic radiograph showing a large radiolucent lesion in the right posterior mandible with an associated impacted third molar. The lesion has also resulted in resorption of the adjacent second and first molar roots and extends into the condyle. Biopsy showed keratocystic odontogenic tumor.) ((A) Pogrel MA. Keratocystic odontogenic tumor. In: Bagheri SC, Bell RB, Khan HA, eds. *Current Therapy in Oral and Maxillofacial Surgery.* Philadelphia, PA: Saunders; 2012:380-383, fig. 48.1. (B) Marx RE. Jaw cysts, benign odontogenic tumors of the jaws, and fibro-osseous diseases. In: Bagheri SC, Bell RB, Khan HA, eds. *Current Therapy in Oral and Maxillofacial Surgery.* Philadelphia, PA: Saunders; 2012:390-410, fig. 50.4.)

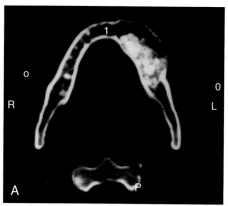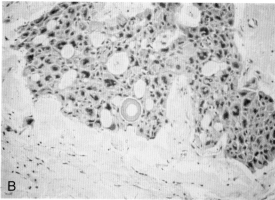

FIGURE 10.5 Calcifying Epithelial Odontogenic Tumor. (**A**) The CEOT (Pindborg tumor) will present as a mixed radiolucent-radiopaque expansile mass. (**B**) The unique histopathology of a CEOT shows large epithelial cells with large bizarre nuclei and prominent intercellular bridges. There is also amyloid and some dystrophic calcifications. (H & E; original magnification ×2.) (Marx RE. Jaw cysts, benign odontogenic tumors of the jaws, and fibro-osseous diseases. In: Bagheri SC, Bell RB, Khan HA, eds. *Current Therapy in Oral and Maxillofacial Surgery*. Philadelphia, PA: Saunders; 2012:390-410, fig. 50.36.)

- Multiple OKCs are seen in nevoid basal cell carcinoma syndrome
- Treatment is based on size
  - Small, accessible cyst: enucleation and curettage with peripheral ostectomy ± cryotherapy
  - Large, inaccessible cyst: decompression—once decompressed, may be amenable to enucleation
  - Recurrent cyst: en bloc or segmental resection

CALCIFYING EPITHELIAL ODONTOGENIC TUMOR (PINDBORG TUMOR) (Fig. 10.5)

- Wide age distribution, but peak incidence is in the fifth decade
- Molar area of mandible > maxilla
- "Driven snow" opacity, can be radiolucent; cortical expansion with "soap bubble appearance"
- Histology: Liesegang rings (concentric calcified ring) and amyloid-like protein
- Treatment: unencapsulated tumor so resection with 1-cm margins decreases recurrence

CLEAR CELL ODONTOGENIC CARCINOMA (CLEAR CELL ODONTOGENIC TUMOR)

- Rare but predominant in older women in their 50s
- 3:1 female to male predilection
- Low-grade malignancy from odontogenic epithelium
- Mandible is most commonly affected
- Large cells with clear cytoplasm histologically (similar to renal cell carcinoma)
- Treatment: wide local excision with 1-cm margins

ADENOMATOID ODONTOGENIC TUMOR

- "2/3" tumor: 2/3 occur in young females; 2/3 are in the anterior maxilla (canine area); and 2/3 are associated with an unerupted tooth
- Can form a sclerotic border on a radiograph
- Histologically, the tumor is encapsulated with gland-like "rosettes," which are small duct-like structures
- Treatment: enucleation

ODONTOGENIC MYXOMA

- Mandible > maxilla

- Predilection for children and young adults, although it can be seen in older adults
- Shows a characteristic trabecular pattern on radiography owing to preservation of medullary bony trabeculae
- Histologically this is a hypocellular tumor that overproduces glycosaminoglycan ground substance (mixoid substance) and can look like a normal dental papilla or follicle
- These are unencapsulated so the treatment is resection with 1-cm margins to avoid recurrence

CALCIFYING ODONTOGENIC CYST (GORLIN CYST) (Fig. 10.6)

- Mandible is more common than maxilla
- No age predilection
- Clinically, the only ondontogenic cyst that produces opacifications on radiographs
- Histologically similar to ameloblastomas with peripheral palisading nuclei with reverse polarity; different in that they contain ghost cells (eosinophilic, glassy, and no nucleus)
- Treatment: enucleation

AMELOBLASTOMA (Fig. 10.7)

- Most common in patients 30-50 years of age
- Typically asymptomatic but can become very large and disfiguring
- Usually benign, but can be life-threatening when large
- Treatment is based on type
  - Clinical subtypes:
    - Unicystic: mural ameloblastoma, unilocular cysts, and tumor is just in the lumen or wall of the cyst; 10% recurrence if truly unicystic and small; pathologist needs entire surgical specimen to diagnose as mural; unicystic ameloblastomas can be treated with enucleation and curettage versus resection
    - Solid or multicystic ameloblastomas require excision with tumor-free margins (at least 1-cm bone margin)
    - Malignant ameloblastoma: benign ameloblastoma that has spread to extragnathic site (most common location is the lung); rare (Some authors think that the spread is due not to true metastatic potential but rather to pieces of large tumors spreading by bulk shedding)

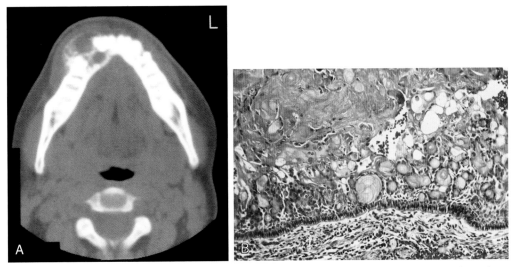

FIGURE 10.6 Calcifying Odontogenic Cyst (Gorlin Cyst). (**A**) A calcified odontogenic cyst with expansion and radiopacities. (**B**) A calcified odontogenic cyst may show keratinized and calcified areas within the lining, as well as clear "ghost" cells. (H & E; original magnification ×10.) (Marx RE. Jaw cysts, benign odontogenic tumors of the jaws, and fibro-osseous diseases. In: Bagheri SC, Bell RB, Khan HA, eds. *Current Therapy in Oral and Maxillofacial Surgery.* Philadelphia, PA: Saunders; 2012:390-410, fig. 50.10.)

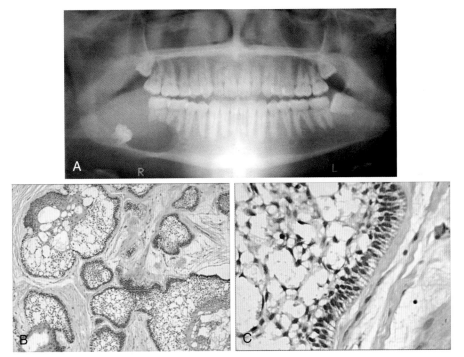

FIGURE 10.7 Ameloblastoma Radiograph and Histology. (**A**) Large unilocular radiolucency of the posterior right mandible with displacement of the third molar to the inferior border and resorption of adjacent molar roots. (**B**) Ameloblastoma (follicular variant). Numerous neoplastic odontogenic islands featuring peripheral columnar cells with reverse polarization surrounding central zone of cells resembling stellate reticulum. (**C**) Higher magnification that shows the reverse polarization of the peripheral columnar cells. ((A-C) Kademani D, Junck DM. Contemporary treatment of ameloblastoma. In: Bagheri SC, Bell RB, Khan HA, eds. *Current Therapy in Oral and Maxillofacial Surgery.* Philadelphia, PA: Saunders; 2012:384-390, figs. 49.9 and 49.4.)

AMELOBLASTIC CARCINOMA

- Very rare
- Behaves clinically as an aggressive malignancy with early metastasis to the lung and brain
- Histologically similar to ameloblastoma but with markers of malignancy such as nuclear pleomorphism and mitotic figures

AMELOBLASTIC FIBROMA

- Occurs in the posterior mandible of children and young adults
- Radiolucent lesions; histologically, appear as cords of odontogenic epithelium with abundant cellular connective tissue
- Some consider these precursor lesions to odontomas
- Treatment: enucleation

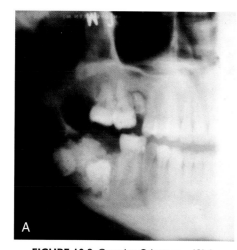
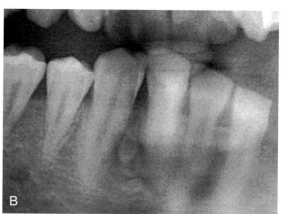

FIGURE 10.8 Complex Odontoma. (**A**) A complex odontoma presents as a diffuse radiopacity. (**B**) A compound odontoma presents with the appearance of small toothlike structures. (Marx RE. Jaw cysts, benign odontogenic tumors of the jaws, and fibro-osseous diseases. In: Bagheri SC, Bell RB, Khan HA, eds. *Current Therapy in Oral and Maxillofacial Surgery.* Philadelphia, PA: Saunders; 2012:390-410, fig. 50.38.)

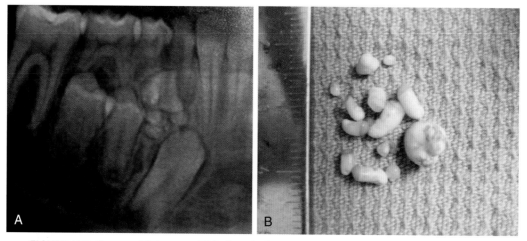

FIGURE 10.9 Compound Odontoma. (**A**) Radiograph of odontoma. (**B**) Odontoma after enucleation. (Abramowicz S, Padwa BL. Pediatric head and neck tumors: benign lesions. In: Bagheri SC, Bell RB, Khan HA, eds. *Current Therapy in Oral and Maxillofacial Surgery.* Philadelphia, PA: Saunders; 2012:813-820, fig. 92.2.)

AMELOBLASTIC FIBRO-ODONTOMA

- Similar pathologically and epidemiologically to ameloblastic fibroma, but the epithelium is more mature and forms tooth product
- Results in a mixed radiopaque/radiolucent lesion clinically
- Treatment: enucleation

ODONTOMA

- Similar pathologically and epidemiologically to ameloblastic fibromas and ameloblastic fibro-odontomas
- Appear on radiograph as either amorphous mixed-density lesions or like balls of tiny teeth
- Subtypes:
  - Complex odontomas (Fig. 10.8) consist of a haphazard arrangement of tooth product
  - Compound odontomas (Fig. 10.9) consist of a more organized arrangement of tooth product and thus resemble tiny teeth
- Treatment: enucleation

FIBRO-OSSEOUS LESIONS[6]

1. Fibrous dysplasia
2. Cherubism
3. Ossifying fibroma
4. Osteoblastoma
5. Periapical cemental dysplasia
6. Cemento-osseous dysplasia

FIBROUS DYSPLASIA

- Pathophysiology
  - Result of a mutation in the GNAS-1 gene during embryogenesis: the effect is pleiotropic
  - If occurs early in embryogenesis → polyostotic (café au lait spots, endocrinopathy: McCune-Albright syndrome)
  - If it occurs late in embryogenesis → polyostotic (café au lait spots, no endocrinopathy: Jaffe-Lichtenstein syndrome) or monostotic (craniofacial fibrous dysplasia)
- Histologic features
  - Woven bone without osteoblastic rimming

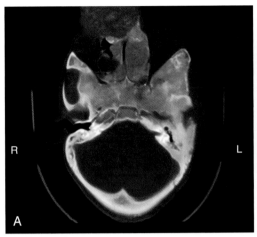
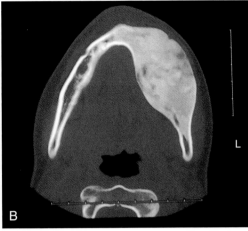

FIGURE 10.10 Fibrous Dysplasia. (**A**) Craniofacial fibrous dysplasia involves contiguous bones of the face and/or base of skull. (**B**) Monostotic fibrous dysplasia involves a single bone with a fusiform, poorly demarcated, ground-glass appearance. (Marx RE. Jaw cysts, benign odontogenic tumors of the jaws, and fibro-osseous diseases. In: Bagheri SC, Bell RB, Khan HA, eds. *Current Therapy in Oral and Maxillofacial Surgery.* Philadelphia, PA: Saunders; 2012:390-410, fig. 50.41.)

- Bone trabeculae are not connected and can form curvilinear shapes → "Chinese script" writing
- Findings are not seen in all specimens or even uniformly throughout a single lesion
- Diagnosis is often made based on the history and physical exam along with radiographic adjuncts
- Clinical features
  - Maxilla > mandible
  - Orbit can also be affected, leading to vision loss
  - Cranial neuropathies associated with foraminal narrowing
  - Painless swelling occurring during the first 2 decades of life
  - Functional deficits related to cranial neuropathies
  - Pain may occur during periods of growth or hormonal changes (eg, pregnancy)
  - Disease usually stable after age 25
- Diagnosis
  - Radiographic changes: may be a multilocular radiolucency with cortical thinning or a mixed "ground glass" appearance (classical appearance) (Fig. 10.10)
  - Markers for metabolic bone disease (calcium, phosphate, alkaline phosphatase, calcitonin, and parathyroid hormone) are usually normal
  - Skin should be examined for pigmentation changes (café au lait spots)
  - Endocrine workup should be initiated to identify endocrinopathy
- Treatment
  - Biopsy for diagnosis (clinical diagnosis, but confirmatory biopsy)
  - Contour resection → in minor cases, should be delayed until after puberty to avoid recurrence and need for further operation
  - Contour resection → in severe cases should be undertaken to prevent sequelae of nasal obstruction, impingement on orbital contents, or cranial neuropathy
  - Therapeutic radiation is not recommended → high rate of sarcomatous transformation

CHERUBISM

- Pathophysiology
  - Autosomal dominant trait with 50-70% penetrance in females and 100% penetrance in males and with three clinical variations

- Type I only affects the ramus and angle of the mandible bilaterally
- Type II involves the ramus, angle, and body of the mandible bilaterally to the mental foramen
- Type III involves both the maxilla and mandible. This form gives the patient the appearance of an upward gaze (Taken together with the symmetrical facial expansion, these individuals resemble cherubs depicted in Renaissance art.)
- Clinical features
  - It is usually first apparent by age 3. Expansion is slow and progresses until adolescence
  - In some cases the expansion involutes, whereas in others it is incomplete
- Diagnosis
  - Radiographs show bilateral multilocular radiolucencies (Fig. 10.11)
  - Histologically, these lesions resemble giant cell lesions consisting of vascular fibrous tissue with variable numbers of multinucleated giant cells
- Treatment
  - Observation in most cases and contour resection in patients who do not achieve spontaneous remission
  - The lesions are highly vascular, and the surgeon should be prepared for intraoperative bleeding

OSSIFYING FIBROMA

- Clinical features
  - Considered a variant of fibrous dysplasia
  - Appears as a localized, painless swelling
  - The mandible is affected more frequently compared with the maxilla
  - Occurs in the third and fourth decades of life but can occur in children and adolescents
- Diagnosis
  - On radiographs these are well-defined radiolucent lesions with increasing radiopacity and less distinct borders as they mature (Fig. 10.12)
  - Histologically similar to fibrous dysplasia but ossifying fibromas have more distinct borders
- Treatment
  - Enucleation is easily performed because these lesions are well encapsulated.

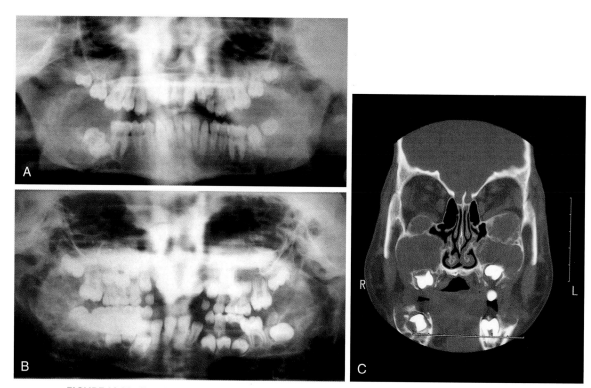

FIGURE 10.11 Cherubism. (A) Type I cherubism is limited to the ramus and posterior mandible. **(B)** Type II cherubism involves the bilateral mandible to the mental foramen and the posterior maxilla. **(C)** The eyes turned toward the heavens in type III cherubism is due to expansion of the maxillary bone's contribution to the orbital floor. (Marx RE. Jaw cysts, benign odontogenic tumors of the jaws, and fibro-osseous diseases. In: Bagheri SC, Bell RB, Khan HA, eds. *Current Therapy in Oral and Maxillofacial Surgery.* Philadelphia, PA: Saunders; 2012:390-410, fig. 50.45.)

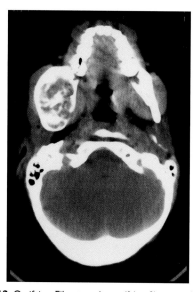

FIGURE 10.12 Ossifying Fibroma. An ossifying fibroma will appear radiographically as a spherical or oval expansion with an expanded but identifiable cortex. (Marx RE. Jaw cysts, benign odontogenic tumors of the jaws, and fibro-osseous diseases. In: Bagheri SC, Bell RB, Khan HA, eds. *Current Therapy in Oral and Maxillofacial Surgery.* Philadelphia, PA: Saunders; 2012:390-410, fig. 50.43.)

OSTEOBLASTOMA

- Clinical features
  - Most commonly seen in the vertebral column, long bones, and sacrum
  - A rare disease of the craniofacial skeleton
- Diagnosis
  - Presents as a chronic swelling with ongoing dull pain

- These lesions occur in ages 5-22 years with a slight male predominance
  - Radiographically appearing as radiolucent lesions with areas of mineralization
  - Histologic examination reveals mineralized material with sheets of irregular trabeculae surrounded by scattered multinucleated osteoclast-like cells
- Treatment
  - En bloc resection because of a propensity to recur

PERIAPICAL CEMENTAL DYSPLASIA

- Clinical features
  - Most commonly seen in middle-aged African women
  - Usually incidental findings on intraoral radiographs or panoramic radiography during routine exam
  - Asymptomatic lesions
- Diagnosis
  - Based on clinical and radiographic findings where lesions are mixed radiolucent-radiopaque or completely radiopaque lesions along the roots of the anterior teeth (Fig. 10.13)
  - Treatment: observation

CEMENTO-OSSEOUS DYSPLASIA

- Clinical features
  - Similar presentation and demographic predilection as periapical cemental dysplasia but can affect teeth and alveolar bone, not limited to the mandibular anterior teeth
- Diagnosis
  - Based on clinical and radiographic findings as in periapical cemental dysplasia but can be seen in any part of the jaw
- Treatment
  - Observation

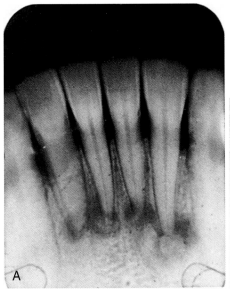

FIGURE 10.13 Periapical Cemental Dysplasia. (A) Periapical cemental dysplasia occurs in the anterior mandible with radiolucencies and radiopacities at the apex of the incisor teeth, usually in an adult of black African descent. (**B**) Histopathology of a periapical cemental dysplasia will show a stromal proliferation of periodontal ligament fibroblasts and islands of bone/cementum. (H & E; original magnification ×4.) (Marx RE. Jaw cysts, benign odontogenic tumors of the jaws, and fibro-osseous diseases. In: Bagheri SC, Bell RB, Khan HA, eds. *Current Therapy in Oral and Maxillofacial Surgery.* Philadelphia, PA: Saunders; 2012:390-410, fig. 50.48.)

VASCULAR MALFORMATIONS[7] (Table 10.1)

SLOW-FLOW MALFORMATIONS

Capillary—also known as "port-wine stain"
- Clinical features
  - Equal sex predilection and 0.3% birth prevalence; enlarged postcapillary venules because of decreased density of precapillary neuromodulation; lesions occur along the trigeminal nerve distribution; Sturge-Weber syndrome consists of capillary malformation and leptomeningeal vascular anomalies
- Diagnosis
  - Lesion is present at birth and blanches with pressure with possible enlargement of underlying soft or hard tissue. MRI and Doppler ultrasound (US) are adjuncts in identifying other associated vascular anomalies deep near the superficial lesion
- Treatment
  - Consists of pulsed-dye light amplification by stimulated emission of radiation (LASER) for the malformation and surgical correction of the underlying surgical deformity

VENOUS MALFORMATION

- Background
  - Autosomal dominant mutation of TIE2/TEK gene; chromosome 9p21-22; 95% are sporadic with an incidence of 1:10,000; 40% occur in the head and neck
- Clinical features
  - Blue, soft, compressible mass; Valsalva causes engorgement; phleboliths and intralesional thrombosis can result in pain; histology shows dilated vascular channels with normal endothelium
- Diagnosis
  - Physical exam with MRI using pre- and postcontrast T1 and T2 images with fat suppression show hyperintensity on T2; phleboliths and thrombi appear as signal voids; plain film or CT may show skeletal deformity

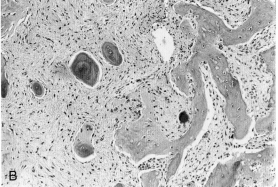

Table 10.1	**Outdated and Current Terms for Circulatory Malformations**	
Outdated Term	**Correct Term**
Port-wine stain, capillary hemangioma	Capillary malformation
Lymphangioma, cystic hygroma	Lymphatic malformation
Cavernous hemangioma	Venous malformation

- Management
  - Intralesional coagulation of large malformations can precipitate disseminated intravascular coagulopathy. Check coags. Daily aspirin therapy prophylaxis against phlebolith formation and intralesional injection of absolute ethanol (large lesions) or 1% sodium tetradecyl sulfate (smaller lesions) can result in sclerosis and shrinkage

LYMPHATIC MALFORMATION

- Background
  - Associated with VEGFR3 mutations; incidence is unknown; histology shows lymphatic spaces walled with eosinophilic and protein-rich fluid; microcystic or macrocystic based on radiographic appearance; large cervicofacial lymphatic malformations can be detected prenatally via US and necessitate surgical airway management at birth (ex utero intrapartum treatment procedure)
- Clinical features
  - Swelling; overlying skin can be normal or have a blue hue; intralesional hemorrhage can cause the vesicles to appear dark red; dermal involvement can cause skin to pucker. Lesions are soft, noncompressible, and result in underlying skeletal enlargement, mandibular overgrowth, malocclusion, and macroglossia
- Diagnosis
  - Physical exam and MRI: malformations are hyperintense on T2-weighted MRI and hypointense on T1-weighted

sequences. Macrocystic lesions can have fluid-fluid levels with large cystic spaces, and microcystic malformations are less well defined and appear as T2 intense infiltrative lesions

- Treatment
  - Macrocystic malformations are treated with sclerosing agents such as a compound of ethanol, doxycycline, bleomycin, and sodium tetradecyl sulfate. OK-432 (killed strain of Group A *Streptococcus pyogenes*) in penicillin suspension is used outside of the United States. Microcystic lesions require surgical excision

HIGH-FLOW MALFORMATIONS

ARTERIOVENOUS MALFORMATIONS

- Clinical features
  - Less common overall, pure arterial malformations are exceedingly rare; 1.5:1 female predilection; associated with Rendu-Osler-Weber syndrome; head and neck involvement is usually intracranial followed by cheek, ear, nose, mandible, and then maxilla. Histologically, arteries and veins communicate without intervening capillary beds
    - A staging system has been formulated, and it consists of four stages of progression:
      - I Quiescent: warm pink lesion
      - II Expansion: an enlarging warm pink lesion with pulsation, thrill, bruit, and tortuous veins
      - III Destruction: physical exam stigmata of a stage II lesion with overlying skin or mucosa changes, ulceration, tissue necrosis, bleeding, and pain
      - IV Decompensation: all of the findings in stage III but with cardiovascular failure

- Diagnosis
  - CT is useful for demonstrating bone destruction, and MRI is useful in assessing the extent of the lesion within the surrounding soft tissues. Doppler US is commonly used to assess the high-flow nature of the lesion
- Treatment
  - Consists of a combined approach of superselective arterial embolization to obliterate the feeding vessels of the AVM nidus followed by surgical excision of the nidus within 2-3 days to avoid re-formation of feeder vessels

REFERENCES

1. Nelson SJ. *Wheeler's Dental Anatomy, Physiology, and Occlusion.* 10th ed. St. Louis, MO: Saunders Elsevier; 2015.
2. Flynn TR. What are the antibiotics of choice for odontogenic infections, and how long should the treatment course last? *Oral Maxillofac Surg Clin North Am.* Nov. 2011;23(4):519–536. http://dx.doi.org/10.1016/j.coms.2011.07.005. v-vi.
3. Wilkes CH. Internal derangements of the temporomandibular joint (pathological variations). *Arch Otolaryngol Head Neck Surg.* 1989;115:469–477.
4. Neville BW. *Oral and Maxillofacial Pathology.* 4th ed. St. Louis, MO: Saunders Elsevier; 2015.
5. Marx RE, Stern D. *Oral and Maxillofacial Pathology: A Rationale for Diagnosis and Treatment.* 2nd ed. Hanover Park, IL: Quintessence; 2012.
6. Kaban LB. *Pediatric Oral and Maxillofacial Surgery.* Philadelphia, PA: Saunders; 1990.
7. Greene AK. Current concepts of vascular anomalies. *J Craniofac Surg.* Jan 2012;23(1):220–224.

Head and Neck Pathology 11

PREFACE

This chapter is a practical, image-based review of common head and neck lesions encountered in routine pathology practice. Included are over 100 histologic images, along with legends that succinctly summarize the key histomorphologic features. In some cases, the legends are expanded to provide a brief description of the pathologic entities and their histologic mimics. We focus on practical pathology for the practicing general otolaryngologist, and unusual and rare entities are not included. The majority of images are of standard hematoxylin and eosin (H & E)-stained slides. Some special stains, including methenamine silver stain for fungal organisms, immunohistochemical stains, and in situ hybridization highlight unique findings. This chapter is structured roughly according to the anatomic regions within the head and neck: oral cavity and oropharynx, osseous jaw, larynx and hypopharynx, nose, paranasal sinuses and nasopharynx, ear, and thyroid and parathyroid glands, with salivary gland lesions separately illustrated. Each section is then arranged into the following themes: non-neoplastic lesions (including infectious, reactive, inflammatory, and hamartomatous lesions), benign tumors, and malignant tumors. This compilation of images should serve as a useful resource for otorhinolaryngology trainees as well as a basic reference for those in practice.

ORAL CAVITY AND OROPHARYNX

DEVELOPMENTAL LESIONS

- Nasopalatine duct cyst (Fig. 11.1)

REACTIVE AND NON-NEOPLASTIC LESIONS

- Fibroepithelial polyp (Fig. 11.2)
- Lobular capillary hemangioma (pyogenic granuloma) (Fig. 11.3)
- Mucocele (Fig. 11.4)
- Reactive lymphoid follicular hyperplasia (Fig. 11.5)
- Necrotizing sialometaplasia (Figs. 11.6 and 11.7)

VASCULAR MALFORMATION

- Lymphangioma (Fig. 11.8)

INFECTIONS

- Candidiasis (Fig. 11.9)
- Granulomatous inflammation (Fig. 11.10)
- Tuberculosis (Fig. 11.11)
- Histoplasmosis (Fig. 11.12)

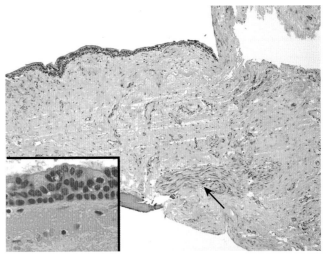

FIGURE 11.1 Nasopalatine Duct Cyst, 200×. The cyst is lined by a ciliated pseudostratified cuboidal to the low columnar epithelium (inset lower left, 400×) with underlying fibroconnective tissue and a prominent nerve (*arrow*). Nasopalatine duct cysts originate from embryonic remnants of the nasopalatine ducts. Although nonodontogenic, when lined by squamous epithelium, the cyst may resemble a periapical (radicular) cyst. Clinical and radiographic information combined with pathology are essential in arriving at the correct diagnosis.

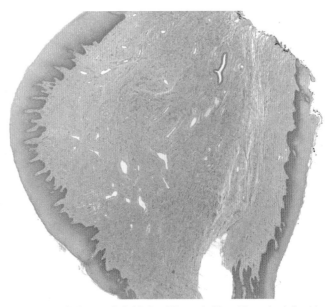

FIGURE 11.2 Fibroepithelial Polyp (Fibroma), 20×. The polyp is lined by an acanthotic, stratified squamous epithelium with a dense fibrovascular tissue stroma. Fibroepithelial polyps are common in the oral cavity and frequently occur in areas that are prone to trauma such as the tongue, buccal mucosa, and lower lip. They may be referred to as "irritation" or "bite" fibromas.

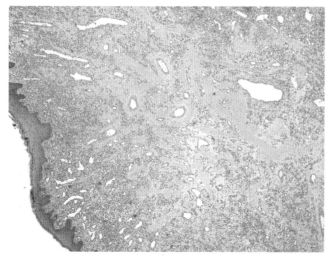

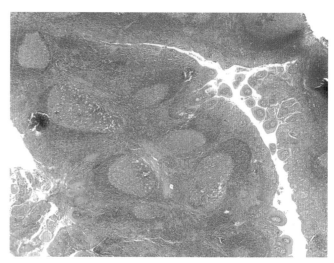

FIGURE 11.3 Pyogenic Granuloma (Lobular Capillary Hemangioma), 40×. The image shows proliferation of small capillary-sized blood vessels in a lobular arrangement with a central small ectatic feeder vessel in each lobule and an inflammatory background. Lobular capillary hemangioma is a common lesion of the oral cavity. When pyogenic granulomas occur during pregnancy, they are commonly referred to as pregnancy epulis or granuloma gravidarum.

FIGURE 11.5 Reactive Lymphoid Follicular Hyperplasia, 20×. This hyperplastic tonsil shows a lymphoid-rich stroma with prominent germinal centers, including tingible-body macrophages. When clinically worrisome, ancillary studies, such as flow cytometry, immunohistochemistry (IHC), and molecular testing for clonal gene rearrangements, are essential to exclude a neoplasia (including lymphoma).

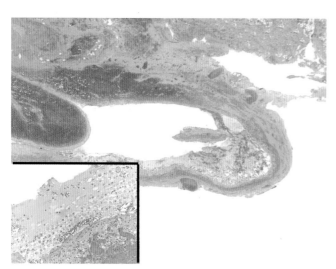

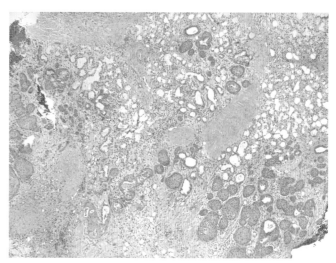

FIGURE 11.4 Mucocele of the Sublingual Gland (Ranula), 20×. The image shows a large area of extravasated mucin. The mucin (which appears gray/pink in color) contains abundant histiocytes with mucin in their cytoplasm (muciphages) (inset lower left, 200×). The extravasated mucin is surrounded by a wall of granulation tissue and as such, mucoceles are pseudocysts (lacking an epithelial cyst lining). Mucoceles are commonly seen in the lower lip because of bite injury to the minor salivary gland ducts. Mucoceles that arise from the sublingual glands push up into the floor of the mouth, forming a noticeable smooth cystic mass, termed *ranula*.

FIGURE 11.6 Necrotizing Sialometaplasia, 20×. The image shows squamous metaplasia of the minor salivary gland ducts in a lobular arrangement. A few open ducts are present; however, many have been obliterated by the squamous metaplastic process. A moderate chronic inflammatory cell infiltrate is seen in the background with marked atrophy and destruction of the minor salivary gland acini (see also Fig. 11.7).

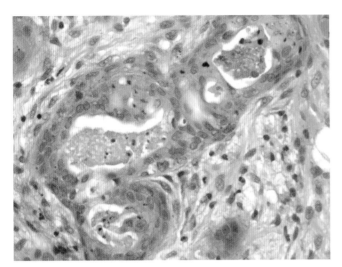

FIGURE 11.7 Necrotizing Sialometaplasia, 400×. Necrotic debris and neutrophils are seen within the lumens of the metaplastic ducts. The metaplastic ductal cells are crowded and show nuclear hyperchromasia. The lesion may mimic a squamous cell carcinoma (SCC) in small biopsy specimens, where the lobular arrangement of the cells is difficult to appreciate. Necrotizing sialometaplasia presents as an ulcerative lesion of the hard palate, and may clinically simulate a carcinoma; however, these lesions usually lack the marked nuclear atypia and increased mitoses seen in a squamous cell carcinoma.

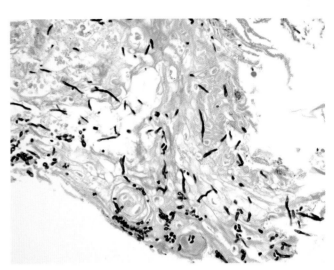

FIGURE 11.9 Candidiasis (Methenamine Silver Stain), 200×. Thickened parakeratotic squamous epithelium containing numerous hyphae, pseudohyphae, and spore forms, consistent with *Candida* spp; some degree of superficial epithelial infiltration with neutrophils is often seen on H & E sections.

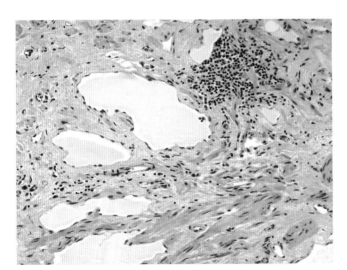

FIGURE 11.8 Lymphangioma, 200×. The image shows large dilated lymphatic vessels lined by a flat, inconspicuous layer of bland endothelial cells. The lymphatic channels contain a pale proteinaceous material (lymph). A dense collection of lymphocytes is seen in the stroma surrounding the vessels. Lymphangiomas are generally seen in the head and neck region of newborns and are treated surgically.

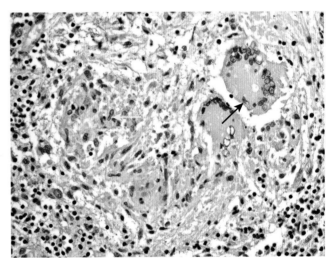

FIGURE 11.10 Granulomatous Inflammation, 200×. The image shows a granuloma consisting of epithelioid histiocytes with elongated, curved nuclei (*yellow arrow*), multinucleated giant cells (*black arrow*), and a peripheral rim of small lymphocytes. The differential diagnosis of granulomatous inflammation is broad and includes a wide range of bacterial (eg, tuberculosis), fungal (eg, histoplasmosis), immunologic (eg, sarcoidosis, Crohn disease) and neoplastic conditions (eg, Hodgkin lymphoma).

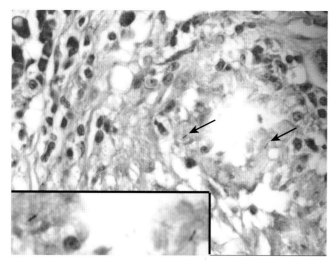

FIGURE 11.11 Tuberculosis (Ziehl-Neelsen Stain), 200×. The image shows acid-fast bacilli (indicated by *arrows* in the image and magnified in the inset lower left). Oral tuberculosis usually presents as an atypical area of ulceration in the oral cavity and may clinically resemble a malignancy. It results from direct inoculation of acid-fast bacilli into the oral tissues.

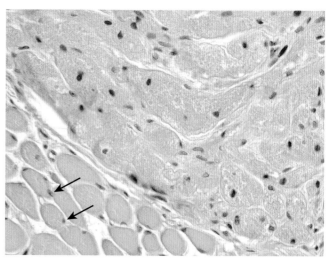

FIGURE 11.13 Granular Cell Tumor of the Tongue, 200×. Cytologically bland large polygonal cells with abundant granular, oncocytic (pink) cytoplasm and centrally located small, dark nuclei. In this image, the granular cells abut skeletal muscle cells (*arrows*). Note the similarity between the two cell types, distinguished by the circumscription of the granular cell tumor with granular, pink fluffy cytoplasm and the skeletal muscle with a glassy/striated cytoplasm. The granular cells react strongly and diffusely with antibodies to S100 protein and are thought to be of Schwannian origin.

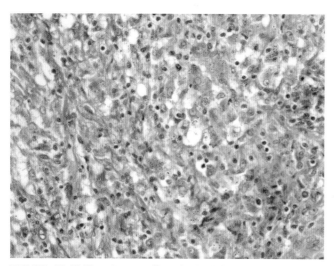

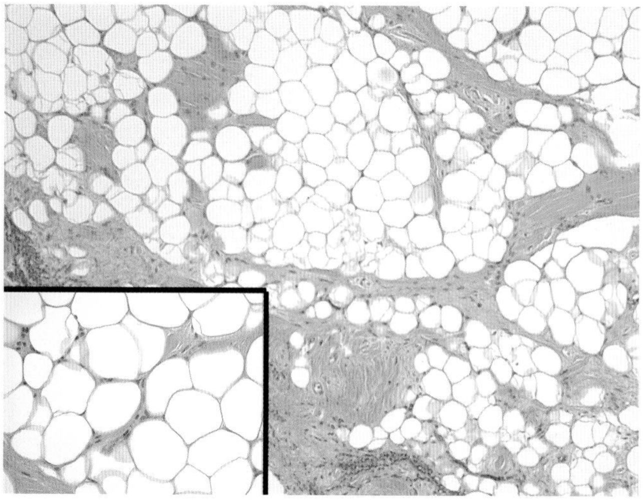

FIGURE 11.12 Histoplasmosis (Periodic Acid Schiff–Stain), 200×. The foamy macrophages possess numerous small fungal spores (1-4 μm) in their cytoplasm surrounded by clear halos.

FIGURE 11.14 Lipoma, 100×. The image shows lobules of mature adipose tissue separated by thick bands of fibrous tissue. The adipocytes are univacuolated with their slender hyperchromatic nuclei located at the periphery of the cell, often not apparent (inset lower left, 400×). Nuclear atypia or marked variation in size might raise the possibility of liposarcoma. Lipomas are usually solitary lesions in adults and commonly involve the oral cavity and the larynx; the degree of cellularity and fibrosis is location-dependent.

BENIGN TUMORS

- Granular cell tumor (Fig. 11.13)
- Lipoma (Fig. 11.14)
- Spindle cell lipoma (Fig. 11.15)

EPITHELIAL PRECURSOR LESIONS

- Mild epithelial dysplasia (Fig. 11.16)
- Severe epithelial dysplasia/carcinoma in situ (Fig. 11.17)
- Verrucous hyperplasia (Fig. 11.18)

MALIGNANT EPITHELIAL LESIONS

- Verrucous carcinoma (Fig. 11.19)
- Keratinizing squamous cell carcinoma (Figs. 11.20 and 11.21)

- Basaloid squamous cell carcinoma (Fig. 11.22)
- Adenosquamous carcinoma (Fig. 11.23)
- Nonkeratinizing squamous cell carcinoma (Fig. 11.24)
- Immunohistochemistry for p16 (Fig. 11.25)

MALIGNANT MESENCHYMAL TUMORS

- Kaposi sarcoma (Fig. 11.26)

IMMUNE-MEDIATED LESIONS

- Pemphigus vulgaris (Fig. 11.27)
- Pemphigoid (Fig. 11.28)

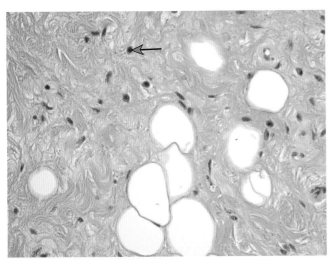

FIGURE 11.15 Spindle Cell Lipoma, **400×**. Spindled fibroblasts, shredded collagen fibers, mast cells (*arrow*), myxoid change, and mature adipocytes characterize this variant of lipoma, commonly seen in the oral cavity.

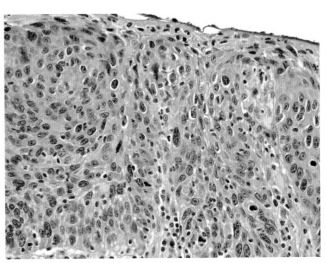

FIGURE 11.17 Severe Epithelial Dysplasia/Carcinoma in Situ, **200×**. There is full-thickness, marked nuclear atypia and pleomorphism, with suprabasilar mitoses and disordered maturation of cells.

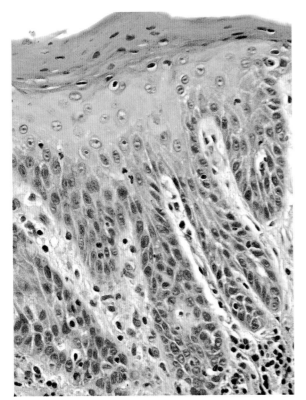

FIGURE 11.16 Mild Epithelial Dysplasia, **200×**. The epithelium shows drop-shaped rete processes and loss of nuclear polarization. Cytologically, there is nuclear hyperchromasia, and prominent nucleoli. The architectural and cytologic features are confined to the lower one-third of the epithelium.

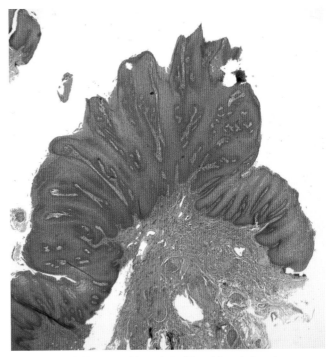

FIGURE 11.18 Verrucous Hyperplasia, **20×**. Although the rete processes appear elongated, they are relatively uniform and do not appear deeper than the surrounding normal epithelium. The lesion lacks significant cytologic atypia. Verrucous hyperplasia is seen in the oral cavity, often in the setting of proliferative verrucous leukoplakia. It has a high recurrence rate and may transform into verrucous carcinoma or invasive SCC. The word *verrucous* reflects the warty appearance of these lesions with pointy, spire-like architecture.

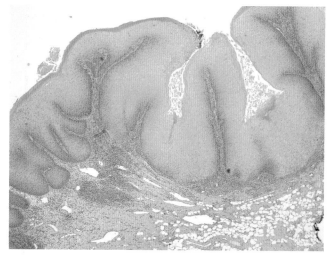

FIGURE 11.19 Verrucous Carcinoma, 20×. Large and broad rete processes push deeply into the submucosa in broad, pushing nests. The folded and thickened epithelium shows marked surface keratinization. A dense chronic inflammatory response may be seen at the advancing front of the lesion, and there is no epithelial atypia. Small and superficial biopsies can create diagnostic difficulties because the base of the lesion may not be visualized.

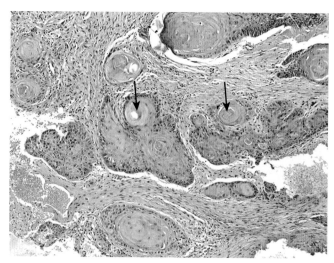

FIGURE 11.20 Keratinizing Squamous Cell Carcinoma, 200×. The image shows a well-differentiated SCC with abundant intralesional keratinization, forming keratin pearls (*arrows*).

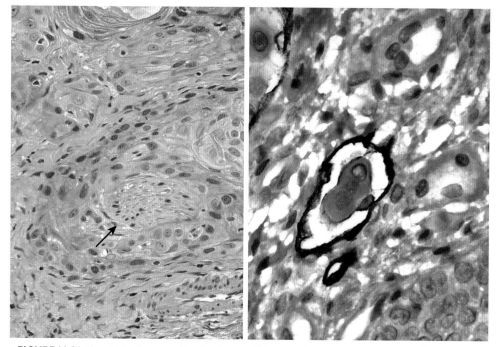

FIGURE 11.21 Keratinizing Squamous Cell Carcinoma with Perineural and Lymphovascular Invasion, 400×. Malignant squamous cells surround a peripheral nerve (*arrow*, left image). Malignant squamous cells in a lymphatic vessel (right image, D2-40 IHC). Perineural invasion and lymphovascular invasion are frequently observed in SCCs.

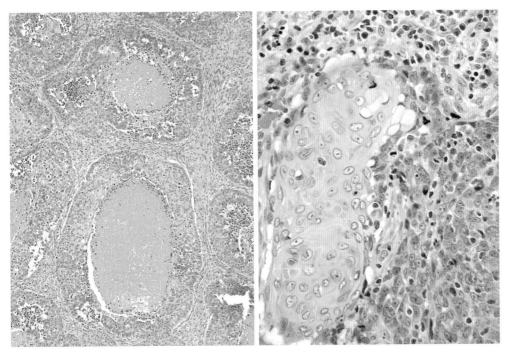

FIGURE 11.22 Basaloid Squamous Cell Carcinoma. Islands of atypical basaloid cells (the term *basaloid* means the cells show a high nuclear to cytoplasmic ratio with small dense hyperchromatic nuclei, similar to basal epithelial cells) with central areas of necrosis (comedo-type necrosis) (left image, 100×). Most basaloid squamous cell carcinomas (BSCCs) show focal areas of high-grade surface dysplasia or keratinizing SCC (right image, 400×). Correctly diagnosing a BSCC can be challenging in small biopsies. The differential diagnosis includes other basaloid lesions such as adenoid cystic carcinoma (ADCC), salivary duct carcinoma, and nonkeratinizing, HPV-related SCC.

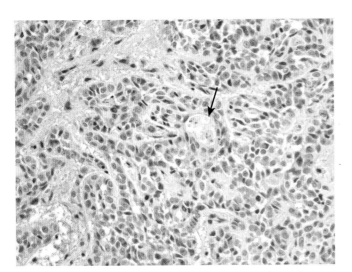

FIGURE 11.23 Adenosquamous Carcinoma, 200×. The image shows an SCC with areas of true glandular differentiation (*arrow*). Adenosquamous carcinomas often behave aggressively.

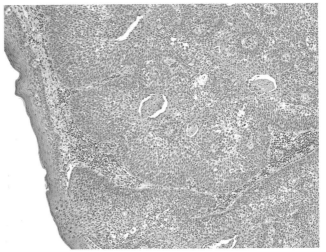

FIGURE 11.24 Nonkeratinizing Oropharyngeal Squamous Cell Carcinoma, 100×. Nests of nonkeratinizing squamous cells with basaloid features, pushing borders, and intraluminal necrosis. Most oropharyngeal cases with this appearance are positive for high-risk (HR) HPV subtypes. They are most frequently found in the base of tongue and palatine tonsils, and careful attention may be needed to distinguish these malignant nests from the normal component lymphoid stroma. Although lacking the typical infiltrative features seen in other carcinomas, these nests of cells are considered to be invasive by nature and likely to metastasize via lymphatic channels within the tonsil if not already metastatic at the time of diagnosis.

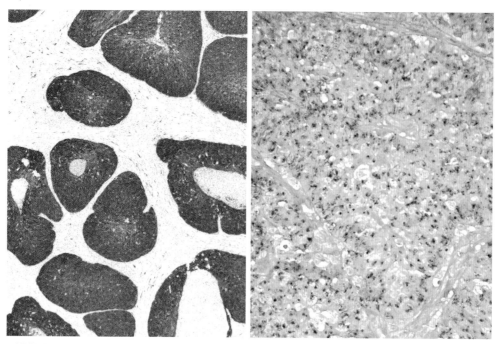

FIGURE 11.25 Human Papillomavirus-Related Nonkeratinizing Oropharyngeal Squamous Cell Carcinoma. P16 IHC and in situ hybridization (ISH) for HR-HPV. Strong cytoplasmic and nuclear staining for P16 (image left, 200×). P16 IHC is a sensitive but nonspecific screening test for HR-HPV. More than 70% of the tumor cells should be positive for this antibody. P16-positive tumors are further evaluated for the presence of HR-HPV by polymerase chain reaction or ISH. The image on the right shows punctate positivity for HR-HPV (ISH, 400×).

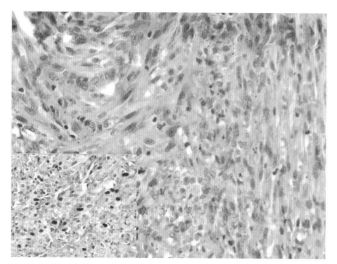

FIGURE 11.26 Kaposi Sarcoma, 400. Moderately pleomorphic spindled cells surround slit-like vascular channels with extravasation of red blood cells. Nuclear reactivity with antibodies to human herpesvirus 8 is seen in most Kaposi sarcomas (inset lower left, 200×).

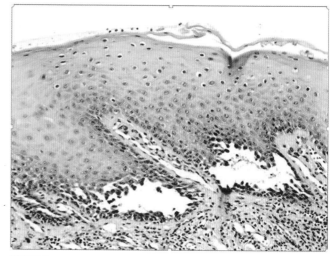

FIGURE 11.27 Pemphigus Vulgaris, 100×. The image shows intraepithelial vesicles. The basal layer is intact. Pemphigus vulgaris is an autoimmune vesiculobullous disease. The IgG antibodies directed against the interepithelial desmosomes cause squamous cells to lose cohesion (acantholysis).

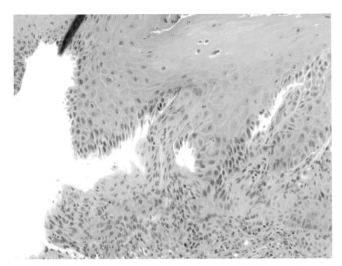

FIGURE 11.28 Pemphigoid, 200×. A sub-basilar cleft is observed. Pemphigoid is an autoimmune vesiculobullous disease with antibodies directed against basement membrane antigens that connect the epithelial cells to the basement membrane.

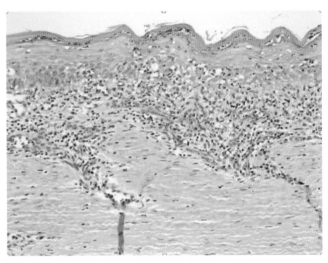

FIGURE 11.29 Lichen Planus, 100×. A dense band-like lymphocytic infiltrate is seen at the epithelial-connective tissue interface, with hydropic (vacuolar) degeneration of epithelial basal cells. The histologic features of lichen planus can be mimicked by a number of conditions, which include lichenoid contact reactions, lichenoid drug eruptions, chronic graft vs. host disease, and lupus erythematosus. Careful clinicopathologic correlation is essential in arriving at the correct diagnosis.

- Lichen planus (Fig. 11.29)
- Sjögren syndrome (Fig. 11.30)

LESIONS OF THE OSSEOUS JAW

- Osteomyelitis (Fig. 11.31)
- Osteoradionecrosis (Fig. 11.32)
- Central giant cell granuloma (Fig. 11.33)
- Osteoma (Fig. 11.34)
- Osteosarcoma (Fig. 11.35)
- Fibrous dysplasia (Fig. 11.36)
- Ossifying fibroma (Fig. 11.37)

SELECTED ODONTOGENIC CYSTS AND TUMORS

ODONTOGENIC CYSTS

- Periapical (radicular) cyst (Fig. 11.38)
- Dentigerous cyst (Fig. 11.39)

BENIGN EPITHELIAL ODONTOGENIC TUMORS

- Solid/multicystic ameloblastoma (Fig. 11.40)
- Calcifying epithelial odontogenic tumor (Fig. 11.41)
- Adenomatoid odontogenic tumor (Fig. 11.42)
- Keratocystic odontogenic tumor (Fig. 11.43)

BENIGN MIXED EPITHELIAL TUMORS

- Odontoma (Fig. 11.44)

BENIGN MESENCHYMAL ODONTOGENIC TUMORS

- Odontogenic myxoma (Fig. 11.45)

LARYNX AND HYPOPHARYNX

NON-NEOPLASTIC LESIONS

- Contact ulcer of the larynx (Fig. 11.46)
- Vocal cord polyp (Fig. 11.47)

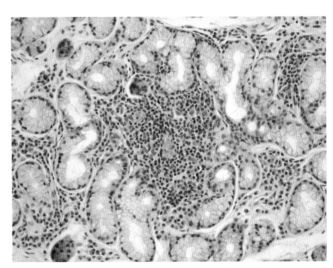

FIGURE 11.30 Sjögren Syndrome, Lip Biopsy, 400×. The image shows a dense lymphoid infiltrate within the parenchyma of the minor salivary gland. More than 50 lymphocytes are seen in one focus. Sjögren syndrome is a systemic autoimmune disease. Patients may present with SICCA syndrome, including dry eyes and dry mouth. The diagnosis is a clinical diagnosis that may be supported by pathologic findings, generally by biopsy of non–bite line minor salivary tissue.

BENIGN EPITHELIAL TUMORS

- Laryngeal papilloma (Fig. 11.48)
- In situ hybridization for human papillomavirus (HPV) (Fig. 11.49)

MALIGNANT EPITHELIAL TUMORS

- Squamous cell carcinoma of the larynx with thyroid cartilage invasion (Fig. 11.50)
- Papillary squamous cell carcinoma (Fig. 11.51)
- Spindle cell (sarcomatoid) carcinoma (Fig. 11.52)

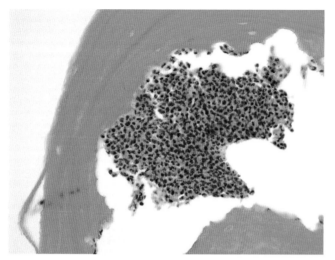

FIGURE 11.31 Osteomyelitis, 400×. The marrow space contains a dense collection of neutrophils. The surrounding nonvital bone shows loss of osteocytes from the lacunae and peripheral "moth-eaten" areas of resorption (an attempt by the osteoclasts to remove the dead bone). Osteomyelitis commonly involves the mandible, and is associated with trauma or spread of infection from an odontogenic focus.

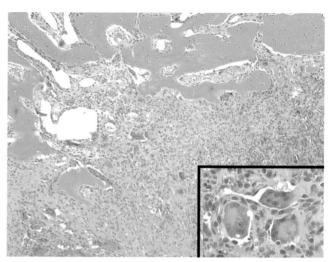

FIGURE 11.33 Central Giant Cell Lesion (Giant Cell Reparative Granuloma), 40×. Plump cytologically bland spindled cells, osteoclast-like multinucleated giant cells, and extravasated red blood cells (inset lower right, 400×). Reactive bone is seen at the advancing front of the lesion. These are commonly seen in young adults and frequently involve the mandible. Before a diagnosis of central giant cell lesion is rendered, other entities with identical histology should be excluded. These include the brown tumor of hyperparathyroidism, cherubism, aneurysmal bone cyst, and peripheral giant cell granuloma.

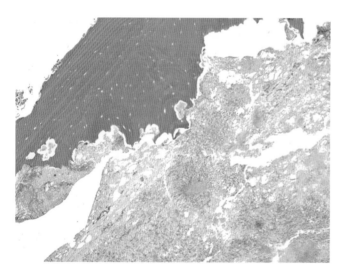

FIGURE 11.32 Osteoradionecrosis, 40×. Necrotic bone with loss of osteocytes from the lacunae and peripheral ragged areas of resorption. The dead bone is surrounded by basophilic bacterial colonies consistent with *Actinomyces* spp. The diagnosis of osteoradionecrosis requires history of prior irradiation because the histologic picture is identical to osteomyelitis of bacterial origin.

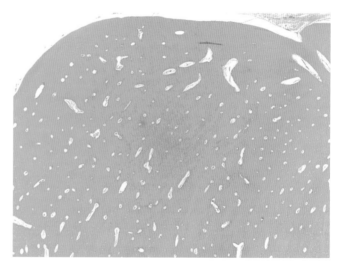

FIGURE 11.34 Osteoma, 20×. The lesion is well circumscribed and consists of dense, mature cortical bone. Osteomas are histologically classified into compact (cortical) and spongy (trabecular) types. Multiple osteomas are seen in the setting of Gardner syndrome, an autosomal-dominant disorder characterized by gastrointestinal (GI) polyps and skin and soft tissue tumors. The GI polyps have a 100% risk of undergoing malignant transformation.

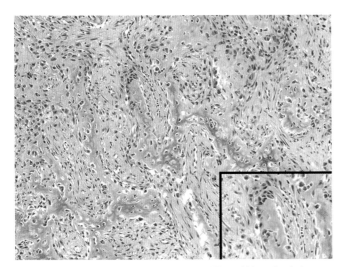

FIGURE 11.35 Osteosarcoma, Osteoblastic Type, 100×. Atypical osteo-blasts with lace-like areas of osteoid (malignant bone) deposition. A few malignant osteoblasts are entrapped within the osteoid (inset lower right, 400×). Osteo-sarcoma is the most common primary malignancy of bone. In the head and neck, osteosarcomas commonly arise in the mandible, and may present as rapidly en-larging painful lesions with loose teeth. Tumors may show extensive fibroblastic or chondroblastic differentiation.

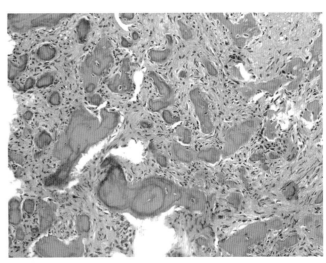

FIGURE 11.37 Ossifying Fibroma, 100×. The image shows dense fibrous tissue, short trabeculae of bone, and numerous rounded psammomatoid (calcified psammoma body-like) deposits. Ossifying fibroma is a neoplastic fibro-osseous lesion. All fibro-osseous lesions (fibrous dysplasia, osseous dys-plasia, and ossifying fibroma) share similar histology and require clinical and radiologic correlation.

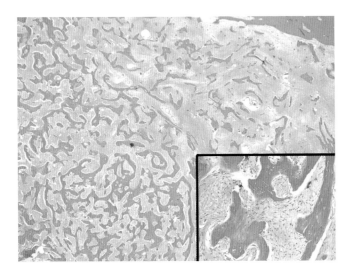

FIGURE 11.36 Fibrous Dysplasia, 20×. Fibrous stroma and irregular trabec-ulae of bone that are said to resemble Chinese characters. The bony trabeculae lack osteoblastic rimming (inset lower right, 400×). Fibrous dysplasia is a devel-opmental fibro-osseous lesion with mutations involving the GNAS-1 gene. It can be monostotic (involving a single bone only) or polyostotic. The polyostotic form can be associated with endocrine disorders, most commonly precocious puberty.

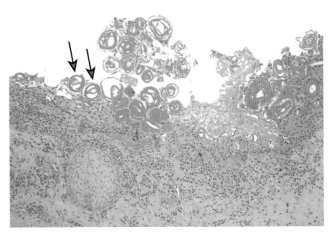

FIGURE 11.38 Periapical (Radicular) Cyst, 100×. The cyst is lined by strati-fied squamous epithelium with Rushton (hyaline) bodies (eosinophilic curved glassy structures, *arrows*). A dense chronic inflammatory cell infiltrate is seen im-mediately beneath the cyst lining. The periapical cyst is an inflammatory odonto-genic cyst, seen at the apex of a non-vital tooth.

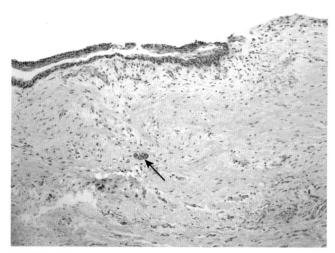

FIGURE 11.39 Dentigerous Cyst, 100×. The cyst is lined by a thin epithelium that resembles the reduced enamel epithelium of a developing tooth. Small islands of odontogenic epithelium (*arrow*) are sometimes seen in the connective tissue wall of the cyst. A dentigerous cyst is a developmental odontogenic cyst and is associated with the crown of an unerupted tooth.

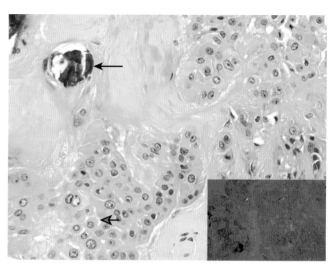

FIGURE 11.41 Calcifying Epithelial Odontogenic Tumor, 200×. Rounded squamoid (squamous-like) cells with dense eosinophilic cytoplasm, hyperchromatic, moderately pleomorphic nuclei, and prominent nucleoli. Intercellular bridges are clearly visible (*arrow*). The cells surround globules of pale acellular eosinophilic material (amyloid) with a focus of calcification (*arrow*). The amyloid demonstrates an apple-green birefringence when viewed under polarized light (inset lower right, 40×).

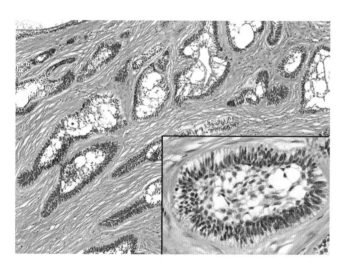

FIGURE 11.40 Solid/Multicystic Ameloblastoma, 100×. The tumor shows a follicular growth pattern. The follicles are bordered by ameloblast-like cells with reverse nuclear polarity (inset lower right, 400×). The center-most areas often demonstrate cystic degeneration and are characterized by loosely connected cells, stellate reticulum-like cells. The stellate cells may display squamous (acanthomatous), granular, or basal cell differentiation.

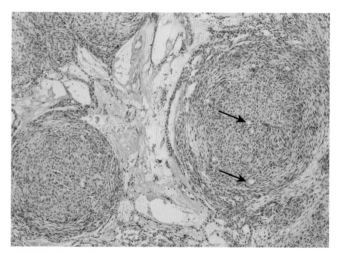

FIGURE 11.42 Adenomatoid Odontogenic Tumor, 100×. Solid nests of spindle-shaped epithelial cells. The solid nests contain duct-like structures (rosettes) lined by a single row of columnar epithelial cells (*arrows*). Adenomatoid odontogenic tumor is considered to be a hamartoma rather than a true neoplasm. It is commonly seen in the anterior segments of the jaw and usually surrounds the crown of an unerupted tooth.

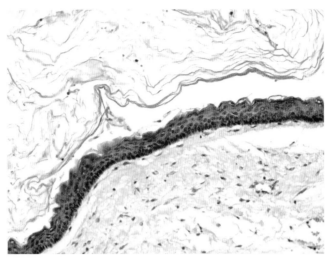

FIGURE 11.43 Keratocystic Odontogenic Tumor, 200×. The cyst is lined by a thin squamous epithelium with a distinct palisaded basal layer and a superficial corrugated layer of parakeratin. The lumen contains abundant laminated keratin. Multiple keratocystic odontogenic tumors occur in the setting of Gorlin (nevoid basal cell carcinoma) syndrome, an autosomal-dominant disorder associated with mutation of the PTCH1 gene.

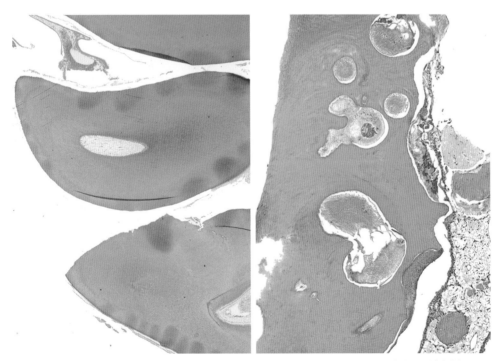

FIGURE 11.44 Compound Odontoma. Formation of two miniature tooth-like structures (odontoids) (left image, 40×). Odontomas are considered to be hamartomatous rather than truly neoplastic. There are two forms, compound odontoma and complex odontoma. When complex, they are composed of a disorganized mass of mineralized material with no resemblance to a tooth (image right, 100×).

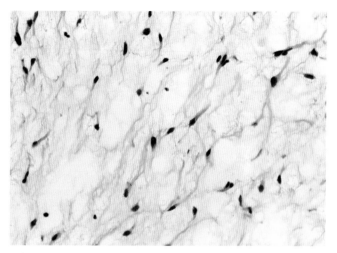

FIGURE 11.45 Odontogenic Myxoma, 400×. The tumor is relatively hypocellular and consists of bland spindle-shaped cells suspended in a myxoid stroma.

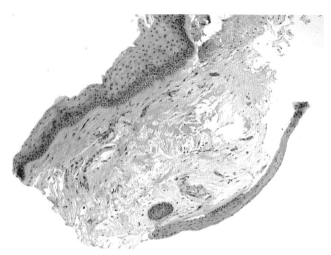

FIGURE 11.47 Vocal Cord Polyp, 40×. Polypoid squamous tissue with an underlying myxoid stroma. The stroma may be hyalinized or hemorrhagic with fibrin. Depending on the chronicity of the lesion, more chronic changes such as ossification or atypical stromal fibroblasts may be seen in longer standing lesions.

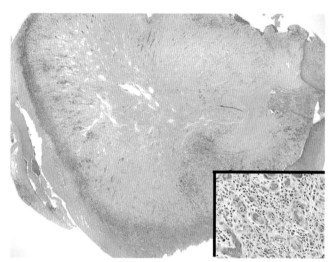

FIGURE 11.46 Contact Ulcer of Larynx (Contact Granuloma), 20×. Polypoid lesion with surface ulceration. The majority of the lesion consists of granulation tissue with vessels arranged in radial spokes (inset lower right, 400×). Contact ulcers form in response to mechanical or chemical trauma.

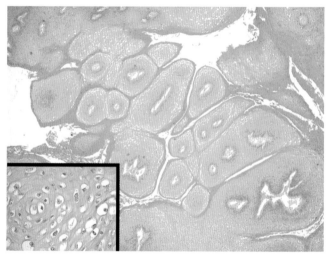

FIGURE 11.48 Laryngeal Papilloma, 20×. Exophytic projections of keratinizing squamous epithelium with fibrovascular cores. Koilocytes, HPV-induced cytopathic changes, are seen in the superficial layers of the epithelium (inset lower left, 400×). They may be binucleated and contain clear cytoplasm and wrinkled, or raisinoid, nuclei. Papillomas are caused by low-risk HPV type 6 or 11. Squamous papillomas of the larynx may be solitary or multiple. Multiple lesions (laryngeal papillomatosis) are more common in young patients. Squamous papillomas are benign and do not generally transform to carcinoma.

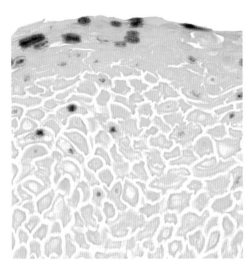

FIGURE 11.49 Human Papillomavirus in Situ Hybridization, 200×. Laryngeal papillomas are caused by infection of the mucosa with HPV types 6 or 11.

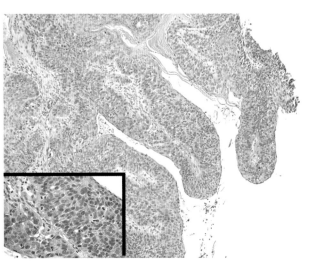

FIGURE 11.51 Papillary Squamous Cell Carcinoma, 40×. The tumor is exophytic and has a papillary architecture, reminiscent of squamous papilloma. However, the papillary fronds are covered by severely stratified squamous epithelium (inset lower left, 400×). This uncommon variant of SCC is most often seen in the larynx, oropharynx, and sinonasal tract, and, in some cases, it is associated with HR-HPV infection.

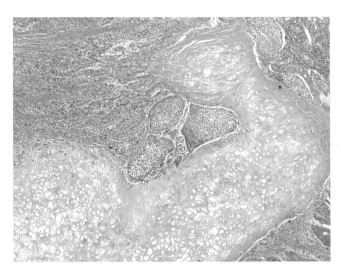

FIGURE 11.50 Squamous Cell Carcinoma of the Larynx, 40×. The image shows invasion of the thyroid cartilage by moderately differentiated islands of SCC.

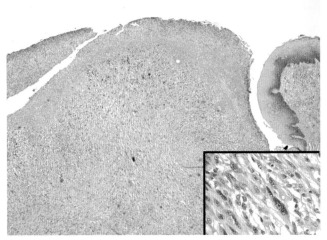

FIGURE 11.52 Spindle Cell (Sarcomatoid) Squamous Cell Carcinoma, 20×. The tumor has a polypoid appearance with surface ulceration, and it contains highly atypical spindled cells in a fascicular arrangement (inset lower right, 400×). Spindle cell SCCs often show foci of squamous differentiation or surface dysplasia. When absent, a definitive diagnosis can be difficult to obtain, and the differential diagnosis includes sarcoma and spindle cell melanoma. In such cases, ancillary testing may be of some assistance, but additional clinical information may be crucial.

NEUROENDOCRINE CARCINOMA

- Poorly differentiated neuroendocrine carcinoma (small cell carcinoma) (Fig. 11.53)

MESENCHYMAL TUMORS

- Low-grade chondrosarcoma (Fig. 11.54)

NOSE, PARANASAL SINUSES, AND NASOPHARYNX

INFLAMMATORY AND INFECTIOUS LESIONS

- Chronic rhinosinusitis (Fig. 11.55)
- Allergic fungal sinusitis (Fig. 11.56)
- Invasive fungal sinusitis (Fig. 11.57)
- Inflammatory nasal polyp (Fig. 11.58)
- Rhinosporidiosis (Fig. 11.59)

HAMARTOMATOUS AND HETEROTOPIC LESIONS

- Nasal glial heterotopia (Fig. 11.60)
- Dermoid cyst (Fig. 11.61)
- Respiratory epithelial adenomatoid hamartoma (Fig. 11.62)

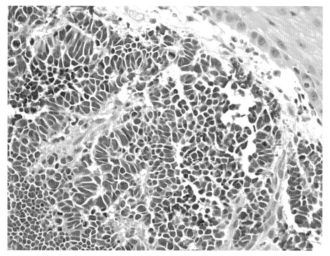

FIGURE 11.53 Small Cell Carcinoma or Poorly Differentiated Neuroendocrine Carcinoma, 200×. Small cell carcinoma located beneath the normal appearing epithelium. The cytomorphologic features are similar to those of pulmonary small cell carcinomas, with nuclear molding, granular chromatin, frequent mitoses, and apoptotic bodies. They are most commonly seen in middle-aged to elderly men and carry a dismal prognosis. The diagnosis is confirmed by immunohistochemical demonstration of neuroendocrine differentiation using markers such as synaptophysin.

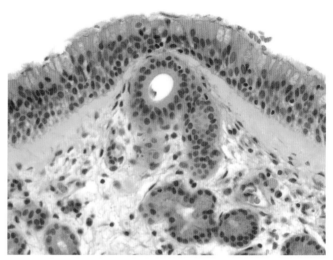

FIGURE 11.55 Chronic Rhinosinusitis, 400×. Stromal edema with chronic inflammatory cells. The chronic nature of the disease is marked by subepithelial hyalinization.

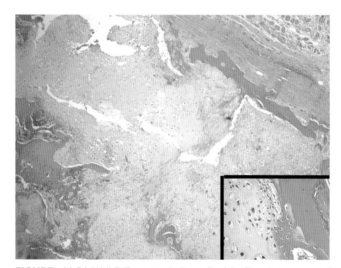

FIGURE 11.54 Well-Differentiated (Low-Grade) Chondrosarcoma of the Thyroid Cartilage, 20×. The tumor is composed of well-formed hyaline cartilage. In comparison with normal cartilage, the tumor is more cellular, with nuclear pleomorphism and hyperchromasia (inset lower right, 400×). Binucleated chondrocytes are frequently observed in laryngeal chondrosarcomas (not shown). Low-grade tumors share similar morphology with chondromas and are essentially diagnosed based on their infiltrative growth pattern.

EPITHELIAL AND NEUROEPITHELIAL TUMORS

- Inverted papilloma (inverted papilloma, Schneiderian type) (Fig. 11.63)
- Schneiderian carcinoma (non-keratinizing sinonasal carcinoma) (Fig. 11.64)
- Nasopharyngeal carcinoma (Fig. 11.65)
- Sinonasal undifferentiated carcinoma (SNUC) (Fig. 11.66)
- Sinonasal adenocarcinoma, intestinal type (ITAC) (Fig. 11.67)
- Olfactory neuroblastoma (esthesioneuroblastoma) (Fig. 11.68)
- Sinonasal meningioma (Fig. 11.69)

MALIGNANT LYMPHOID AND MELANOCYTIC LESIONS

- NK/T-cell lymphoma, nasal type (Fig. 11-70)
- Sinonasa melanoma (Fig. 11-71)

MESENCHYMAL LESIONS

- Angiofibroma (Fig. 11.72)
- Glomangiopericytoma (Fig. 11.73)
- Chordoma (Fig. 11.74)
- Rhabdomyosarcoma (Figs. 11.75 and 11.76)

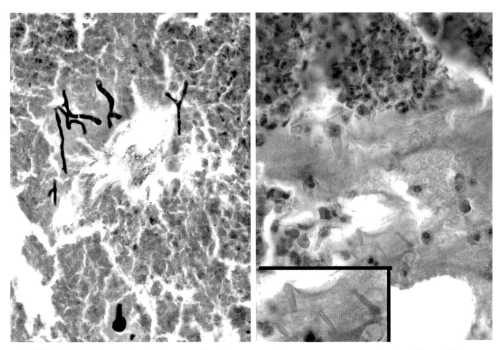

FIGURE 11.56 Allergic Fungal Sinusitis. Abundant mucus with numerous entrapped eosinophils and Charcot-Leyden crystals (allergic mucus) (right image, 200×). The silver stain shows occasional fungal hyphae (left image, 400×).

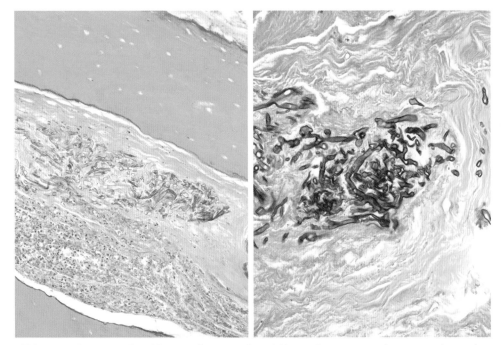

FIGURE 11.57 Invasive Fungal Sinusitis. Fragments of nonvital bone adjacent to a necrotic marrow cavity containing granular debris, neutrophils, and thick nonseptate fungal hyphae, consistent with Mucor (left, 100×). Thick non-septate fungal hyphae are seen within the lumen of a blood vessel (methenamine silver stain, right, 400×). Vascular invasion is often associated with necrosis, hemorrhage, and inflammation. The condition is generally seen in immuno-compromised patients (eg, in the setting of diabetes, human immunodeficiency virus [HIV] or lymphoid malignancies), often caused by fungi of the order Mucorales (eg, Rhizopus and Mucor).

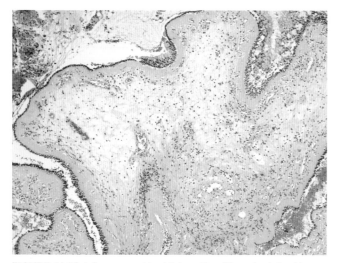

FIGURE 11.58 Inflammatory Nasal Polyp, 40×. The polyp is lined by respiratory epithelium, with marked subepithelial hyalinization and stromal edema with an inflammatory background.

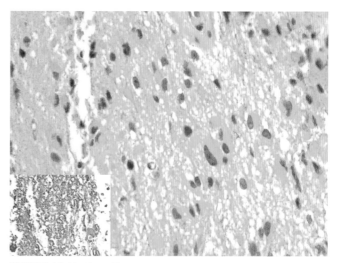

FIGURE 11.60 Nasal Glial Heterotopia, 400×. Non-neoplastic glial tissue found within the nasal cavity separate from the central nervous system. The glial tissue can be difficult to appreciate on H & E sections. Immunostaining with antibodies to S100 protein or glial fibrillary acidic protein can be helpful in identifying the glial component (inset lower left, 400×).

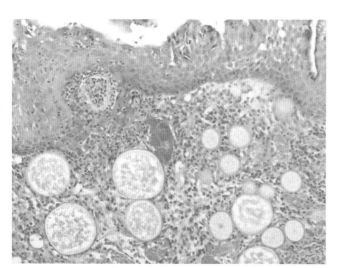

FIGURE 11.59 Rhinosporidiosis, 200×. Thick-walled rounded variably sized cyst-like structures (sporangia) (10-200 μm in diameter), filled with small spores. Rhinosporidiosis is caused by the fungus *Rhinosporidium seeberi* and is endemic to South India and Sri Lanka. The disease usually presents as a unilateral polypoid lesion.

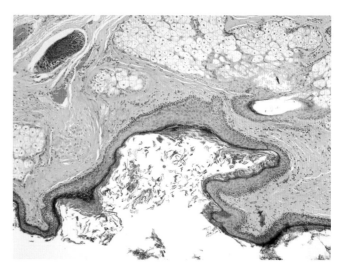

FIGURE 11.61 Dermoid Cyst, 100×. The cyst is lined by keratin, producing squamous epithelium with a prominent granular cell layer. The cyst wall contains hair follicles and sebaceous glands. Dermoid cysts are usually midline cysts and occur in a number of locations within the head and neck region. They contain ectodermal and mesodermal elements. Nasal dermoids are often seen at the dorsum of the nose.

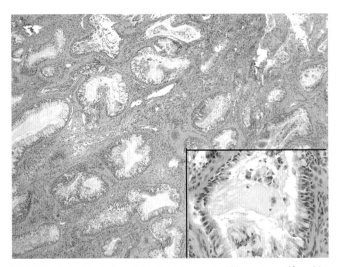

FIGURE 11.62 Respiratory Epithelial Adenomatoid Hamartoma, 40×. Numerous glandular structures lined by ciliated columnar cells and occasional mucus cells (inset lower right, 400×). The glands contain mucus. The stroma exhibits dense chronic inflammation. Clinically, the lesions are polypoid and usually involve the posterior nasal septum.

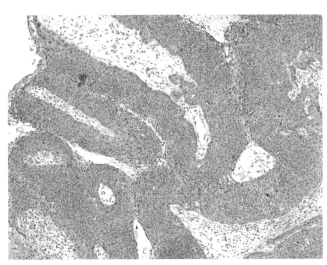

FIGURE 11.64 Sinonasal Squamous Cell Carcinoma, Nonkeratinizing Type (Schneiderian Carcinoma), 100×. The tumor shows a plexiform or ribbon-like growth pattern and full-thickness severe epithelial atypia, and it lacks keratinization. Tumors may be positive for HR-HPV.

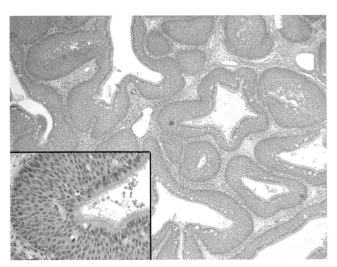

FIGURE 11.63 Inverted Papilloma, 40×. The tumor exhibits an endophytic growth with islands of transitional-type epithelium containing occasional mucus cells and small collections of neutrophils. Respiratory cells overlie the transitional epithelium (inset lower left, 400×). A distinct basal layer is observed, and there is rarely atypia.

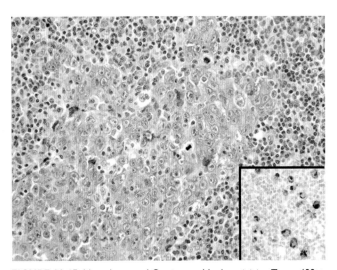

FIGURE 11.65 Nasopharyngeal Carcinoma, Nonkeratinizing Types, 400×. An island of undifferentiated cells with indistinct cell borders (syncytial pattern) associated with dense lymphoid stroma. The tumor cells have large nuclei with open chromatin and prominent nucleoli. Almost all nonkeratinizing nasopharyngeal carcinomas are radiosensitive and Epstein-Barr early mRNA (EBER)-positive (inset lower right, 400×).

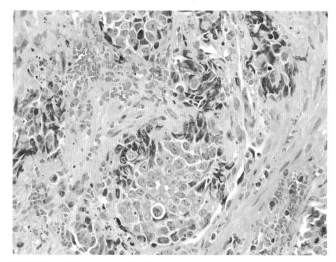

FIGURE 11.66 Sinonasal Undifferentiated Carcinoma, 400×. Nests of undifferentiated medium-sized to large-sized cells. The hyperchromatic nuclei are round to oval shaped and pleomorphic, and they show prominent nucleoli. SNUC is a rare, highly aggressive malignancy arising in the sinonasal tract. Patients usually present with signs and symptoms secondary to local invasion (eg, proptosis, pain, anosmia, and diplopia). Because many tumors in this region appear histologically similar, the diagnosis of SNUC, a diagnosis of exclusion, is generally conferred following a battery of immunohistochemical stains.

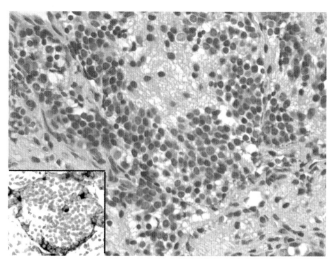

FIGURE 11.68 Olfactory Neuroblastoma, 400×. Small cells with minimal cytoplasm are suspended in an eosinophilic fibrillary background. The nuclei are monomorphic and round with fine granular chromatin. Prominent nucleoli and mitotic figures are not seen. Immunostaining with S100 protein is confined to the slender sustentacular (supporting) cells that surround the groups of neoplastic cells (inset lower left, 400×). Olfactory neuroblastomas develop in the upper nasal cavity in the region of the olfactory epithelium near the cribriform plate.

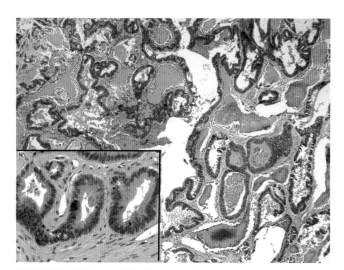

FIGURE 11.67 Intestinal-Type Sinonasal Adenocarcinoma, 40×. The tumor has a papillary-tubular architecture, similar to the pattern seen in many colorectal adenocarcinomas (inset, 400×). Glands are lined by tall columnar cells with elongated hyperchromatic nuclei that appear stratified. ITACs have been linked to exposure to hardwood and dust particles and show an exceptionally high recurrence rate (here shown infiltrating bone).

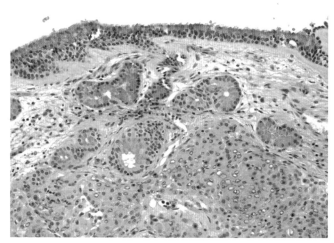

FIGURE 11.69 Sinonasal Meningioma, 100×. Whorled nodules of bland spindled cells are seen within the nasal mucosa. The spindled cells have abundant eosinophilic cytoplasm and oval nuclei with intranuclear pseudoinclusions. Sinonasal meningiomas are rare and usually involve the nasal cavity and paranasal sinuses.

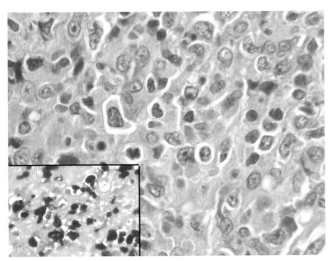

FIGURE 11.70 Extranodal NK/T-Cell Lymphoma, Nasal Type, 400×. Atypical lymphoid cells with irregular nuclear contours and prominent nucleoli. Positive ISH for EBER is seen with this extranodal NK/T-cell lymphoma (inset lower left, 400×). NK/T-cell lymphomas usually present as midline nasal septal destructive lesions. Angioinvasion and angiocentricity are frequently seen with large areas of necrosis. NK/T-cell lymphoma is an aggressive malignancy that carries a poor prognosis.

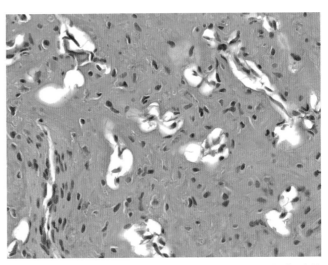

FIGURE 11.72 Angiofibroma, 400×. The tumor is composed of variably sized blood vessels and moderately cellular fibrous tissue, with bland spindled cells. Angiofibromas predominantly affect male adolescents, arise from the posterior lateral nasal wall, and often present with nasal obstruction and epistaxis. Patients with familial adenomatous polyposis are more likely to have angiofibromas, suggesting that mutations of the APC gene may be involved in the pathogenesis of these lesions.

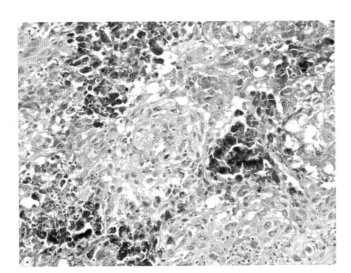

FIGURE 11.71 Sinonasal Melanoma, 200×. Highly atypical epithelioid and spindled cells with abundant intracytoplasmic melanin pigment (*dark-brown*). Sinonasal melanomas arise from melanocytes resident within the nasal epithelium. Clinically, they may present as a nasal polyp. Unlike skin melanomas, the depth of invasion does not correlate with biological behavior. Immunohistochemical stains for S-100, HMB-45 and other markers are used to confirm the diagnosis, but often MiTF is the most useful.

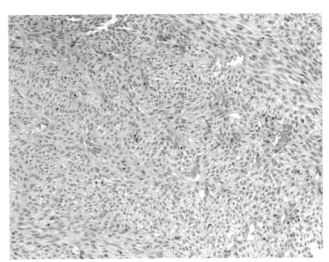

FIGURE 11.73 Glomangiopericytoma, 200×. Sheet-like arrangement of monotonous rounded cells without distinct cell borders (syncytial pattern). The cells surround irregular vascular structures. In some areas, the cells are spindled, and they demonstrate a fascicular growth (upper right and lower left). Glomangiopericytomas arise within the nasal cavity or paranasal sinuses and show a smooth muscle phenotype. This is a benign lesion usually cured by excision but can exhibit aggressive behavior, rarely.

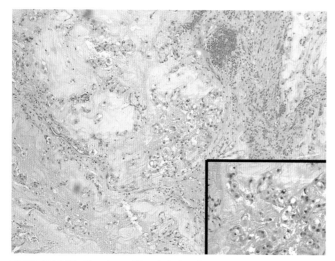

FIGURE 11.74 Chordoma, 40×. Lobules of myxoid material containing characteristic vacuolated (physaliferous) cells (inset lower right, 400×). Chordomas are believed to be of notochordal origin. In the head and neck, they develop in the skull base and may extend to involve the nasopharynx, nasal cavity, paranasal sinuses, or maxilla secondarily.

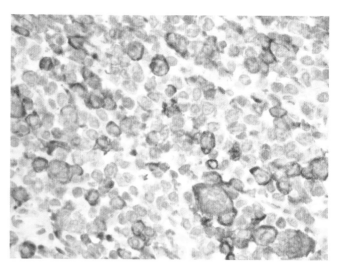

FIGURE 11.76 Embryonal Rhabdomyosarcoma, Desmin Immunohistochemistry, 400×. Embryonal rhabdomyosarcomas are more common in children, and they display skeletal muscle differentiation. Tumor cells are positive for antibodies to muscle-specific proteins: desmin, myogenin, myoglobin, and myo-D1, with the latter three being more specific for skeletal muscle differentiation.

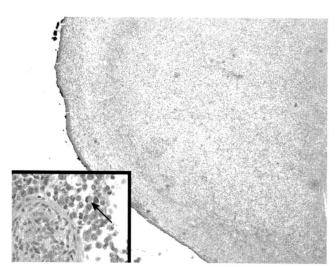

FIGURE 11.75 Embryonal Rhabdomyosarcoma, Botryoid Type, 400×. The tumor presents as a nasal polyp, covered with respiratory-type epithelium. The polyp contains a solid growth of small blue cells with minimal cytoplasm that are concentrated at the periphery of the polyp, immediately beneath the epithelium (cambium layer). A cell with abundant eosinophilic cytoplasm, a "differentiating" rhabdomyoblast, is seen in a background of cells with little cytoplasm (arrow, inset lower left).

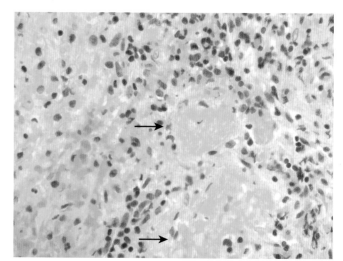

FIGURE 11.77 Wegener Granulomatosis (Granulomatosis with Polyangitis), 400×. The walls of the blood vessels seen in this image are largely destroyed by the inflammatory process (arrows). This is an immune-mediated systemic vasculitic process, and patients often have elevated serum antineutrophil cytoplasmic antibodies (C-ANCA).

IMMUNE-MEDIATED LESIONS

- Wegener granulomatosis (Figs. 11.77 and 11.78)

SALIVARY GLANDS

VASCULAR MALFORMATION

- Hemangioma (Fig. 11.79)

INFLAMMATORY AND LYMPHOID LESIONS

- Lymphoepithelial cyst (Fig. 11.80)
- Mucosa-associated lymphoid tissue lymphoma (Fig. 11.81)
- Chronic sclerosing sialadenitis associated with IgG4 disease (Mikulicz disease) (Fig. 11.82)

BENIGN TUMORS

- Pleomorphic adenoma (Fig. 11.83)
- Basal cell adenoma (Fig. 11.84)
- Warthin tumor (Fig. 11.85)

MALIGNANT TUMORS

- Adenoid cystic carcinoma (Fig. 11.86)
- Polymorphous low-grade adenocarcinoma (Fig. 11.87)
- Mucoepidermoid carcinoma (Fig. 11.88)
- Mucoepidermoid carcinoma (mucicarmine stain) (Fig. 11.89)
- Acinic cell carcinoma (Figs. 11.90 and 11.91)
- Epithelial-myoepithelial carcinoma (Fig. 11.92)
- Carcinoma ex-pleomorphic adenoma (Fig. 11.93)
- Salivary duct carcinoma (Fig. 11.94)

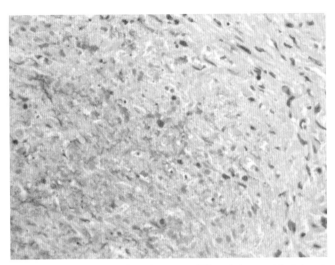

FIGURE 11.78 Wegener Granulomatosis, 400×. A characteristic feature is fibrinoid/granular degeneration of collagen.

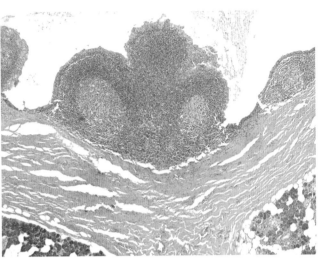

FIGURE 11.80 Lymphoepithelial Cyst of the Parotid Gland, 40×. The cyst is lined by a thin squamous epithelium. Dense lymphoid tissue with lymphoid follicles is seen directly beneath the epithelial lining. A separate and distinct pattern of multiple small lymphoepithelial cysts is a widely recognized cause of parotid swelling in HIV-infected patients.

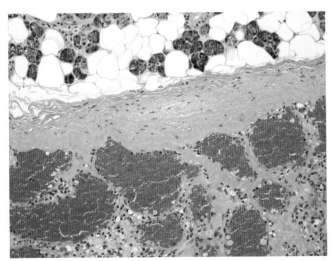

FIGURE 11.79 Hemangioma of the Parotid Gland, 200×. The image shows benign parotid tissue and densely packed blood-filled vascular channels. Hemangiomas are generally classified into capillary and cavernous types, depending on the size of the blood vessels.

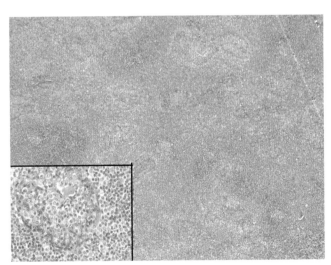

FIGURE 11.81 Extranodal Marginal Zone Lymphoma, 20×. Destruction of the parotid gland architecture by a diffuse lymphoid infiltrate. The lymphoepithelial islands (consisting of neoplastic lymphoid cells and metaplastic parotid gland ducts) are widely separated by the neoplastic lymphoid infiltrate. The inset shows an epithelial island being surrounded and infiltrated by malignant lymphoid cells with pale cytoplasm and small irregular, folded nuclei (400×). The tumors occur more frequently in older women and in patients with a prior history of Sjögren syndrome.

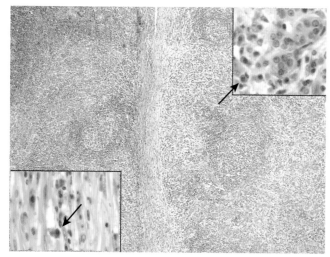

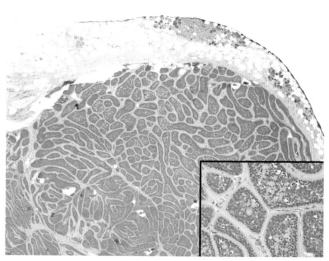

FIGURE 11.82 IgG4-Related Sialadenitis. This low-power image shows marked cellular fibrosis and chronic inflammation with follicle formation and loss of submandibular gland acini. The residual ducts (inset upper right) and the fibrotic areas (inset lower left, 40×) show an increased number of plasma cells (*arrows*, 400×). The plasma cells showed strong cytoplasmic staining with IgG4 antibody. The lesion formerly referred to as chronic sclerosing sialadenitis (Kuttner tumor) was treated by excision. IgG4-related sialadenitis is a systemic immune-mediated disease that responds to corticosteroid therapy.

FIGURE 11.84 Basal Cell Adenoma, 20×. The tumor is well circumscribed and is composed of variably shaped nests of cytologically bland basaloid cells arranged in a "jigsaw puzzle" pattern. The tumor cell nests are surrounded by an acellular eosinophilic basement-membrane-like material (inset lower right, 400×). Nuclear palisading is noted at the periphery of tumor cell nests. Basal cell adenomas are primarily distinguished from basal cell adenocarcinomas by their lack of invasion.

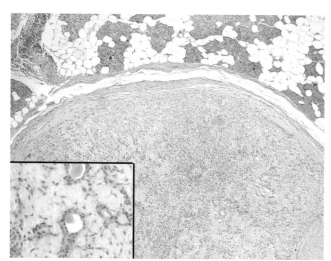

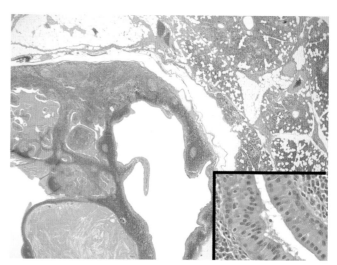

FIGURE 11.83 Pleomorphic Adenoma, 40×. The tumor is well circumscribed by a fibrous capsule and is sharply demarcated from the adjacent parotid gland tissue. The tumor consists of a combination of myoepithelial cells and small ducts within a chondromyxoid stroma (inset lower left, 400×). The myoepithelial cells can be spindled, epithelioid, plasmacytoid, or have clear cytoplasm. Pleomorphic adenoma is the most common benign salivary gland tumor.

FIGURE 11.85 Warthin Tumor, 40×. A papillary projection can be seen protruding into a cystic space. The papillary projections are lined by a double layer of cuboidal to columnar oncocytic epithelial cells, with ample pink, granular cytoplasm and nuclei with central, prominent nucleolus and an underlying lymphoid stroma (inset lower right, 400×). This pattern is very characteristic of this tumor.

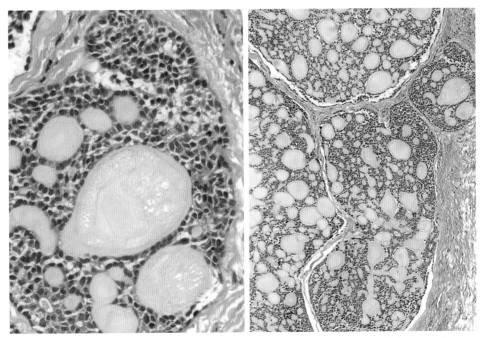

FIGURE 11.86 Adenoid Cystic Carcinoma, **40×**. ADCCs typically show a cribriform, or "Swiss cheese," pattern (right image). The neoplastic myoepithelial cells with their hyperchromatic small angulated nuclei surround rounded spaces containing acid mucopolysaccharidoses (left image, 200×). ADCC is the second most common malignant neoplasm of the seromucinous glands of the upper aerodigestive tract. They are often painful lesions because of their frequent perineural invasion. The disease follows a protracted course, with poor long-term survival.

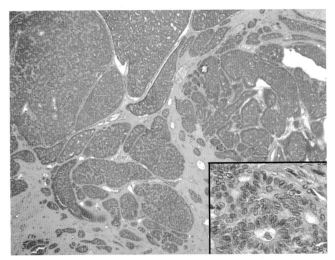

FIGURE 11.87 Polymorphous Low-Grade Adenocarcinoma, 20×. The tumor shows polymorphous growth with solid, cribriform, and tubular architectural growth patterns. Despite the architectural diversity, individual tumor cells are monomorphic, and they display bland round-to-oval nuclei with vesicular chromatin and inconspicuous nucleoli (inset lower right, 400×). The tumor occurs almost exclusively in minor salivary glands and most commonly involves the junction of the hard and soft palate in middle-aged women.

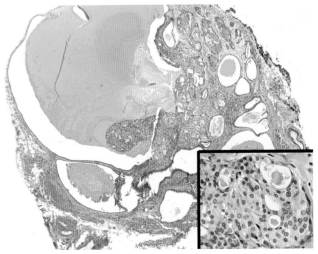

FIGURE 11.88 Mucoepidermoid Carcinoma, Low Grade, 20×. Low-grade mucoepidermoid carcinomas are cystic with mucus and epidermoid cells (inset lower right, 400×). Mucoepidermoid carcinoma is the most common salivary gland malignancy in both children and adults. A majority of cases show a characteristic chromosomal translocation t(11;19) (q21;p13), which creates the MECT1/MAML2 fusion protein.

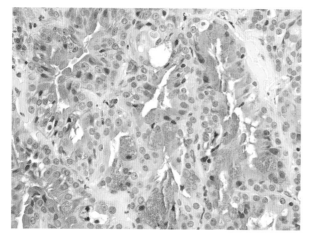

FIGURE 11.89 Mucoepidermoid Carcinoma, Mucicarmine Stain, 400×. A mucicarmine stain is used to highlight goblet-shaped mucus cells containing intracellular mucin in mucoepidermoid carcinoma.

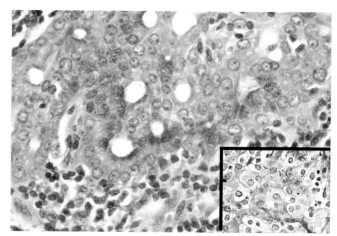

FIGURE 11.91 Acinic Cell Carcinoma, 400×. The tumor exhibits distinct acinar differentiation, with neoplastic acinar cells having numerous blue-purple zymogen secretory granules. The zymogen granules are periodic acid Schiff–positive and diastase resistant (inset lower right, 400×). Lymphocytes are sometimes seen in acinic cell carcinoma.

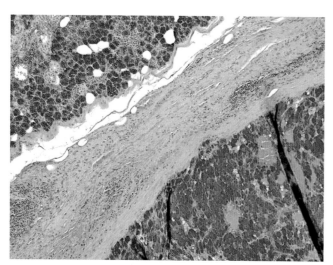

FIGURE 11.90 Acinic Cell Carcinoma, 40×. Acinic cell carcinomas show acinar differentiation and closely recapitulate the acinar tissue of a normal salivary gland. The image shows the tumor (lower right) in relation to the normal parotid gland tissue (upper left). Note a normal lobular pattern is not found within the tumor, an important clue to the diagnosis.

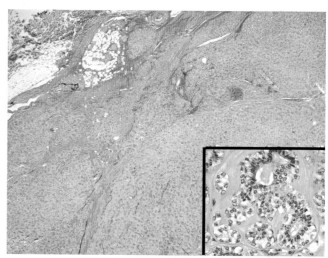

FIGURE 11.92 Epithelial-Myoepithelial Carcinoma, 20×. The tumor is invasive and shows tubular growth. The tubules are lined by an inner layer of eosinophilic ductal cells and an outer layer of myoepithelial cells that exhibit abundant clear cytoplasm and large round eccentrically located nuclei with prominent nucleoli (inset lower right, 400×).

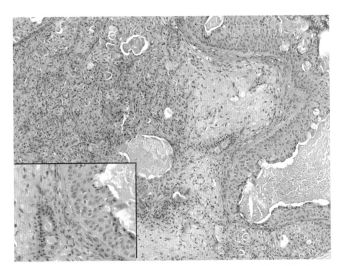

FIGURE 11.93 Carcinoma Ex-Pleomorphic Adenoma, 20×. The image shows a mixture of pleomorphic adenoma with chondromyxoid stroma and benign glandular elements, along with highly atypical glands of a carcinoma (in this case a mucoepidermoid carcinoma; inset lower left, 400×). The type of carcinoma developing in a pleomorphic adenoma is not always classifiable (carcinoma, not otherwise specified) and is often high grade. Salivary duct carcinoma is the most common malignant component. Carcinoma ex-pleomorphic adenoma is further classified into in situ, minimally invasive, and invasive.

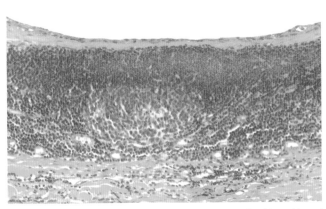

FIGURE 11.95 Branchial Cleft Cyst, 200×. The cyst is lined by a thin and flattened squamous epithelium that overlies a dense lymphoid infiltrate with lymphoid follicles. First branchial cleft cysts are usually seen anterior to the tragus and sometimes contain cartilage.

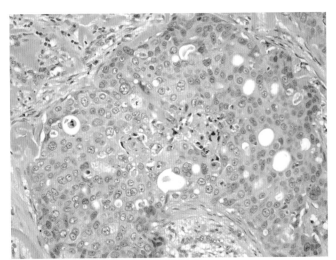

FIGURE 11.94 Salivary Duct Carcinoma, 400×. Salivary duct carcinomas are histologically similar to infiltrating ductal carcinomas of the breast. The image shows a nest of tumor cells with comedo-type necrosis and rounded cystic spaces. The cells have abundant eosinophilic cytoplasm and exhibit large pleomorphic round nuclei with prominent nucleoli. Salivary duct carcinomas are high-grade malignancies that most commonly involve the parotid glands of elderly men.

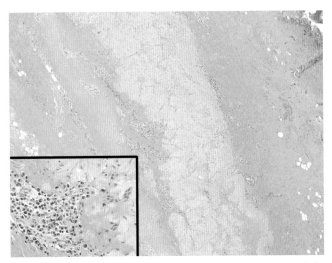

FIGURE 11.96 Chondrodermatitis Nodularis Helicis, 20×. A chronic inflammatory cell infiltrate extends from the skin surface and surrounds the auricular cartilage. The inflammatory cell infiltrate consists predominantly of plasma cells (inset lower left, 400×).

EAR

EXTERNAL EAR

- Branchial cleft cyst (Fig. 11.95)
- Chondrodermatitis nodularis chronicus helicis (Fig. 11.96)
- Basal cell carcinoma (Fig. 11.97)
- Ceruminous adenoma (Fig. 11.98)

MIDDLE EAR

- Otic polyp (Fig. 11.99)
- Cholesteatoma (Fig. 11.100)
- Encephalocele (Fig. 11.101)

- Middle ear adenoma/carcinoid (Fig. 11.102)
- Paraganglioma (Fig. 11.103)

INNER EAR

- Vestibular schwannoma (Fig. 11.104)

THYROID AND PARATHYROID GLANDS

NON-NEOPLASTIC LESIONS

- Thyroglossal duct cyst (Fig. 11.105)
- Hashimoto thyroiditis (Fig. 11.106)
- Graves disease (Fig. 11.107)

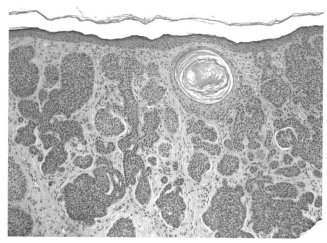

FIGURE 11.97 Basal Cell Carcinoma, 100×. Nests of basaloid cells with peripheral clefting. Nuclear palisading is seen at the periphery of the nests. The tumor is focally attached to the overlying epidermis (upper right). (Courtesy of Mrs. Michelle Forestall Lee, MGH.)

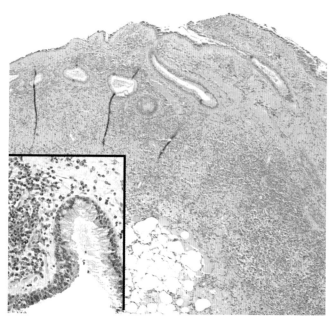

FIGURE 11.99 Otic Polyp, 40×. The polyp contains granulation tissue, small blood vessels, lymphocytes, and plasma cells. The epithelium covering the polyp may be squamous or columnar (inset lower left, 400×). Otic polyps are usually secondary to otitis media.

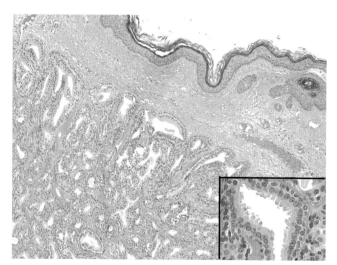

FIGURE 11.98 Ceruminous Adenoma, 100×. The tumor is well circumscribed, and it shows solid proliferation of cystically dilated glandular structures. The glands are lined by an inner layer of eosinophilic ductal cells that exhibit apical snouting (apocrine differentiation) and an outer layer of basal cells that rest on a thick acellular hyalinized basement membrane (inset lower right, 100×).

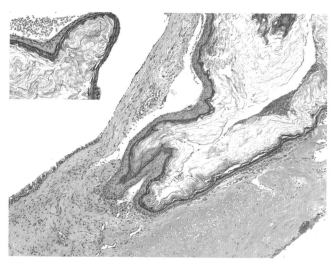

FIGURE 11.100 Cholesteatoma. The cholesteatoma is an outpouching of the squamous epithelium on or near the tympanic membrane into the middle ear mucosa, similar to an epidermal inclusion cyst (lower right, 40×). It is composed of keratin debris and stratified squamous epithelium (inset upper left, 400×). Although histologically benign, cholesteatomas are often aggressive and destructive, eroding middle ear ossicles.

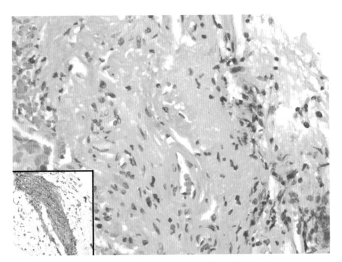

FIGURE 11.101 Middle Ear Encephalocele, 400×. The image shows neural tissue. An encephalocele is herniation of brain tissue into the middle ear covered by meninges. Encephaloceles contain neurons, highlighted by S100 immunostain (inset lower left, 400×). They arise because of a bony defect in the skull.

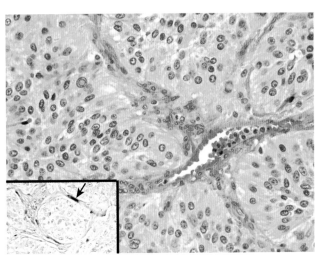

FIGURE 11.103 Paraganglioma, 400×. Well-developed nests of epithelioid cells (Zellballen arrangement), surround delicate vascular channels. The round-to-ovoid nuclei exhibit fine granular chromatin and small nucleoli. Supporting the cell nests are the inconspicuous sustentacular cells, best appreciated with S100 immunostain (*arrow*, inset lower left, 400×). Paragangliomas are negative for epithelial markers such as keratin, helping to distinguish them from neuroendocrine carcinomas.

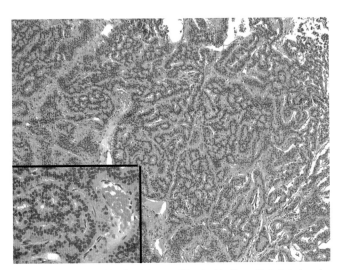

FIGURE 11.102 Middle Ear Adenoma/Carcinoid, 40×. Orderly trabeculae of eosinophilic cells with ovoid nuclei. Glandular spaces are readily observed. The nuclei exhibit fine granular chromatin ("salt and pepper") characteristics of neuroendocrine tumors (inset lower left, 200×).

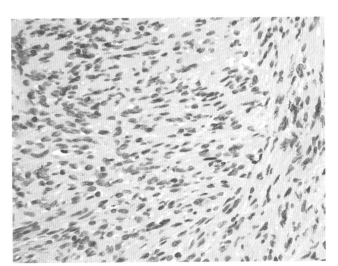

FIGURE 11.104 Vestibular Schwannoma, 400×. The neoplastic spindled Schwann cells exhibit slender wavy or buckled nuclei. Vestibular schwannomas arise from the eighth cranial nerve. Unilateral lesions are commonly seen in adults, whereas bilateral lesions frequently occur in younger patients with neurofibromatosis type 2.

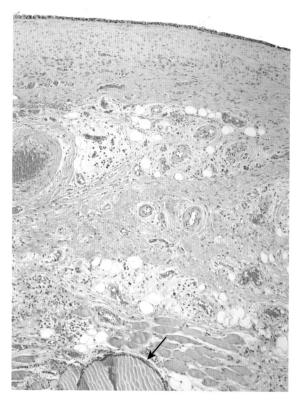

FIGURE 11.105 Thyroglossal Duct Cyst, 100×. The cyst is lined by ciliated, cuboidal, or squamous epithelium. Skeletal muscle and a few thyroid follicles (*arrow*) are present in the connective tissue wall of the cyst. Thyroglossal duct cysts present as midline neck masses that are closely associated with the hyoid bone. Lesions move vertically upon swallowing.

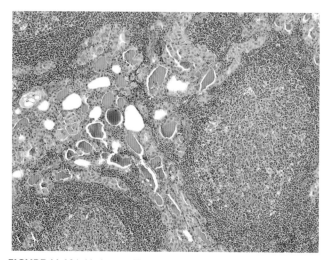

FIGURE 11.106 Hashimoto Thyroiditis, 200×. The follicular cells show oncocytic features and are surrounded by a dense lymphoid stroma with prominent lymphoid follicles.

BENIGN THYROID TUMORS

- Follicular adenoma (Fig. 11.108)

MALIGNANT THYROID TUMORS

- Papillary thyroid carcinoma, classical type (Fig. 11.109)
- Papillary thyroid carcinoma, follicular variant (Fig. 11.110)
- Papillary thyroid carcinoma, tall-cell variant (Fig. 11.111)

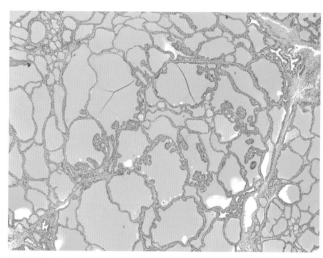

FIGURE 11.107 Graves Disease, 40×. Hyperplastic and hypersecretory thyroid tissue with irregularly shaped thyroid follicles. Small poorly formed papillary projections extend into the irregular thyroid follicles.

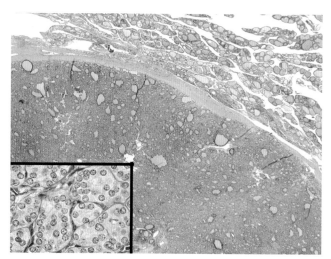

FIGURE 11.108 Follicular Adenoma, 20×. A well-defined capsule separates the tumor from the surrounding thyroid gland. There is no evidence of invasion. The follicular epithelial cells are arranged in small follicles (inset lower right, 400×). The follicular cells have uniform small round nuclei with fine granular chromatin and small inconspicuous nucleoli.

- Papillary thyroid carcinoma, diffuse sclerosing variant (Fig. 11.112)
- Follicular carcinoma (Fig. 11.113)
- Oncocytic (Hurthle cell) carcinoma (Fig. 11.114)
- Poorly differentiated carcinoma (Fig. 11.115)
- Medullary thyroid carcinoma (Fig. 11.116)
- Anaplastic thyroid carcinoma (Fig. 11.117)

PARATHYROID

- Parathyroid adenoma (Fig. 11.118)
- Parathyroid carcinoma (Fig. 11.119)

ACKNOWLEDGMENTS

The authors wish to thank Stephen Conley, director of the Massachusetts General Hospital Pathology Photo Laboratory, for photo editorial assistance.

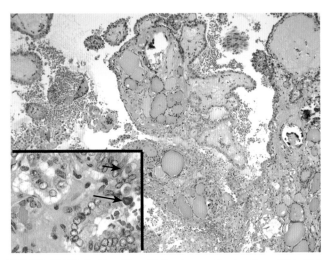

FIGURE 11.109 Papillary Thyroid Carcinoma, Classical Type, 40×. Well-formed papillae with fibrovascular cores. The papillary structures are lined by cells that show enlarged pale overlapping nuclei. There are nuclear grooves and pseudoinclusions (inset lower right, *arrows*, 400×) and psammoma bodies (right).

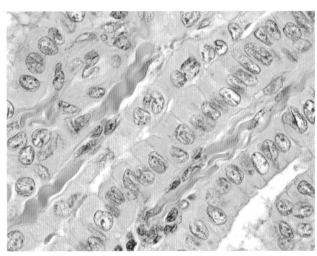

FIGURE 11.111 Papillary Thyroid Carcinoma, Tall-Cell Variant, 400×. Papillary carcinomas that demonstrate a predominance of tall columnar cells, whose height is at least 2-3 times their width, are termed *tall-cell variants*. The columnar cells in this image are tightly packed, and they show pronounced nuclear features of papillary carcinoma. Note the nuclear grooves and irregular nuclear membranes. The tall-cell variant has typically been associated with a more advanced stage at presentation than classical papillary carcinomas, but patients generally still have a very favorable outcome.

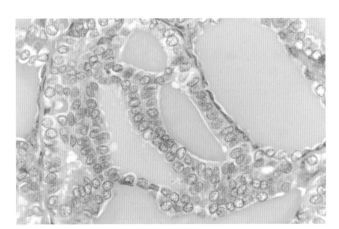

FIGURE 11.110 Papillary Thyroid Carcinoma, Follicular Variant, 400×. The image shows follicular architecture lacking true/architectural papillae. The follicular cells contain nuclei that are enlarged and pale with elongation and nuclear overlap. There are nuclear grooves and the colloid has a thick, dense appearance (eosinophilic or bubble gum colloid).

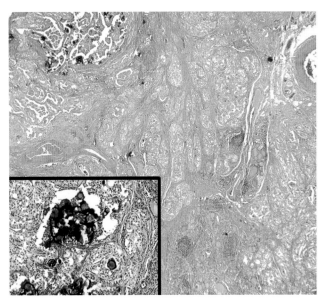

FIGURE 11.112 Papillary Thyroid Carcinoma, Diffuse Sclerosing Variant, 20×. Extensive fibrotic areas separate the tumor cell nests in this papillary thyroid carcinoma variant. They often arise in a background that shows marked lymphocytic thyroiditis, as is seen here. Numerous psammoma bodies are present (inset lower right, 200×). These lesions typically occupy an entire lobe of the thyroid or the entirety of the gland with no discrete mass noted grossly or by imaging.

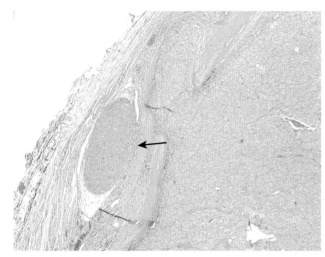

FIGURE 11.113 Follicular Carcinoma, 100×. This follicular neoplasm has a thick capsule, penetrated by tumor cells with mushrooming capsular invasion. Additionally, tumor cells penetrate a thick-walled vein in the lesional capsule (angioinvasion, *arrow*).

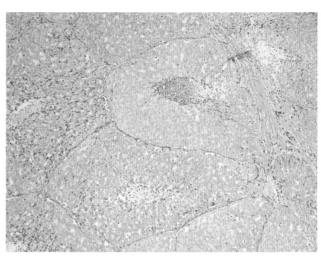

FIGURE 11.115 Poorly Differentiated Thyroid Carcinoma, 100×. In this image, nests of tumor cells with small round hyperchromatic nuclei are separated by thin bands of fibrous tissue (insular growth pattern). Comedo-type necrosis is seen as a small, well-defined focus located in the center of solid nests or insulae.

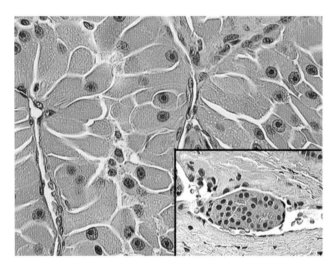

FIGURE 11.114 Follicular Thyroid Carcinoma, Oncocytic (Hurthle Cell) Type, 400×. A follicular carcinoma of the thyroid, and yet the cells have abundant granular cytoplasm and round to oval nuclei with prominent nucleoli (oncocytes). As in other follicular carcinomas, the diagnosis of malignancy requires the identification of capsular and/or vascular invasion. In this case, the tumor invaded a blood vessel within the capsule (inset lower right, 400×).

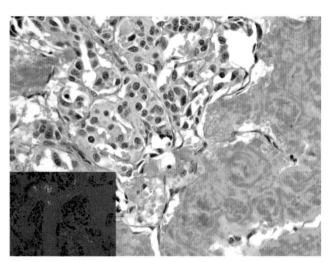

FIGURE 11.116 Medullary Thyroid Carcinoma, 400×. Nests of plasmacytoid cells associated with an acellular eosinophilic material (amyloid). The cells have round, eccentrically located nuclei with granular chromatin. The amyloid has an apple-green birefringence when stained with Congo red and viewed under polarized light (inset lower left, 200×). Medullary thyroid carcinoma is a malignant neoplasm of parafollicular C cells.

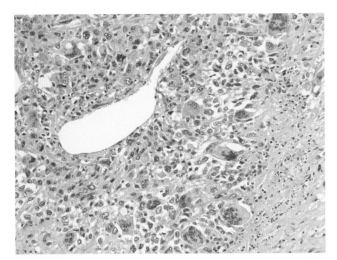

FIGURE 11.117 Undifferentiated (Anaplastic) Thyroid Carcinoma, 400×. Atypical spindle cells surround a residual vascular channel. Tumor giant cells demonstrate multiple large hyperchromatic nuclei with prominent nucleoli. Necrosis is present (*right*), and there are often several atypical mitotic figures (not shown).

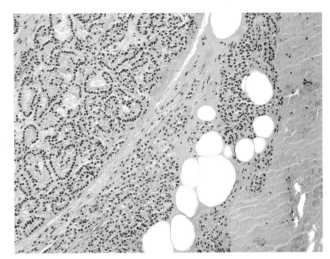

FIGURE 11.118 Parathyroid Adenoma, 200×. A thin capsule separates the adenoma from the surrounding normal parathyroid tissue. The adenoma is devoid of intercellular (stromal) fat. Parathyroid adenomas can be multiple. Multiple parathyroid adenomas may be seen in patients with multiple endocrine neoplasia type 1 syndrome.

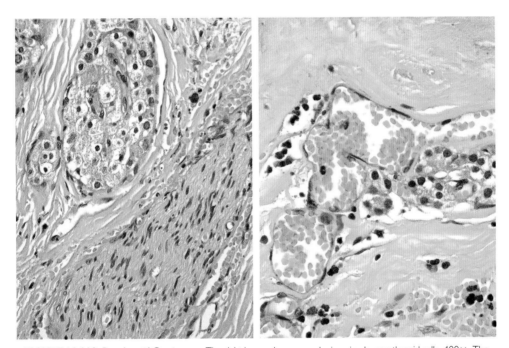

FIGURE 11.119 Parathyroid Carcinoma. The right image shows vascular invasion by parathyroid cells, 400×. The left image shows a nest of parathyroid cells extending into a vessel located close to a nerve (*arrow*), 400×. The diagnosis of parathyroid carcinoma is difficult to make and often occurs after the development of metastatic disease.

SUGGESTED READINGS

Bamba R, Sweiss NJ, Langerman AJ, Taxy JB, Blair EA. The minor salivary gland biopsy as a diagnostic tool for Sjogren syndrome. *Laryngoscope.* 2009;119(10):1922–1926.

Barnes L. Intestinal-type adenocarcinoma of the nasal cavity and paranasal sinuses. *Am J Surg Pathol.* 1986;10(3):192–202.

Batsakis JG, el-Naggar AK. Rhinoscleroma and rhinosporidiosis. *Ann Otol Rhinol Laryngol.* 1992;101(10):879–882.

Bishop JA, Lewis Jr JS, Rocco JW, Faquin WC. HPV-related squamous cell carcinoma of the head and neck: an update on testing in routine pathology practice. *Semin Diagn Pathol.* 2015;32(5):344–351. pii:S0740-2570(15)00014-3.

Cancer Genome Atlas Research Network. Integrated genomic characterization of papillary thyroid carcinoma. *Cell.* October 23, 2014;159(3):676–690.

Deshpande V. IgG4 related disease of the head and neck. *Head Neck Pathol.* 2015;9(1):24–31.

El-Mofty SK, Patil S. Human papillomavirus (HPV)-related oropharyngeal nonkeratinizing squamous cell carcinoma: characterization of a distinct phenotype. *Oral Surg Oral Med Oral Pathol Oral Radiol Endod.* 2006;101(3):339–345.

Furlong MA, Fanburg-Smith JC, Childers EL. Lipoma of the oral and maxillofacial region: site and subclassification of 125 cases. *Oral Surg Oral Med Oral Pathol Oral Radiol Endod.* 2004;98(4):441–450.

Gomes CC, Diniz MG, Gomez RS. Review of the molecular pathogenesis of the odontogenic keratocyst. *Oral Oncol.* 2009;45(12):1011–1014.

Guertl B, Beham A, Zechner R, Stammberger H, Hoefler G. Nasopharyngeal angiofibroma: an APC-gene-associated tumor? *Hum Pathol.* 2000;31(11):1411–1413.

Kanavaros P, Lescs MC, Brière J, et al. Nasal T-cell lymphoma: a clinicopathologic entity associated with peculiar phenotype and with Epstein-Barr virus. *Blood.* 1993;81(10):2688–2695.

Lin BM, Wang H, D'Souza G, et al. Long-term prognosis and risk factors among patients with HPV-associated oropharyngeal squamous cell carcinoma. *Cancer.* 2013;119(19):3462–3471.

Mazur MT, Shultz JJ, Myers JL. Granular cell tumor. Immunohistochemical analysis of 21 benign tumors and one malignant tumor. *Arch Pathol Lab Med.* 1990;114(7):692–696.

Mervyn Shear, Paul Speight. *Cysts of the Oral and Maxillofacial Regions.* 4th ed. Oxford: Wiley-Blackwell; 2007.

Muzyka BC, Epifanio RN. Update on oral fungal infections. *Dent Clin North Am.* 2013;57:561–581.

Slootweg PJ. Odontogenic tumours—an update. *Current Diagnostic Pathology.* 2006;12(1):54–65.

Scully C, Carrozzo M. Oral mucosal disease: lichen planus. *Br J Oral Maxillofac Surg.* 2008;46(1):15–21.

Scully C, Lo Muzio L. Oral mucosal diseases: mucous membrane pemphigoid. *Br J Oral Maxillofac Surg.* 2008;46(5):358–366.

Scully C, Mignogna M. Oral mucosal disease: pemphigus. *Br J Oral Maxillofac Surg.* 2008;46(4):272–277.

Seethala RR, Dacic S, Cieply K, Kelly LM, Nikiforova MN. A reappraisal of the MECT1/MAML2 translocation in salivary mucoepidermoid carcinomas. *Am J Surg Pathol.* 2010;34(8):1106–1121.

Tabareau-Delalande F, Collin C, Gomez-Brouchet A, et al. Diagnostic value of investigating GNAS mutations in fibro-osseous lesions: a retrospective study of 91 cases of fibrous dysplasia and 40 other fibro-osseous lesions. *Mod Pathol.* 2013;26(7):911–921.

Triantafillidou K, Venetis G, Karakinaris G, Iordanidis F. Ossifying fibroma of the jaws: a clinical study of 14 cases and review of the literature. *Oral Surg Oral Med Oral Pathol Oral Radiol.* 2012;114(2):193–199.

van der Waal I. Potentially malignant disorders of the oral and oropharyngeal mucosa; terminology, classification and present concepts of management. *Oral Oncol.* 2009;45(4-5):317–323.

Voz ML, Aström AK, Kas K, Mark J, Stenman G, Van de Ven WJ. The recurrent translocation t(5;8)(p13;q12) in pleomorphic adenomas results in upregulation of PLAG1 gene expression under control of the LIFR promoter. *Format Oncogene.* 1998;16(11):1409–1416.

West RB, Kong C, Clarke N, et al. MYB expression and translocation in adenoid cystic carcinomas and other salivary gland tumors with clinicopathologic correlation. *Am J Surg Pathol.* 2011;35(1):92–99.

Williams L, Thompson LD, Seethala RR, et al. Salivary duct carcinoma: the predominance of apocrine morphology, prevalence of histologic variants, and androgen receptor expression. *Am J Surg Pathol.* 2015;39(5):705–713.

Barnes L, Eveson JW, Reichart P, Sidransky D. *World Health Organization classification of tumours. Pathology and Genetics of Head and Neck Tumours.* Lyon: IARC; 2005.

TEMPORAL BONE

CASE 1: MONDINI MALFORMATION (Fig. 12.1)

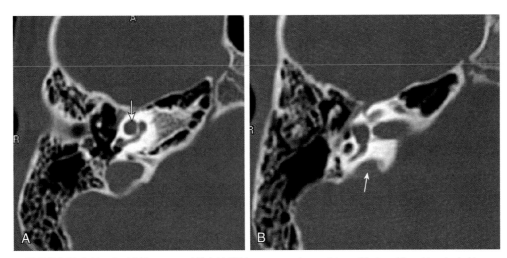

FIGURE 12.1 Mondini Malformation. (**A**) Axial CT demonstrates incomplete partitioning of the mid and apical turn of the right cochlea with deficient modiolus (arrow). (**B**) Axial CT one slice superior demonstrates an enlarged vestibular aqueduct (arrow).

Imaging findings: A congenital malformation of the cochlea with a well-formed basal turn and incomplete partitioning of the mid and apical turns. In addition, modiolar deficiency is present with loss of the normal "Christmas tree" appearance of the modiolus and spiral lamina on the axial images. The normal 2½ turns are absent with >1½ turns of the cochlea present. There may also be enlargement of the vestibular aqueduct because of dilatation of the endolymphatic duct and sac.

Differential diagnosis: Cochlear dysplasia (<1½ turns of the cochlea) or branchial–oto-renal syndrome (elongation of the basal turn and small middle and apical turns of the cochlea).

Refer to Cummings chapter 192 for more details.

Further Reading

Jackler RK, Luxford WM, House WF. Congenital malformation of the inner ear: a classification based on embryogenesis. *Laryngoscope.* 1987;97(suppl 40):2–14.

Sennaroglu L, Saatci I. Unpartitioned versus incompletely partitioned cochleae: radiologic differentiation. *Otol Neurotol.* 2004;25(4):520–529.

CASE 2: CHOLESTEROL GRANULOMA (Fig. 12.2)

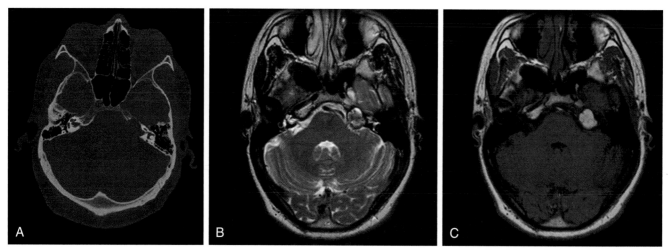

FIGURE 12.2 Cholesterol Granuloma. (A) Axial noncontrast CT images demonstrate an expansile lucent lesion in the left petrous apex. **(B)** The lesion is increased in signal on T2-weighted imaging. **(C)** There is also T1-weighted hyperintensity characteristic of the cholesterol crystals and hemorrhagic material within a cholesterol granuloma.

Imaging findings: Expansile unilocular cystic lesion most commonly present in the petrous apex. These lesions may also occur in the mastoid portion of temporal bone and in the middle ear cavity.

Computed tomography (CT): Well-circumscribed unilocular expansile lesion with sclerotic smooth margin, sharp zone of transition, and most commonly posterior to the horizontal aspect of the petrous internal carotid artery.

Magnetic resonance imaging (MRI): Classically, these lesions are hyperintense on both T1- and T2-weighted images and do not demonstrate enhancement or diffusion abnormality.

Differential diagnosis: Petrous apex mucocele, petrous cephalocele, or congenital epidermoid.

Refer to Cummings chapter 177 for more details.

Further Reading

Clifton AG, Phelps PD, Brookes GB. Cholesterol granuloma of the petrous apex. *Br J Radiol.* 1990;63(753):724–726.

Sanna M, Dispenza F, Mathur N, De Stefano A, De Donato G. Otoneurological management of petrous apex cholesterol granuloma. *Am J Otolaryngol.* 2009;30(6):407–414.

CASE 3: PETROUS APEX MUCOCELE (Fig. 12.3)

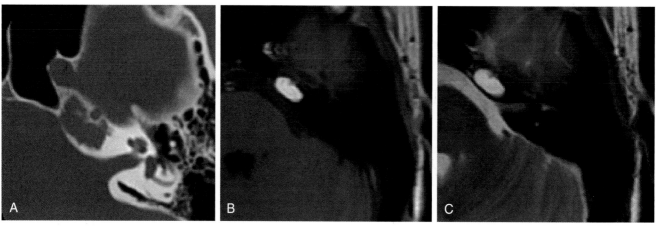

FIGURE 12.3 Petrous Apex Mucocele. (A) Axial CT demonstrates an expansile fluid-filled air cell without septations at the left petrous apex with a sharp zone of transition along its periphery. **(B)** T1-weighted axial image demonstrates a unilocular homogeneously hyperintense lesion at the petrous apex. **(C)** T2-weighted image also demonstrates the lesion to be hyperintense in signal intensity. Differential diagnosis would include a petrous apex cholesterol granuloma. This was pathologically proven to be a mucocele.

Imaging findings: Expansile unilocular cystic lesion related to a pneumatized petrous apex. Smoothly marginated, well-circumscribed cystic lesion.

CT: Well-circumscribed unilocular expansile lesion with a sclerotic smooth margin with a sharp zone of transition. Typically, these are hypoattenuating lesions, but they may be higher than CSF attenuation because of the presence of proteinaceous material.

MRI: Variable signal intensity because of the presence of proteinaceous material on both T1- and T2-weighted images;

typically demonstrating minimal rim enhancement because of mucosal enhancement.

Differential diagnosis: Cholesterol granuloma, petrous cephalocele, or congenital epidermoid.

Further Reading

Larson TL, Wong ML. Primary mucocele of the petrous apex: MR appearance. *AJNR.* 1992;13(1):203–204.

Le BT, Roehm PC. Petrous apex mucocele. *Otol Neurotol.* 2008;29(1):102–103.

CASE 4: EXTERNAL AUDITORY CANAL ATRESIA (Fig. 12.4)

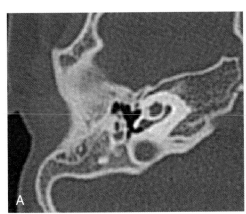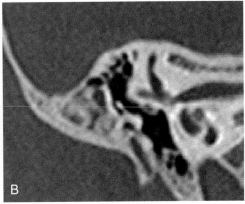

FIGURE 12.4 External Auditory Canal Atresia. (**A**) Axial CT at the level of the right EAC demonstrates a bony plate replacing the EAC. Note that this is solid bone and without air cells. (**B**) Coronal CT in the same patient demonstrates the absence of the EAC and low tegmen. Note that the malleus is fused to the atresia plate.

Imaging findings: Hypoplastic or absent pinna and absence of the EAC. The EAC is located posterior and superior to the condylar fossa. The atresia plate may or may not be pneumatized. The middle ear cleft, measured from the medial aspect of the atresia plate to the cochlear plate, normally should measure >3 mm; <3 mm is not amenable to surgical repair. The position of the middle cranial fossa relative to the atresia plate may be of importance. A low-lying middle cranial fossa relative to the atresia plate should be noted. The ossicular chain is typically abnormal. The manubrium should be partially fused to the atresia plate. Malleoincudal or incudostapedial fusion may be present. Assess ossicles for their integrity. The stapes superstructure is perhaps the most important structure to identify. In addition, determine the presence of the oval and round windows. The facial nerve may take an anomalous course. The vertical/mastoid segment should be

identified and is typically in an anterior location. The position of this segment relative to the oval window on coronal images should be determined. If at the level of the oval window on coronal images, the patient may not be amenable to surgery.

Differential diagnosis: None

Refer to Cummings chapter 194 for more details.

Further Reading

El-Begermy MA, Mansour OI, El-Makhzangy AM, El-Gindy TS. Congenital auditory meatal atresia: a numerical review. *Ear Arch Otorhinolaryngol.* 2009;266(4):501–506.

Mayer TE, Brueckmann H, Siegert R, Witt A, Weerda H. High-resolution CT of the temporal bone in dysplasia of the auricle and external auditory canal. *AJNR.* 1997;18(1):53–65.

CASE 5: CHOLESTEATOMA (Fig. 12.5)

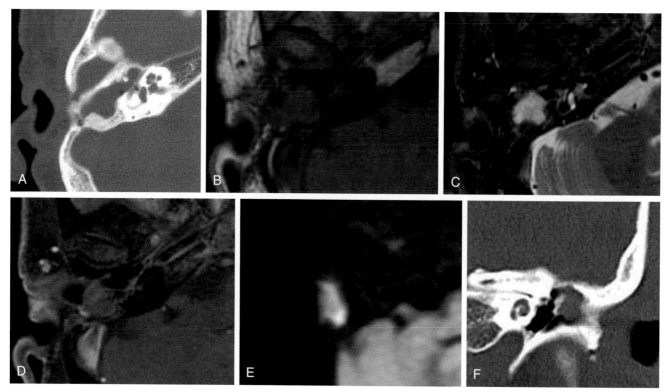

FIGURE 12.5 Cholesteatoma. (**A**) Axial CT demonstrates opacification of the right middle ear cavity at the level of the epitympanum, as well as the aditus ad antrum and the mastoid antrum, which is also expanded. Note absence of the body and short process of the incus. (**B**) MRI, T1-weighted axial image demonstrates that the mastoid antrum, aditus ad antrum, and epitympanum are filled with hypointense material. (**C**) The corresponding area demonstrates hyperintense material on T2-weighted imaging. (**D**) Postcontrast axial image demonstrates enhancement within the middle ear cavity consistent with chronic otitis media. However, the material within the mastoid antrum demonstrates mucosal enhancement. (**E**) Trace diffusion image demonstrates restricted diffusion of the contents of the mastoid antrum consistent with cholesteatoma. (**F**) In another patient, coronal CT demonstrates a mass in the left Prussak space, with erosion of the scutum consistent with a pars flaccida–type cholesteatoma.

Imaging findings: Representing keratinized squamous epithelium forming mass-like tissue, these lesions are destructive in nature, causing ossicular/bony erosion, a hallmark of these lesions. Cholesteatomas may be congenital or acquired. The congenital type most commonly occurs at the petrous apex. The second most common location is in the attic of the epitympanum. Cholesteatomas in this location are often congenital in origin. The acquired cholesteatomas include the pars flaccida and pars tensa types. The pars flaccida type is located in the Prussak space, which is found between the head of the malleus and the scutum, and, classically, causes erosions of the scutum. The pars tensa type occurs in the middle ear cavity away from the Prussak space.

CT: Soft-tissue mass in the middle ear cavity causing bony or ossicular erosion. A small early cholesteatoma may not demonstrate bony/ossicular erosion. Soft-tissue mass in the Prussak space will cause blunting or erosion of the scutum. At the petrous apex, these lesions will cause bony erosion of the petrous apex.

MRI: All cholesteatomas demonstrate hypointense signal intensity on T1-weighted images, hyperintense signal intensity on T2-weighted images, and no enhancement. All cholesteatomas demonstrate restricted diffusion on the diffusion-weighted images.

Differential diagnosis: Middle ear cavity mass—glomus tympanicum tumor, schwannoma, or middle ear cavity adenoma/adenocarcinoma.

Petrous apex: Cholesterol granuloma, petrous apex mucocele, and petrous apex cephalocele.

Refer to Cummings chapter 139 for more details.

Further Reading

Nelson M, Roger G, Koltai PJ, et al. Congenital cholesteatoma: classification, management, and outcome. *Arch Otolaryngol Head Neck Surg.* 2002;128(7):810–814.

Potsic WP, Korman SB, Samadi DS, Wetmore RF. Congenital cholesteatoma: 20 years experience at the Children's Hospital of Philadelphia. *Otolaryngol Head Neck Surg.* 2002;12(6):409–414.

CASE 6: COALESCENT MASTOIDITIS (Fig. 12.6)

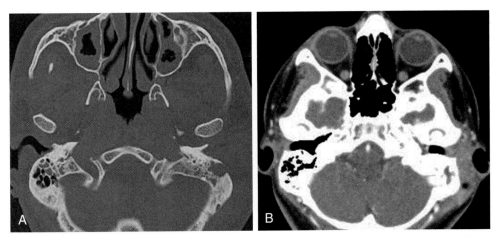

FIGURE 12.6 Coalescent Mastoiditis. (A) Axial noncontrast CT, bone windows demonstrates opacification of the left mastoid air cells with expansion of an air cell with loss of normal mastoid architecture and erosion of the lateral mastoid cortex. **(B)** Soft-tissue windows demonstrate adjacent soft-tissue thickening in the preauricular region.

Imaging findings: Opacification of the mastoid air cells with loss of the normal lacy architecture of the mastoid air cells. Because of the infectious/inflammatory process, destructive changes of the walls of the mastoid air cells occur with coalescence of the mastoid air cells into larger opacified air cells. Deossification of the adjacent bone may occur with acute osteomyelitis, and sclerosis in chronic osteomyelitis.

CT: Opacification of the mastoid air cells with coalescence of the mastoid air cells to form larger opacified mastoid air cells with adjacent deossification or sclerosis.

MRI: Variable signal intensity of the mastoid air cell contents because of the presence of purulent material on both T1- and T2-weighted images with associated mucosal enhancement within the air cells. Diffusion abnormality may be present because of exudate.

Refer to Cummings chapter 139 for more details.

Further Reading

Holliday RA, Reede DL. MRI of middle ear and mastoid disease. *Radiol Clin North Am.* 1989;27:283–299.

Mafee MF, Singleton EL, Valvassori GE, Espinosa GA, Kumar A, Aimi K. Acute otomastoiditis and its complications: role of CT. *Radiology.* 1985;155:391–397.

CASE 7: GRADENIGO SYNDROME/PETROUS APICITIS (Fig. 12.7)

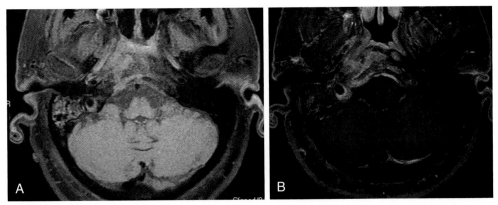

FIGURE 12.7 Gradenigo Syndrome/Petrous Apicitis. (A) Axial precontrast T1-weighted image with fat saturation demonstrates abnormal intermediate signal intensity at the right petrous apex with thickening of the adjacent dura. Involvement of the prevertebral musculature below the skull base is also present. Mastoid airspace disease is also seen. **(B)** Postcontrast T1-axial image demonstrates enhancement of the right petrous apex, adjacent dura, and prevertebral musculature.

Imaging findings: Opacification of the petrous apex air cells with destructive change and enhancement of the petrous apex and adjacent dura.

CT: Opacification of the petrous apex air cells with erosion or permeative change of the adjacent bone. Gradenigo syndrome classically consists of the triad of otorrhea, periorbital pain (involvement of the trigeminal nerve), and diplopia (involvement of the abducens nerve).

MRI: Opacification of the petrous apex air cells, which may demonstrate variable signal intensity on T1- and T2-weighted images because of the presence of exudate/proteinaceous material. Postcontrast images demonstrate enhancement of the mucosa of the petrous air cells, as well as exuberant dural enhancement around the petrous apex. Adjacent cranial nerve enhancement may also be seen.

Differential diagnosis: Tumor of the petrous apex, such as metastatic disease.

Refer to Cummings chapter 139 for more details.

Further Reading

Dave AV, Diaz-Marchan PJ, Lee AG. Clinical and magnetic resonance imaging features of Gradenigo syndrome. *Am J Ophthalmol.* 1997;124(4):568–570.

Contrucci RB, Sataloff RT, Myers DL. Petrous apicitis. *Ear Nose Throat J.* 1985;64(9):427–431.

CASE 8: VASCULAR LOOP COMPRESSION (Fig. 12.8)

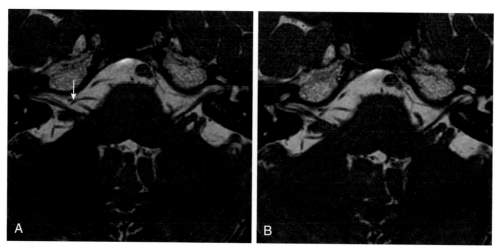

FIGURE 12.8 Vascular Loop Compression. (A) Thin-section T2-weighted axial (FIESTA sequence) at the level of the right VII/VIIIth nerve complex demonstrates a vessel representing the AICA displacing the cisternal segment of the nerve complex posteriorly (arrow). **(B)** Adjacent axial slice again demonstrates posterior displacement of the nerve complex.

Imaging findings: Most common vessel is the anterior inferior cerebellar artery (AICA), although a high-riding posterior inferior cerebellar artery or vertebral artery may also be the cause. The vessel may impinge at the root entry zone of the seventh/eighth nerve complex at the level of the brainstem. The vessel may displace the cisternal segment of the nerve or it may extend into the internal auditory canal or IAC (in cases of AICA loop). If the AICA loop extends laterally past the midpoint of the IAC, vascular loop compression may be present because of the lack of space within the IAC. Though veins may also be a causative agent, the pulsatile motion of the artery is suspected as the more common cause of the symptoms.

MRI: Thin-section T2-weighted images are used to determine the relationship of the vascular loop to the nerve complex. Axial as well as reformatted images along the long and short axis of the nerve complex should be examined. The source images from a three-dimensional magnetic resonance angiography (MRA) of the vessels of the skull base may also be of utility to determine whether there is arterial or venous compression.

Further Reading

Gultekin S, Celik H, Akpek S, Oner Y, Gumus T, Tokgoz N. Vascular loops at the cerebellopontine angle: Is there a correlation with tinnitus? *AJNR.* 2008;29(9):1746–1749.

Wuertenberger CJ, Rosahl SK. Vertigo and tinnitus caused by vascular compression of the vestibulocochlear nerve, or intracanalicular vestibular schwannoma: review and case presentation. *Skull Base.* 2009;19(6):417–424.

CASE 9: FACIAL NEURITIS (Fig. 12.9)

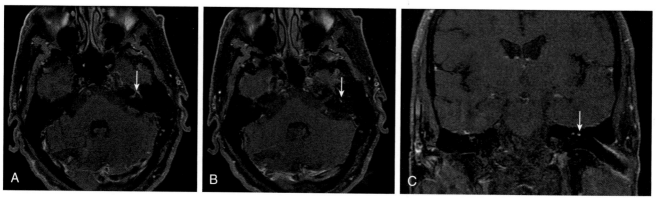

FIGURE 12.9 Facial Neuritis. (A) On axial postcontrast T1-weighted imaging with fat suppression, there is abnormal enhancement of the left facial nerve from the labyrinthine segment to the geniculate ganglion to the tympanic segment (arrow). **(B)** Increased enhancement of the left facial nerve extends to the mastoid segment (arrow). **(C)** Coronal images show the asymmetric nature of the left facial nerve enhancement (arrow).

Imaging findings: In the normal facial nerve, any segment of the intratemporal facial nerve may have enhancement except the labyrinthine segment. The most common area of normal facial nerve enhancement is the geniculate fossa. The mastoid segment is the second most common area of potentially normal intratemporal enhancement. The canalicular segment of the facial nerve should not enhance. In facial neuritis, there is asymmetric and increased enhancement of the facial nerve compared with the normal opposite side. In Bell palsy, there is fusiform enhancement of all segments of the intratemporal facial nerve. Enhancement of the main trunk of the facial nerve below the skull base may also be seen.

CT: Typically negative.

MRI: Asymmetric and increased enhancement of the facial nerve on the affected side compared with the opposite asymptomatic side. In Bell palsy, there is fusiform enhancement and enlargement of the intratemporal facial nerve. Facial neuritis may also manifest as enhancement of the canalicular segment or enhancement of the fundal aspect of the IAC. IAC enhancement in neuritis tends to be indistinct or have a brush-like pattern on postcontrast images.

Differential diagnosis: Facial schwannoma, perineural spread of tumor, metastatic disease, tuberculosis, granulomatous disease, or Guillain-Barré syndrome.

Refer to Cummings chapter 170 for more details.

Further Reading

Engstrom M, Abdsaleh S, Ahlström H, Johansson L, Stålberg E, Jonsson L. Serial gadolinium-enhanced magnetic resonance imaging and assessment of facial nerve function in Bell's palsy. *Otolaryngol Head Neck Surg.* 1997;117(5):559–566.

Saatci I, Sahintürk F, Sennaroğlu L, Boyvat F, Gürsel B, Besim A. MRI of the facial nerve in idiopathic facial palsy. *Eur Radiol.* 1996;6(5):631–636.

CASE 10: VESTIBULAR SCHWANNOMA (Fig. 12.10)

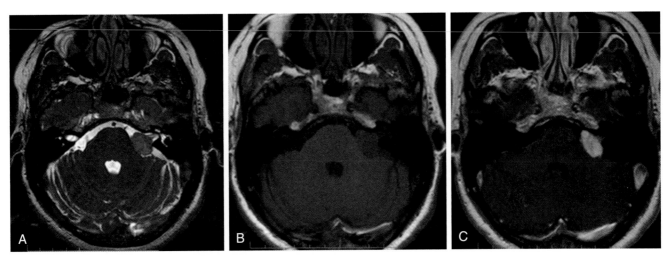

FIGURE 12.10 Vestibular Schwannoma. (**A**) Axial thin-section heavily T2-weighted image shows an extra-axial mass in the left CPA. (**B**) T1-weighted imaging shows the lesion to be lower in signal intensity than normal brain parenchyma. (**C**) Postcontrast T1-weighted imaging shows avid enhancement of the lesion; note the ice cream cone–like appearance characteristic of vestibular schwannoma. There is no visible dural tail, a finding more typical for meningioma.

Imaging findings: These are the most common tumors to develop in the IAC/CPA cistern. Originating from the vestibular component of the vestibulocochlear nerve, these masses arise at the Schwann cell-glial cell interface. Small lesions are seen within the IAC. The relationship to the crista falciformis is somewhat important to determine before surgery. As these lesions grow, they extend concentrically outward and have a classic "ice cream cone" appearance in the IAC/CPA cistern. Points to determine are the relationship of the mass to the brainstem, as well as to the space remaining in the fundal area of the IAC. Schwannomas follow the nerve of origin, and if there is penetration into the otic capsule, this should be into the vestibule for vestibular schwannoma. Penetration of the cochlea indicates the presence of cochlear schwannoma. Extension into the facial canal indicates a facial schwannoma.

CT: Used to determine bony remodeling. CT may be negative for small lesions. Larger lesions may demonstrate expansion of the IAC, blunting of the porous acousticus, or remodeling of the otic capsule if penetration has occurred.

MRI: These masses are classically hypointense on T1-weighted images and iso- or heterogeneously hyperintense on T2-weighted images, and they demonstrate heterogeneous, moderate to avid enhancement on postcontrast images. Lesions usually do not restrict on diffusion-weighted images. Local mass effect is seen on the brainstem if large, but because of the slow growing nature of these lesions, there are no signal changes of the adjacent brain parenchyma.

Differential diagnosis: Other schwannomas (facial/cochlear), meningioma, metastatic disease, lymphoma, tuberculoma, or granulomatous disease.

Refer to Cummings chapter 177 for more details.

Further Reading

Selesnick SH, Rebol J, Heier LA, Wise JB, Gutin PH, Lavyne MH. Internal auditory canal involvement of acoustic neuromas: surgical correlates to magnetic resonance imaging findings. *Otol Neurotol.* 2001;22:912–916.

Nutick SL, Babb MJ. Determinants of tumor size and growth in vestibular schwannomas. *J Neurosurg.* 2001;94:922–926.

CASE 11: CEREBELLOPONTINE ANGLE MENINGIOMA (Fig. 12.11)

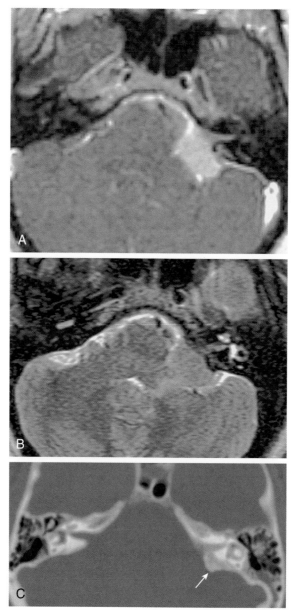

FIGURE 12.11 Cerebellopontine Angle Meningioma with Classic Features on MRI and CT. (**A**) Post-gadolinium T1-weighted MRI: The tumor is eccentric to the IAC and broadly dura based with obtuse angles at the bone-tumor interface. This hemispherical tumor shows uniform enhancement. Note the lack of IAC involvement. (**B**) T2-weighted MRI. The tumor is homogeneously isointense to gray matter. (**C**) CT bone windows. The tumor shows extensive hyperostosis underlying the dural base (arrow). (From Flint PW, Haughey BH, Lund VJ, et al. *Cummings Otolaryngology—Head and Neck Surgery*. 6th ed. Philadelphia, PA: Saunders; 2015.)

Imaging findings: Magnetic resonance (MR) and CT are imaging modalities that allow for differentiation of these tumors from other CPA lesions, such as acoustic neuromas. These tumors represent 3% of tumors at this location. Unlike acoustic neuromas, 60% of CPA meningiomas extend to the middle fossa. Meningiomas are typically hemispheric because of the attachments to the posterior petrous wall. A dural tail is often visualized.

MRI: On MRI, meningiomas are variable on T2-weighted images and isointense or slightly hypointense on T1-weighted images. Surface-flow voids may be present, and calcifications and cystic foci cause heterogeneity on MRI images of meningiomas.

CT: Approximately two-thirds are hyperintense relative to the brain. Unlike acoustic neuromas, meningiomas are homogeneous and occasionally calcified. They show homogeneous enhancement to contrast. Hyperostosis of adjacent bone is infrequent but characteristic of meningiomas.

Differential diagnosis: Acoustic neuroma or epidermoid.

Refer to Cummings chapter 177 for more details.

Further Reading

Choudhri AF, Parmar HA, Morales RE, Gandhi D. Lesions of the skull base: imaging for diagnosis and treatment. *Otolaryngol Clin North Am.* 2012;45(6):1385–1404.

Friedmann DR, Grobelny B, Golfinos JG, Roland Jr JT. Nonschwannoma tumors of the cerebellopontine angle. *Otolaryngol Clin North Am.* 2015 Jun;48(3):461–475.

CASE 12: FACIAL HEMANGIOMA (Fig. 12.12)

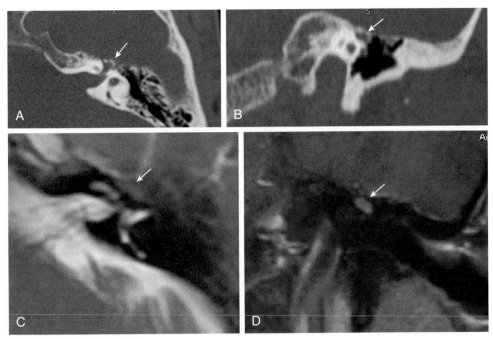

FIGURE 12.12 Facial Hemangioma. (**A**) Axial CT at the level of the anterior genu of the left facial canal demonstrates a bony lesion involving the geniculate segment of the facial canal (arrow). (**B**) Coronal CT at the level of the geniculate segment of the facial canal demonstrates a bony lesion superior to and involving the facial canal (arrow). (**C**) Axial T2-weighted image demonstrates that this lesion is hypointense in signal intensity demonstrating the bony nature of this lesion (arrow). (**D**) Postcontrast coronal T1-weighted image demonstrates moderate enhancement of this mass (arrow).

Imaging findings: These lesions are not true tumors but represent venous vascular malformations. They are classically associated with the facial nerve and most commonly occur at the geniculate fossa. Another less common location is the internal auditory canal. Unlike facial schwannoma, patients develop facial nerve symptoms early in the course of the disease process, and early surgical intervention is often required.

CT: As these lesions arise from the adjacent bone, bony proliferation with spicules of bone is seen on CT, which is why these lesions are also named ossifying hemangiomas. The lesions may demonstrate the presence of phleboliths; therefore, calcifications in the IAC should suggest a venous vascular malformation.

MRI: These lesions are typically hypointense on T1-weighted images and markedly hyperintense on T2-weighted images. On the T2-weighted images, focal areas of signal drop-off may be seen, which may represent phleboliths. On postcontrast images, the lesions demonstrate variable patterns of enhancement, from minimal to avid enhancement.

Differential diagnosis: Facial schwannoma or perineural spread of tumor.

Further Reading

Greene AK, Rogers GF, Mulliken JB. Intraosseous "hemangiomas" are malformations and not tumors. *Plast Reconstr Surg.* 2007;119(6):1949–1950.

Friedman O, Neff BA, Willcox TO, Kenyon LC, Sataloff RT. Temporal bone hemangiomas involving the facial nerve. *Otol Neurotol.* 2002;23(5):760–766.

CASE 13: SUPERIOR SEMICIRCULAR CANAL DEHISCENCE (Fig. 12.13)

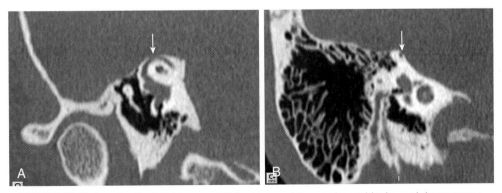

FIGURE 12.13 Superior Canal Dehiscence. (**A**) Poschl view of the superior semicircular canal demonstrates a defect associated with the roof of the superior semicircular canal (arrow). (**B**) Stenver plane also demonstrates a defect associated with the roof of the superior semicircular canal (arrow).

Imaging findings: Bony defect associated with the superior semicircular canal is best demonstrated on high-resolution CT. Patients with this abnormality present with Tullio phenomenon, which is vertigo in response to loud sounds. In addition, rotatory nystagmus, also called oscillopsia, may be present. These findings are the result of the "third window phenomenon" with abnormal processing of the aberrant fluid wave within the perilymph. High-resolution CT best demonstrates the defect of the superior semicircular canal on both sagittal and coronal images. Multiplanar reformatting of the temporal bone may also be performed in the Stenver and Poschl plane.

Differential diagnosis: Petrous apex mucocele, petrous cephalocele, or congenital epidermoid.

Refer to Cummings chapter 135 for more details.

Further Reading

Zhou G, Gopen Q, Poe DS. Clinical and diagnostic characterization of canal dehiscence syndrome: a great otologic mimicker. *Otol Neurotol.* 2007 Oct;28(7):920–926.

Ceylan N, Bayraktaroglu S, Alper H, Savaş R, Bilgen C, Kirazli T, Güzelmansur I, Ertürk SM. CT imaging of superior semicircular canal dehiscence: added value of reformatted images. *Acta Otolaryngol.* 2010 Sep;130(9):996–1001.

SKULL BASE

CASE 14: JUGULAR FORAMEN MENINGIOMA (Fig. 12.14)

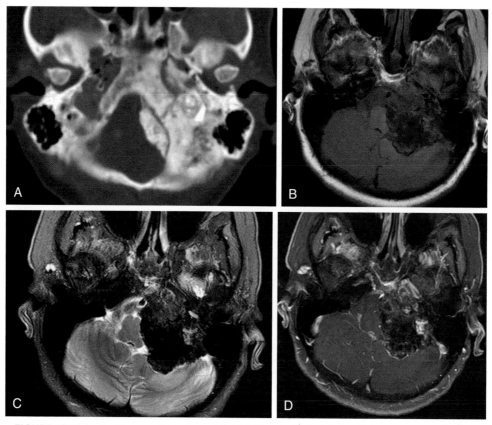

FIGURE 12.14 Jugular Foramen Meningioma. (**A**) Axial CT at the level of the jugular foramen demonstrates extensive bony proliferation of the left lateral skull base with effacement of the jugular foramen. (**B**) Axial T1-weighted image demonstrates bony expansion of the lateral skull base and areas of isointense signal centered at the lateral skull base. (**C**) Axial T2-weighted image demonstrates the hypointense signal of the expanded lateral skull base with areas of intermediate signal intensity on the T1-weighted image. (**D**) Postcontrast T1-weighted axial image demonstrates mild enhancement of this lesion. The extensive periosteal reaction is typical for meningiomas in this location.

Imaging findings: Arising from meningothelial rests within the dura, these masses induce a markedly proliferative hyperostosis of bone. There may be expansion of the jugular foramen, and additional foramina of the skull base may be involved. Both intracranial and extracranial extension of the meningioma above and below the skull base may be present.

CT: Soft tissue mass at the level of the jugular foramen with the presence of bony hyperostosis around the jugular foramen.

MRI: Typically isointense to the gray matter cortex on both T1- and T2-weighted images. These masses demonstrate homogeneous avid enhancement on postcontrast images. A dural tail is typically associated with these masses. One-third of the lesions demonstrate diffusion restriction on diffusion-weighted images.

Differential diagnosis: Jugular foramen schwannoma, glomus jugulare tumor, metastatic disease, lymphoma, or plasmacytoma.

Further Reading

Hamilton BE, Salzman KL, Patel N, et al. Imaging and clinical characteristics of temporal bone meningioma. *AJNR.* 2006;27(10):2204–2209.

Kaye AH, Hahn JF, Kinney SE, Hardy Jr RW, Bay JW. Jugular foramen schwannomas. *J Neurosurg.* 1984;60(5):1045–1053.

CASE 15: GLOMUS JUGULARE TUMOR (Fig. 12.15)

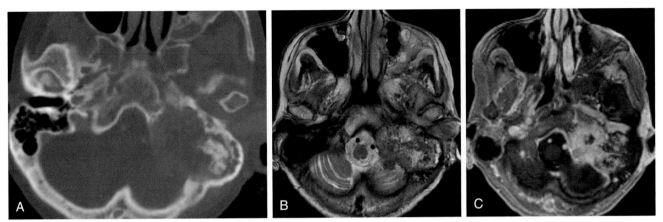

FIGURE 12.15 Glomus Jugulare. (**A**) CT imaging shows a destructive left temporal bone mass that involves the left jugular foramen. (**B**) The mass is primarily hyperintense on axial T2-weighted imaging with smaller areas of hypointensity. (**C**) The mass shows primarily avid enhancement on the postcontrast T1-weighted imaging.

Imaging findings: Arising from the glomus bodies at the dome of the jugular foramen, these masses are lesions with permeative change and destruction of the adjacent bone.

CT: Soft tissue mass that demonstrates avid enhancement with associated destruction and permeative change of the adjacent bone. Superior extension of this mass may destroy the jugular plate with extension of the mass into the middle ear cavity.

MRI: "Salt-and-pepper" appearance on both T1- and T2-weighted images. On T1-weighted images, these lesions are hypointense with focal areas of hyperintense signal, which may represent hemorrhage. On T2-weighted images, these lesions are hyperintense with focal areas of signal drop-off representing the presence of arterial vessels within the lesion. On postcontrast images, these lesions demonstrate avid heterogeneous enhancement.

Nuclear medicine: These masses show radiotracer uptake on an octreotide scan.

Differential diagnosis: Jugular foramen schwannoma, meningioma, lymphoma, plasmacytoma, or metastatic disease.

Refer to Cummings chapter 177 for more details.

Further Reading

Chakeres DW, LaMasters DL. Paragangliomas of the temporal bone: high resolution CT studies. *Radiology.* 1984;150(3):749–753.

Olsen WL, Dillon WP, Kelly WM, Norman D, Brant-Zawadzki M, Newton TH. MR Imaging of paragangliomas. *AJR.* 1984;148(1):201–204.

CASE 16: JUGULAR FORAMEN SCHWANNOMA (Fig. 12.16)

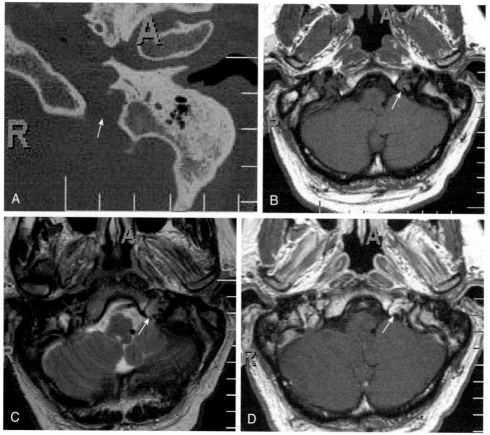

FIGURE 12.16 Jugular Foramen Schwannoma. (**A**) CT axial image of the lateral skull base demonstrates subtle erosion of the jugular spine on the left. The walls of the jugular foramen are smooth and sclerotic in appearance (arrow). (**B**) T1-weighted axial image demonstrates intermediate signal intensity within the left jugular foramen (arrow). (**C**) T2-weighted axial image demonstrates heterogeneously hyperintense signal intensity (arrow). (**D**) Postcontrast T1-weighted axial image demonstrates heterogeneous moderate to avid enhancement (arrow). This was a pathologically proven schwannoma.

Imaging findings: These masses arise from cranial nerves IX-XI, most commonly the vagus nerve (X). The lesions present as a soft-tissue mass with expansion and smooth remodeling of the jugular foramen.

CT: Soft-tissue mass, which demonstrates moderate to avid heterogeneous enhancement. There is smooth remodeling of the jugular foramen with sclerotic margins and a sharp zone of transition.

MRI: Typically hypointense on T1-weighted images, heterogeneously hyperintense on T2-weighted images, and demonstrating heterogeneous moderate to avid enhancement on postcontrast images.

Differential diagnosis: Jugular foramen meningioma, glomus jugulare tumor, metastatic disease, lymphoma, or plasmacytoma.

Refer to Cummings chapter 177 for more details.

Further Reading

Song MH, Lee HY, Jeon JS, Lee JD, Lee HK, Lee WS. Jugular foramen schwannoma: analysis on its origin and location. *Otol Neurotol.* 2008;29(3):384–391.

Wilson MA, Hillman TA, Wiggins RH, Shelton C. Jugular foramen schwannomas: diagnosis, management, and outcomes. *Laryngoscope.* 2005;115(8):1486–1492.

CASE 17: CHONDROSARCOMA (Fig. 12.17)

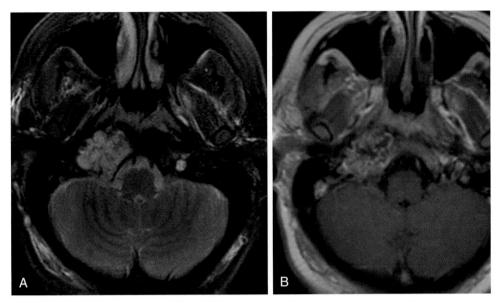

FIGURE 12.17 Chondrosarcoma. (A) Axial T2-weighted image shows a hyperintense mass in the right petroclival region of the skull base. The T2-weighted hyperintensity is characteristic of a chondroid tumor. **(B)** Patchy enhancement is present on axial postcontrast T1-weighted imaging. Note the off-midline location of this mass, which is more typical for chondrosarcoma rather than chordoma.

Imaging findings: These tumors arise from the chondroid elements of the central skull base; the most common location is the petro-occipital fissure between the anterior basiocciput of the clivus and the petrous temporal bone. A second common location is a midline mass at the spheno-occipital synchondrosis between the basisphenoid and the anterior basiocciput.

CT: Typically an off-midline lesion at the central skull base centered at the petro-occipital fissure with adjacent erosion and permeative change of the adjacent bone. Punctate calcifications may be present and represent chondroid calcifications. As these lesions extend superiorly to involve the petrous temporal bone, they classically displace the horizontal petrous internal carotid artery superiorly and anteriorly.

MRI: These lesions are hypointense on T1-weighted images and markedly hyperintense on T2-weighted images with low-signal-intensity foci, which may represent calcifications. These lesions demonstrate variable patterns of enhancement. On MRA, there is superior and anterior displacement of the horizontal petrous internal carotid artery.

Differential diagnosis: Typically pathognomonic; however, metastatic disease, chordoma, lymphoma, and plasmacytoma may also be considered.

Refer to Cummings chapter 118 for more details.

Further Reading

Cho YT, Kim JH, Khang SK, Lee JK, Kim CJ. Chordomas and chondrosarcomas of the skull base: comparative analysis of clinical results in 30 patients. *Neurosurg Rev.* 2008;31(1):35–43.

Sbaihat A, Bacciu A, Pasanisi E, Sanna M. Skull base chondrosarcomas: surgical treatment and results. *Ann Otol Rhinol Laryngol.* 2013;22(12):763–770.

CASE 18: FIBROUS DYSPLASIA. (Fig. 12.18)

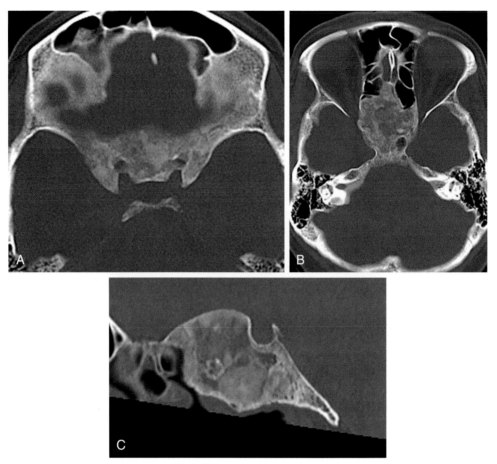

FIGURE 12.18 Fibrous Dysplasia. (**A**) Axial CT image at the level of the anterior clinoid processes shows diffuse expansile change extending laterally toward the lesser sphenoid wings bilaterally. (**B**) More inferiorly, this osseous change shows a "ground glass" appearance into the sphenoid and ethmoid sinuses. (**C**) Sagittal CT imaging shows the changes of fibrous dysplasia in the sphenoid bone in the central skull base below the sella turcica.

These lesions are developmental lesions and are not neoplastic. Representing immature bone, fibrous dysplasia has a classic "ground glass" appearance on CT with associated bone expansion in larger lesions. A cystic form may also occur. The monostotic form is typically sporadic in etiology. Polyostotic fibrous dysplasia may be associated with McCune-Albright syndrome.

CT: Geographic bone lesion, which demonstrates "ground glass" appearance with or without cystic change. There is no evidence of bony erosion or destruction. Larger lesions may cause neural foraminal narrowing because of mass effect and expansile change.

MRI: Hypointense on T1-weighted images and markedly hypointense on T2-weighted images. The cystic areas may be hyperintense in T2-weighted signal intensity. These lesions demonstrate moderate to avid enhancement on postcontrast images.

Differential diagnosis. CT is pathognomonic. On MRI, also consider other osteofibrous lesions or sclerotic lesions such as metastatic disease.

Refer to Cummings chapter 41 for more details.

Further Reading

Chong VF, Khoo JB, Fan YF. Fibrous dysplasia involving the base of the skull. *AJR*. 2002;178(3):717–720.

Wei YT, Jiang S, Cen Y. Fibrous dysplasia of skull. *J Craniofac Surg*. 2010;21(2): 538–452.

CASE 19: ABERRANT INTERNAL CAROTID ARTERY (Fig. 12.19)

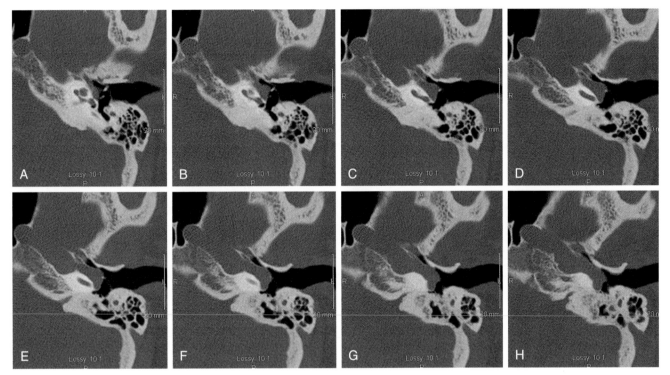

FIGURE 12.19 Aberrant Internal Carotid Artery. (**A-H**) Consecutive axial CT images progressing from superior to inferior from A to H demonstrate a mass overlying the cochlear promontory. Following the consecutive slices, note that this lesion enters the posterior genu of the petrous internal carotid artery and gives the horizontal segment of the petrous internal carotid artery an elongated appearance. Not shown is that the internal carotid artery enters the skull base at a more posterior location and turns laterally to enter the middle ear cavity.

Imaging findings: Congenital anomalous course of the internal carotid through the petrous temporal bone. The anomalous inferior cerebellar artery (ICA) enters the skull base in a posterior location and makes a hairpin loop laterally to enter the middle ear cavity. Crossing the cochlear promontory, the anomalous ICA then enters the horizontal petrous ICA canal in a lateral position with apparent elongation of the horizontal petrous ICA.

CT: Course of the aberrant ICA as described above. The vertical carotid canal is seen in a posterior location. The ICA then enters the middle ear cavity and extends into a lateralized horizontal petrous ICA canal.

MRI/MRA. Best demonstrated on MRA with course as described previously. Compression view from above on the MRA maximum intensity projection image demonstrates the posterior position of the vertical petrous ICA, the hairpin loop laterally, and the elongated horizontal petrous ICA segment.

Differential diagnosis: Pathognomonic on imaging. On physical examination, persistent stapedial artery or hypervascular tumor (glomus tumor or schwannoma).

Refer to Cummings chapter 192 for more details.

Further Reading

Lo WW, Solti-Bohman LG, McElveen Jr JT. Aberrant carotid artery: radiologic diagnosis with emphasis on high resolution computed tomography. *Radiographics*. 1985;5(6):985–993.

Swartz JD, Bazarnic ML, Naidich TP, Lowry LD, Doan HT. Aberrant internal carotid artery lying within the middle ear. High resolution CT diagnosis and differential diagnosis. *Neuroradiology*. 1985;27(4): 322–326.

CASE 20: STAPEDIAL ARTERY (Fig. 12.20)

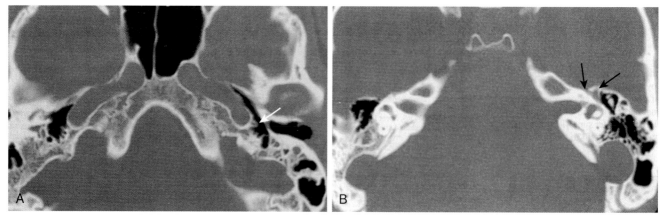

FIGURE 12.20 Persistent Stapedial Artery. (**A**) CT axial image demonstrates a small defect of the bony canal at the posterior genu of the left internal carotid artery with an apparent mass. This represents the persistent stapedial artery (arrow). (**B**) CT axial image at the level of the geniculate fossa demonstrates the classic "Y configuration" of the geniculate fossa (arrows). One channel represents the facial hiatus for the greater superficial petrosal nerve. The second channel represents the persistent stapedial artery, which continues as the middle meningeal artery.

Imaging findings: In most patients, this is not seen on imaging and found during surgery only. The persistent stapedial artery results from failure of regression of the embryonal stapedial artery. This vessel arises from the petrous ICA at the posterior genu, enters the middle ear cavity, and travels through the obturator foramen of the stapes. The vessel then enters the horizontal segment of the facial canal, travels anteriorly, and exits at the geniculate fossa, which may be a channel separate from the facial hiatus.

CT: Typically negative. May demonstrate a soft-tissue mass at the level of the stapes, expansion of the tympanic facial canal, and a "Y" configuration of the geniculate fossa, representing the facial hiatus for the greater superficial petrosal nerve and the channel for the persistent stapedial artery, which becomes the middle meningeal artery. The foramen spinosum in these cases is absent.

MRI/MRA: Typically normal. On MRA, may demonstrate an anomalous vessel arising from the posterior genu of the petrous internal carotid artery, which may be followed to the geniculate fossa and become the middle meningeal artery. The middle meningeal artery at the level of the foramen spinosum is absent.

Differential diagnosis: Pathognomonic on imaging. On physical examination, aberrant internal carotid artery, or hypervascular tumor (glomus tumor or schwannoma).

Further Reading

Silbergleit R, Quint DJ, Mehta BA, Patel SC, Metes JJ, Noujaim SE. The persistent stapedial artery. *AJNR.* 2000;21(3):572–577.

Yilmaz T, Bilgen C, Savas R, Alper H. Persistent stapedial artery: MR angiographic and CT findings. *AJNR.* 2003;24(6):1133–1135.

SINONASAL CAVITY

CASE 21: INVERTED PAPILLOMA (Fig. 12.21)

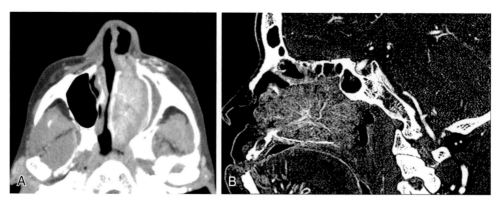

FIGURE 12.21 Inverted Papilloma. (**A**) There is a polypoid-enhancing soft-tissue mass from the left nasal cavity projecting through the left posterior choana to the nasopharynx. Peripheral cerebriform enhancement is sometimes seen. (**B**) On sagittal reconstruction, spiculated calcification is seen at the origin on the papilloma.

Imaging finding: Most common type of papilloma (most common benign tumor of the sinonasal cavity) that typically arises from the lateral wall of the nasal cavity centered at the middle meatus and may extend into the antrum of the maxillary sinus.

CT: Soft-tissue mass in the nasal cavity without bone erosion or destruction. Typically centered at the level of the middle meatus and may demonstrate hyperostosis of bone, which may be the point of attachment/origin of the mass. Because of its location, this mass may cause sinus obstruction.

MRI: Alternating hyperintense and hypointense lines on T2-weighted images with curvilinear striations described as a cerebriform or convoluted pattern. Postcontrast images may show a similar cerebriform enhancement pattern with alternating hyperenhancing and hypoenhancing layers.

Differential diagnosis: Sinonasal polyp, squamous cell carcinoma, or sinonasal polyposis.

Refer to Cummings chapter 48 for more details.

Further Reading

Maroldi R, Farina D, Palvarini L, Lombardi D, Tomenzoli D, Nicolai P. Magnetic resonance imaging findings of inverted papilloma: differential diagnosis with malignant sinonasal tumors. *Am J Rhinol.* 2004;18(5):305–310.

Yousem DM, Fellows DW, Kennedy DW, Bolger WE, Kashima H, Zinreich SJ. Inverted papilloma: evaluation with MR imaging. *Radiology.* 1992;185(2):501–505.

CASE 22: NASAL MENINGOCELE (Fig. 12.22)

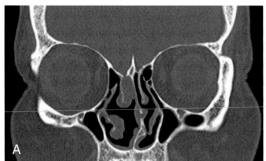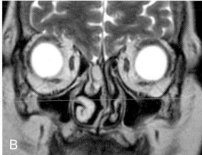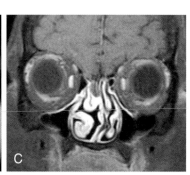

FIGURE 12.22 Nasal Meningocele. (**A**) Coronal CT of the nasal cavity demonstrates a mass in right superior nasal cavity medial to the vertical strut of the middle turbinate. Note the small defect of the right cribriform plate. (**B**) Coronal T2-weighted image demonstrates this lesion to be increased in signal intensity. (**C**) Coronal postcontrast T1-weighted image demonstrates that this lesion does not enhance, consistent with a nasal meningocele.

Nasal meningocele occurs because of a defect along the anterior skull base and herniation of the meninges containing CSF through the defect. CSF leak may be associated with this. The most common cause is prior trauma. Dehiscence of the cribriform plate may also be a cause.

CT: Cystic lesion within the nasal cavity that extends from the anterior skull base. This lesion has a thin wall and demonstrates no enhancement.

MRI: Cystic lesion iso- or hyperintense to CSF signal intensity on T1- and T2-weighted images. Because of the CSF pulsations, flow-related artifacts may be associated with a nasal meningocele, resulting in central-signal drop-off. After the administration of contrast, there is no enhancement centrally.

Differential diagnosis: Imaging is usually pathognomonic. If the defect along the anterior skull base is not seen, this lesion may be mistaken for a dermoid, epidermoid, or cystic neoplasm.

Further Reading

Mukerji SS, Parmar HA, Gujar S, Passamani P. Intranasal meningoencephalocele presenting as a nasal polyp—a case report. *Clin Imaging.* 2011;35(4):309–311.

Zinreich SJ, Borders JC, Eisele DW, Mattox DE, Long DM, Kennedy DW. The utility of magnetic resonance imaging in the diagnosis of intranasal meningoencephaloceles. *Arch Otolaryngol Head Neck Surg.* 1992;118(11):1253–1256.

CASE 23: POLYPOSIS (Fig. 12.23)

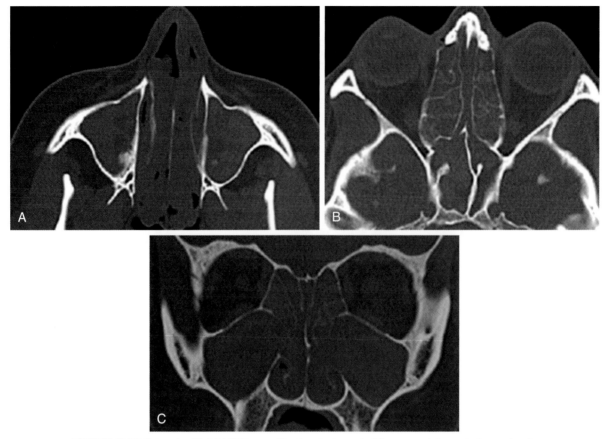

FIGURE 12.23 Polyposis. (**A**) Axial CT image without contrast reveals diffuse mucosal disease in the nasal cavity and visualized sinuses. There is polypoid tissue projecting through the posterior choanae. (**B**) Areas of hyperdensity are seen among the opacification indicative of inspissated secretions. Fungal colonization in allergic sinusitis can often appear similarly. (**C**) In the coronal plane, the extensive nature of the polyposis causes near complete opacification of bilateral nasal cavities and sinuses.

Imaging findings: Polypoid masses within the nasal cavity and sinuses. There may be bony remodeling without bone erosion/destruction. Sinus opacification with or without mucocele formation may be present.

CT: Polypoid or lobulated lesions within the sinonasal cavity. These lesions are hypoattenuating in appearance, higher than CSF but lower than soft-tissue density. Sinus obstruction and mucocele formation may be present.

MRI: Peripheral rim enhancement of the sinonasal polyps is seen. Mucosal enhancement of the sinus mucosa is seen with or without fluid. Mucocele formation may also be seen.

Differential diagnosis: Squamous cell carcinoma, lymphoma, or granulomatous disease.

Further Reading

Gosepath J, Mann WJ. Current concepts in therapy of chronic rhinosinusitis and nasal polyposis. *ORJ J Otorhinolaryngol Relat Spec.* 2005;67(3):125–136.

Pearlman AN, Chandra RK, Chang D. Relationships between severity of chronic rhinosinusitis and nasal polyposis, asthma, and atopy. *Am J Rhinol Allergy.* 2009;23(2):145–148.

CASE 24: ESTHESIONEUROBLASTOMA (Fig. 12.24)

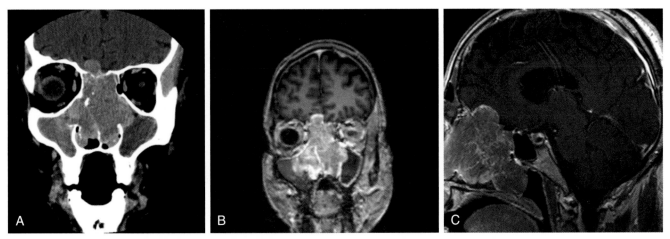

FIGURE 12.24 Esthesioneuroblastoma. (**A**) There is an extensive soft-tissue mass involving the right greater than left paranasal sinuses and nasal cavity with extension through the anterior skull base on coronal CT. Calcifications are not seen in the mass in this case but have been associated with esthesioneuroblastoma along with peritumoral cyst formation. (**B**) On postcontrast T1-weighted imaging, there is enhancement of the mass. Note the involvement of the olfactory recesses, which is characteristic for esthesioneuroblastoma. (**C**) Sagittal postcontrast T1-weighted imaging shows the intracranial and extracranial components of the mass.

Imaging findings: Arising from the olfactory nerves, this mass has often extended superiorly to the level of the cribriform plate at the time of presentation and into the subfrontal area. These are destructive tumors with associated bony erosion and permeative change. Large lesions are often "dumbbell" in shape, with the waist at the level of the anterior skull base. Macrocysts may be present at the tumor-brain interface and may be pathognomonic for this entity.

CT: Sinonasal mass in the superior half of the nasal cavity with associated bone erosion/destruction.

MRI: Hypointense on T1-weighted images, iso- to hyperintense on T2-weighted images, and heterogeneous moderate to avid enhancement on postcontrast images. These masses are diffusion positive on diffusion-weighted images. Macrocysts may be seen at the tumor-brain interface. Sinus obstruction may also be present.

Refer to Cummings chapter 82 for more details.

Further Reading

Schuster JJ, Phillips CD, Levine PA. MR of Esthesioneuroblastoma (olfactory neuroblastoma) and appearance after craniofacial resection. *AJNR.* 1994;15(6):1169–1177.

Yu T, Xu YK, Li L, et al. Esthesioneuroblastoma methods of intra cranial extension: CT and MR imaging findings. *Neuroradiology.* 2009;51(12):841–850.

CASE 25: ALLERGIC FUNGAL RHINOSINUSITIS (Fig. 12.25)

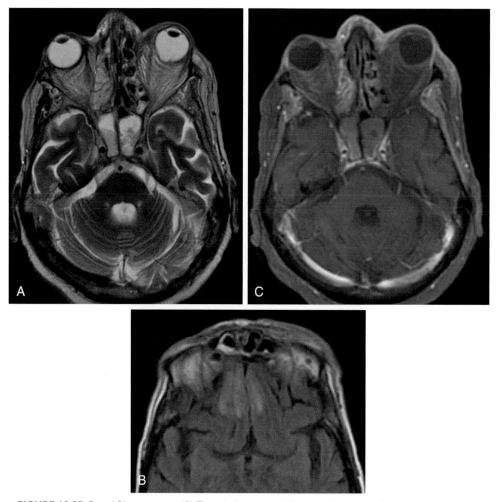

FIGURE 12.25 Fungal Rhinosinusitis. (**A**) There is sinus mucosal disease with invasive inflammatory edema in the bilateral orbits on this T2-weighted image. Note the deformity of the left globe contour. (**B**) Edema extends through the anterior skull base into the inferior frontal lobes on axial T2-FLAIR (T2 Fluid Attenuated Inversion Recovery) imaging. (**C**) There is decreased enhancement of the soft tissues in the orbits and sinuses on postcontrast T1-weighted imaging with fat suppression. The decreased or absent enhancement is a result of tissue devascularization, a key sign of invasive fungal disease.

Imaging findings: Rhinosinusitis complicated by noninvasive fungal hyphae.

CT: Sinus inflammatory changes with high-density material within the sinus cavities on noncontrast CT scan. The sinuses may be expanded in appearance.

MRI: Variable T1-weighted signal intensity because of the presence of water, protein, and fungal elements. Presence of heavy metals in the fungal elements, as well as proteinaceous concretions, may cause T1-weighted hypointensity similar to air.

Differential diagnosis: Blood products within the sinuses or presence of proteinaceous concretions related to chronic sinus obstruction.

Refer to Cummings chapter 41 for more details.

Further Reading

Aribandi M, McCoy VA, Bazan 3rd C. Imaging features of invasive and noninvasive fungal sinusitis: a review. *Radiographics*. 2007;27(5):1283–1296.

Wise SK, Rogers GA, Ghegan MD, Harvey RJ, Delgaudio JM, Schlosser RJ. Radiologic staging system for allergic fungal rhinosinusitis (AFRS). *Otolaryngol Head Neck Surg*. 2009;140(5):735–740.

CASE 26: CEREBROSPINAL FLUID LEAK CAUSED BY A DEFECT OF THE CRIBIFORM PLATE (Fig. 12.26)

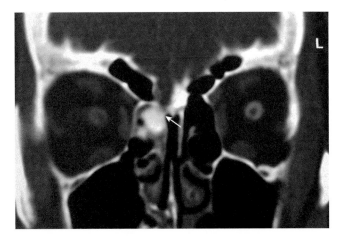

FIGURE 12.26 Cerebrospinal Fluid Leak Caused by a Defect of the Cribriform Plate. Coronal CT of the anterior skull base after a cisternogram procedure. High-density material is seen within the subarachnoid spaces, intracranially. Note the contrast below the anterior skull base within the right ethmoid air cell caused by a defect of the cribriform plate (arrow).

Imaging findings: Most common cause of CSF leak is due to trauma and fracture. Spontaneous leak may be due to dehiscence related to thinning of the bone, and increased incidence is noted in obesity.

CT: Best method to evaluate for CSF leak. Defect of the cribriform plate on thin-section imaging. Presence of fluid within the adjacent sinuses or nasal cavity. Post-cisternogram CT demonstrates presence of contrast within the sinuses or nasal cavity in patients actively leaking (Fig. 12.24).

MRI: Thin-section T2-weighted coronal images may demonstrate a channel: communication between the CSF space and nasal cavity.

Nuclear medicine: Indium DTPA (diethylenetriamine pentaacetic acid) may be used to help determine the presence of a leak but may not accurately determine the precise location of the leak.

Refer to Cummings chapter 41 for more details.

Further Reading

Lloyd KM, DelGaudio JM, Hudgins PA. Imaging of skull base cerebrospinal fluid leaks in adults. *Radiology*. 2008;248(3):725–736.

CASE 27: DACRYOCYSTITIS (Fig. 12.27)

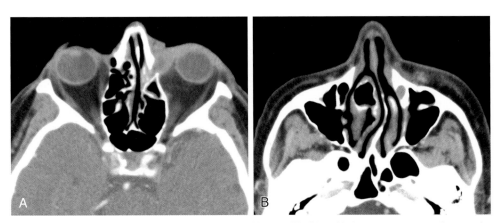

FIGURE 12.27 Dacryocystitis with Dacryocystocele. (**A**) Axial CT of the orbit demonstrates a mass adjacent and anterior to the medial canthus of the left orbit. The central portion is hypoattenuating and appears to arise from the nasolacrimal sac. (**B**) Axial CT inferior to A demonstrates soft-tissue material filling the nasolacrimal canal without bony erosion. Note the subtle stranding of the premaxillary soft tissue.

Dacryocystitis is inflammation of the nasolacrimal apparatus. Drainage of tears from the orbit occurs along the inferior and superior colliculus of the lids, which converge to the nasolacrimal sac and through the nasolacrimal duct draining into the inferior meatus of the nasal cavity. Because of an

underlying stricture, a dacryolith or mass obstruction of the nasolacrimal apparatus may occur with secondary inflammation. Increased attenuation of the contents of the nasolacrimal canal may be seen with dilatation of the nasolacrimal sac, which forms a diverticulum from the superior aspect of the nasolacrimal canal, and may be seen as a cystic lesion adjacent to the medial canthus. Surrounding inflammation or an inflammatory mass may be seen adjacent to the medial canthus.

CT: Soft-tissue mass and/or cystic lesion adjacent to the medial canthus with surrounding stranding of the adjacent fat.

MRI: Cystic lesion adjacent to the medial canthus, which follows fluid signal intensity with stranding of the adjacent fat. Enhancement may be seen with the solid component, as well as enhancement within the nasolacrimal canal.

Differential diagnosis: Mass arising from the nasolacrimal apparatus, including adenocarcinoma and adenoid cystic carcinoma, lymphoma, and metastatic disease.

Refer to Cummings chapter 53 for more details.

Further Reading

Asheim J, Spickler E. CT demonstration of dacryolithiasis complicated by dacryocystitis. *AJNR*. 2005;26(10):2640–2641.

Vaidhyanath R, Kirke R, Brown L, Sampath R. Lacrimal fossa lesions: pictorial review of CT and MRI features. *Orbit*. 2008;27(6):410–418.

PHARYNX

CASE 28: TORNWALDT CYST (Fig. 12.28)

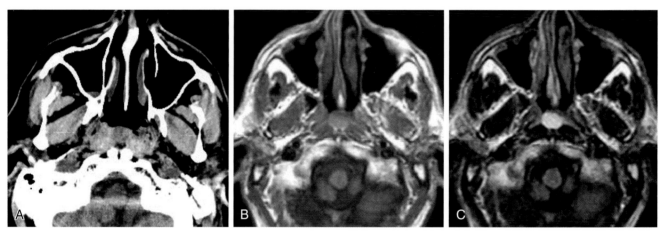

FIGURE 12.28 Tornwaldt Cyst. (**A**) Axial CT at the level of the nasopharynx demonstrates a midline cystic lesion in the posterior superior aspect of the nasopharynx. (**B**) T1-weighted axial image at the level of the nasopharynx demonstrates the cyst to be slightly hyperintense relative to muscle signal intensity. (**C**) T2-FLAIR axial image demonstrates the cyst to be homogeneously hyperintense in signal intensity.

Imaging findings: A pseudocyst found in the superior posterior aspect of the midline nasopharynx and related to closure of the Tornwaldt diverticulum. Represents the site at which the embryonic notochord and endoderm of the primitive pharynx came in contact.

CT: Midline cystic lesion of the superior posterior nasopharynx. Typically demonstrates no enhancement or minimal wall enhancement unless infected.

MRI: Variable signal intensity because of the presence of proteinaceous material on T1- and T2-weighted images.

Differential diagnosis: Mucous retention cyst, adenoidal cyst from minor salivary gland, benign mixed tumor, or NP carcinoma.

Refer to Cummings chapter 101 for more details.

Further Reading

Ikushima I, Korogi Y, Makita O, et al. MR imaging of Tornwaldt's cysts. *AJR*. 1999;172(6):1663–1665.

Moody MW, Chi DH, Mason JC, Phillips CD, Gross CW, Schlosser RJ. Tornwaldt's cyst: incidence and a case report. *Ear Nose Throat J*. 2007;86(1):45–47.

CASE 29: OROPHARYNGEAL LYMPHOMA (Fig. 12.29)

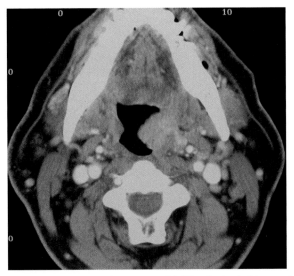

FIGURE 12.29 Oropharyngeal Lymphoma. Postcontrast axial CT at the level of the oropharynx demonstrates a bulky mildly enhancing mass in the left tonsillar fossa. This may be difficult to distinguish from squamous cell carcinoma.

Imaging findings: Waldeyer ring, comprising the adenoids, palatine and lingual tonsils, and the posterior margin of the soft palate, is the most common location for extranodal form of lymphoma. Separating squamous cell carcinoma from lymphoma may be difficult on CT imaging and easier on MRI. Lymphoma is isointense to muscle signal intensity on T1-weighted images, iso- to mildly hyperintense on T2-weighted images, and demonstrating moderate to avid enhancement. The nodal disease is typically well circumscribed without extracapsular extension or cystic change. This may also be diffusion positive on diffusion-weighted images.

Further Reading

Kato H, Kanematsu M, Kawaguchi S, Watanabe H, Mizuta K, Aoki M. Evaluation of imaging findings differentiating extranodal non-Hodgkin's lymphoma from squamous cell carcinoma in naso- and oropharynx. *Clin Imaging.* 2013;37(4):657–663.

Zhang CX, Liang L, Zhang B, et al. Imaging anatomy of Waldeyer's ring and PET/CT and MRI findings of oropharyngeal non-Hodgkin's lymphoma. *Asian Pac J Cancer Prev.* 2015;16(8):3333–3338.

CASE 30: OROPHARYNGEAL SQUAMOUS CELL CARCINOMA (Fig. 12.30)

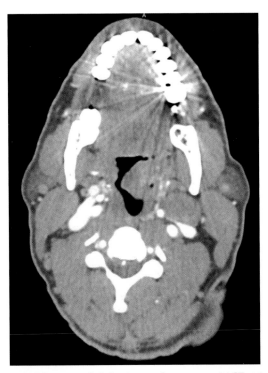

FIGURE 12.30 Oropharyngeal Squamous Cell Carcinoma. Postcontrast axial CT at the level of the oropharynx demonstrates a mass in the left tonsillar fossa. Associated cystic lymph node is seen in level II on the left in this patient with human papillomavirus–related OP squamous cell carcinoma.

Imaging findings: Unilateral tonsillar enlargement and presence of a neck mass in level II is usually pathognomonic for OP squamous cell carcinoma. This may be difficult to distinguish from lymphoma as described previously. Some imaging findings that may be useful are the presence of extracapsular extension within the lymphadenopathy, as well as cystic change or necrosis. On MRI, squamous cell cancer is mildly hyperintense on T2-weighted images and is not diffusion positive.

Refer to Cummings chapter 101 for more details.

Further Reading

Cophan DM, Popat S, Kaplan SE, Rigual N, Loree T, Hicks Jr WL. Oropharyngeal cancer: current understanding and management. *Curr Opin Otolaryngol Head Neck Surg.* 2009;17(2):88–94.

Kato H, Kanematsu M, Kawaguchi S, Watanabe H, Mizuta K, Aoki M. Evaluation of imaging findings differentiating extranodal non-Hodgkin's lymphoma from squamous cell carcinoma in naso- and oropharynx. *Clin Imaging.* 2013;37(4):657–663.

CASE 31: SUBGLOTTIC STENOSIS AND TRACHEAL STENOSIS (Fig. 12.31)

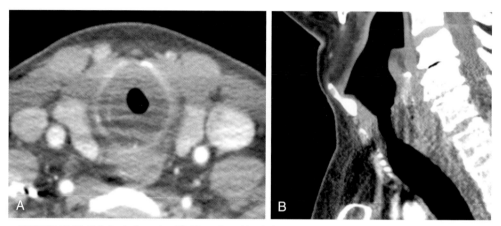

FIGURE 12.31 Subglottic Stenosis. (**A**) Circumferential soft-tissue thickening of the subglottic larynx is present on axial postcontrast CT of the neck. (**B**) In the sagittal plane, the resulting narrowing of the airway can be appreciated.

Imaging findings: Typically caused by prolonged intubation and associated pressure necrosis of the mucosa related to the balloon of the endotracheal tube with subsequent scar formation; obstructive granulation and scar tissue in the subglottic region or trachea can lead to dyspnea. Greater than 25% narrowing of the airway results in dyspnea.

CT/MRI: CT without contrast is sufficient to make a radiologic diagnosis. The mucosal surface of the subglottic region and trachea are not seen on CT. Any soft tissue identified is abnormal. The percentage of stenosis is determined by degree of patency relative to the normal lumen size.

Differential diagnosis: Granulomatous disease, papilloma, or squamous cell cancer

Refer to Cummings chapter 68 for more details.

Further Reading

Lorenz RR. Adult laryngotracheal stenosis: etiology and surgical management. *Curr Opin Otolaryngol Head Neck Surg.* 2003;11(6):467–472.

Sarper A, Ayten A, Eser I, Ozbudak O, Demircan A. Tracheal stenosis after tracheostomy or intubation: review with special regard to cause and management. *Tex Heart Inst J.* 2005;32(2):154–158.

CASE 32: TRUE VOCAL FOLD PARALYSIS (Fig. 12.32)

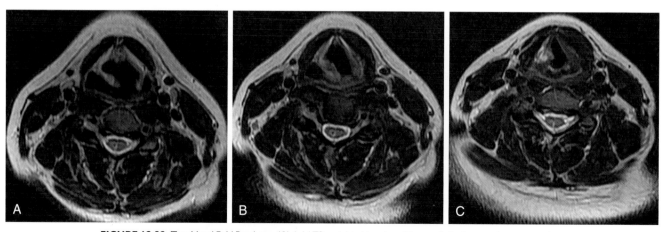

FIGURE 12.32 True Vocal Fold Paralysis. (**A**) Axial T2-weighted imaging of the cervical spine was done on a patient who had extensive injury to the right medulla and cervical spinal cord. Notice the enlargement of the right piriform sinus compared with the left. (**B**) The right aryepiglottic fold is turned inward. (**C**) The right true vocal fold is medialized and shows fatty atrophy from chronic denervation and paralysis.

Imaging findings: True vocal fold paralysis may be divided into acute, subacute, and chronic forms. In acute vocal fold paralysis, the true vocal fold is medialized and may be identified on both CT and MRI. In subacute true vocal fold paralysis, the true vocal fold begins to lose volume without loss of the normal density on CT. This diagnosis is made on MRI of the larynx, which demonstrates hyperintense signal intensity of the affected true vocal fold on T2-weighted images. In chronic true vocal fold paralysis, there is lateralization of the true vocal fold with fatty replacement, which is well demonstrated on both CT and MRI.

Imaging on CT or MR should extend from the skull base to the level of the pulmonary artery to encompass the jugular foramen and the course of the vagus nerve and recurrent laryngeal nerve.

Differential diagnosis: Glottic squamous cell carcinoma.

Further Reading

Myssiorek D. Recurrent laryngeal nerve paralysis: anatomy and etiology. *Otolaryngol Clin North Am.* 2004;37(1):25–44.

Chin SC, Edelstein S, Chen CY, Som PM. Using CT to localize side and level of vocal cord paralysis. *AJR.* 2003;180(4):1165–1170.

CASE 33: LARYNGEAL CHONDROSARCOMA (Fig. 12.33)

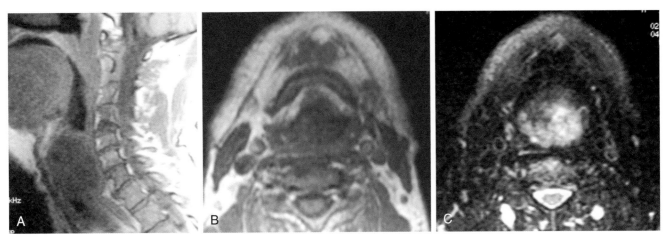

FIGURE 12.33 Chondrosarcoma of the Epiglottis. (**A**) Sagittal T1-weighted image demonstrates a bulky mass in the supraglottic larynx. Note that this mass is predominantly hypointense. (**B**) T1-weighted axial image demonstrates the large mass filling the supraglottic larynx. (**C**) T2-weighted axial image with fat suppression demonstrates that this lesion is markedly hyperintense with low-signal-intensity foci, which may represent calcifications.

Imaging findings: The cartilaginous portions of the larynx include the epiglottis, arytenoid, cricoid, and thyroid cartilage. These are the sites for laryngeal chondrosarcoma, a rare malignancy of the larynx.

CT: Soft-tissue mass centered on one of the cartilaginous structures of the larynx. Calcifications may be present. This mass may demonstrate variable patterns of enhancement.

MRI: Hypointense on T1-weighted images, markedly hyperintense on T2-weighted images with foci of signal drop-off, which may represent calcifications. Variable degree of enhancement on postcontrast studies.

Differential diagnosis: Laryngeal squamous cell carcinoma, lymphoma, or granulomatous disease.

Refer to Cummings chapter 106 for more details.

Further Reading

Wang Q, Chen H, Zhou S. Chondrosarcoma of the larynx: report of two cases and review of the literature. *Int J Clin Exp Pathol.* 2015;8(2):2068–2073.

Policarpo M, Taranto F, Aina E, Aluffi PV, Pia F. Chondrosarcoma of the larynx: a case report. *Acta Otorhinolaryngol Ital.* 2008;28(1):38–41.

CASE 34: NASOPHARYNGEAL MASS (Fig. 12.34)

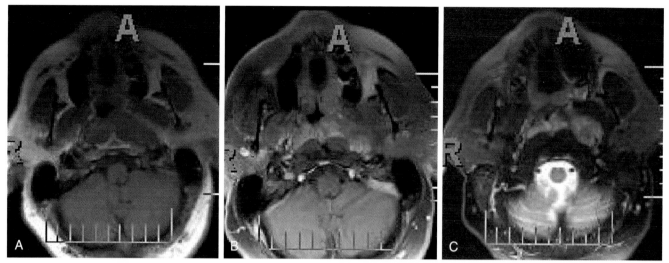

FIGURE 12.34 Nasopharyngeal Mass, Squamous Cell Cancer. (**A**) T1-weighted axial image demonstrates a mass associated with the posterior wall of the nasopharynx and the fossa of Rosenmuller bilaterally. Additionally, note the left retropharyngeal lymph node. (**B**) Postcontrast T1-weighted axial image demonstrates moderate heterogeneous enhancement of the NP mass and the left retropharyngeal lymph node. (**C**) T2-weighted axial image with fat suppression demonstrates the mass and adenopathy to be heterogeneous and moderately hyperintense in signal intensity.

Imaging findings: The most common malignancies of the nasopharynx are squamous cell carcinoma and lymphoma, which comprise up to 90% of all malignancies in this location. As mentioned above, it may be difficult to distinguish squamous cell carcinoma (SCCA) and lymphoma on CT, although MRI may be useful. Lymphoma tends to be intermediate in signal intensity on T2-weighted images and is diffusion positive. The appearance of lymphadenopathy may also help separate these two entities as extracapsular extension and necrosis are more commonly seen in SCCA. Minor salivary gland malignancies may also occur in this location, including mucoepidermoid carcinoma and adenocarcinoma. For the determination of skull-base involvement, intracranial extension, and perineural spread of tumor, MR is superior to CT.

Refer to Cummings chapter 96 for more details.

Further Reading

Glastonbury CM. NP carcinoma: the role of magnetic resonance imaging in diagnosis, staging, treatment, and follow-up. *Top Magn Reson Imaging.* 2007;18(4):225–235.

CASE 35: TONSILLITIS (Fig. 12.35)

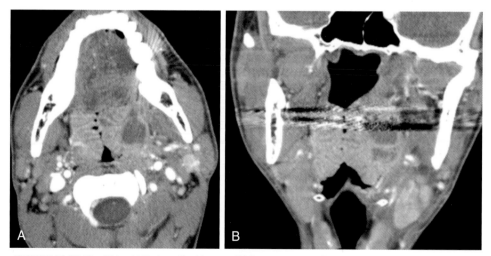

FIGURE 12.35 Tonsillitis with Peritonsillar Abscess. (**A**) Postcontrast axial CT images reveal enlarged bilateral palatine tonsils with a striated enhancement pattern consistent with tonsillitis. On the left, there is an adjacent rim-enhancing fluid collection consistent with peritonsillar abscess formation. (**B**) On coronal reconstruction, the tonsillitis with left peritonsillar abscess formation can again be seen with additional left cervical lymphadenopathy.

Imaging findings: Inflammation of the tonsils may be seen as enlargement of the tonsils with a striated or striped appearance because of the presence of crypts within the tonsils. Mucosal enhancement with submucosal edema gives the inflamed tonsils this striped appearance. Edema of the muscular wall of the oropharynx may also be seen. Development of a tonsillar abscess may be seen within the tonsil or a peritonsillar abscess, which lies in the peritonsillar recess of the pharyngeal mucosal space. On CT, enhancement of the mucosal surface with submucosal edema is present. On MRI, the tonsil is hypointense on T1-weighted images and hyperintense on T2-weighted images.

On postcontrast MRI, the tonsil again demonstrates a striated or striped appearance.

Refer to Cummings chapter 101 for more details.

Further Reading

Suzumoto M, Hotomi M, Billal DS, Fujihara K, Harabuchi Y, Yamanaka N. A scoring system for management of acute pharyngo-tonsillitis in adults. *Auris Nasus Larynx.* 2009;36(3):314–320.

Tewfik TL, Al Garni M. Tonsillopharyngitis: clinical highlights. *J Otolaryngol.* 2005;34(suppl 1):S45–S49.

SALIVARY GLANDS

CASE 36: RANULA (Fig. 12.36)

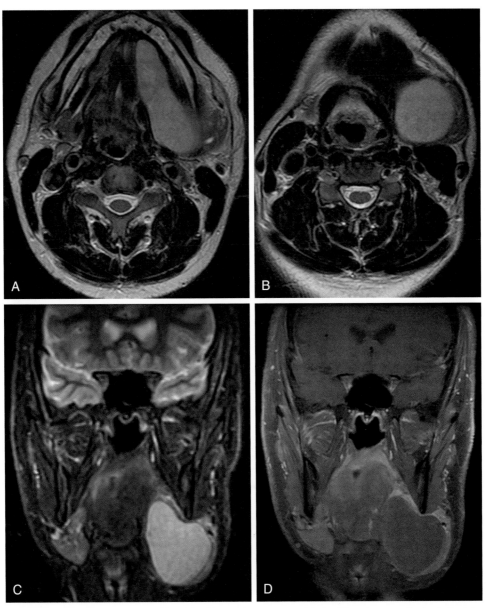

FIGURE 12.36 Ranula. (**A**) Axial T2-weighted image demonstrates a lobulated hyperintense collection in the left floor of the mouth. (**B**) The lesion is again seen on this axial T2-weighted image with extension inferiorly to the left submandibular space. (**C**) Coronal STIR (Short Tau Inversion Recovery) imaging shows this lesion from the left sublingual space to the submandibular space, consistent with a diving or plunging ranula. (**D**) There is no enhancement of the ranula on postcontrast T1-weighted imaging given its cystic nature.

Imaging findings: A ranula is a pseudocyst of the floor of the mouth, arising from the sublingual glands or minor salivary glands. Typically midline in location, these are unilocular, well-circumscribed cystic lesions. Simple ranulas are confined to the floor of the mouth. When these extend through the mylohyoid muscle into the submental region or posteriorly and inferiorly into the submandibular space, they are called plunging or diving ranulas.

CT: Well-circumscribed unilocular cystic lesion with a thin wall, which demonstrates enhancement.

MRI: These lesions are typically hypointense lesions on T1-weighted images and hyperintense on T2-weighted images.

On postcontrast images, the wall will enhance. If proteinaceous material is present, a variable signal is seen on MRI.

Differential diagnosis: Abscess, dermoids, or epidermoid.

Refer to Cummings chapter 8 for more details.

Further Reading

Kurabayashi T, Ida M, Yasumoto M, et al. MRI of ranulas. *Neuroradiology.* 2000;42(12):917–922.

Rosa PA, Hirsch DL, Dierks EJ. Congenital neck masses. *Oral Maxillofac Surg Clin North Am.* 2008;20(3):339–352.

CASE 37: PAROTITIS (Fig. 12.37)

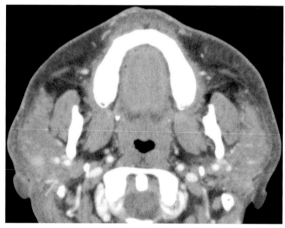

FIGURE 12.37 Parotitis in Patient with Systemic Lupus Erythematosus. Postcontrast CT at the level of the parotid glands demonstrates increased enhancement and stranding of the parotid parenchyma on the left side in this patient with left parotitis. Right parotitis is also present.

Imaging findings: Parotitis is sialadenitis of the parotid gland. The earliest finding is increased size and attenuation of the parotid gland. The parenchyma may demonstrate stranding or reticulation. Thickening of the capsule of the gland may be seen. Associated stranding of the adjacent fat, thickening of the skin, and abscess formation may be present. The draining salivary (Stenson) duct should be assessed for an obstructive process such as a stone, stricture, or mass. Associated dilatation of the salivary duct with thickening and enhancement of the wall of the salivary duct is sialodochitis, or ductal sialadenitis.

Differential diagnosis: Sjögren syndrome, sialosis, lymphoma, or leukemia.

Refer to Cummings chapter 85 for more details.

Further Reading

Cascarini L, McGurk M. Epidemiology of salivary gland infections. *Oral Maxillofac Surg Clin North Am.* 2009;21(3):353–370.

Yousem DM, Kraut MA, Chalian AA. Major salivary gland imaging. *Radiology.* 2000;216(1):19–29.

CASE 38: SIALOLITH (Fig. 12.38)

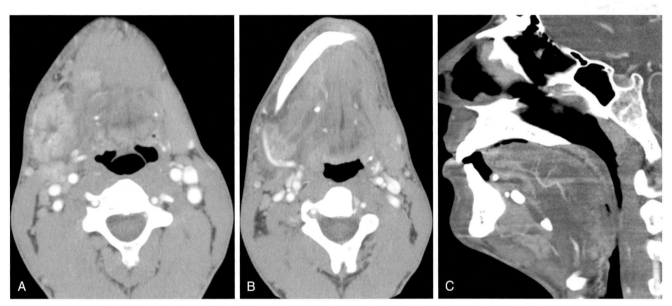

FIGURE 12.38 Sialolith. (**A**) There is inflammatory change and edema within and surrounding the right submandibular gland with intraglandular ductal dilatation seen on this axial postcontrast CT image. (**B**) Wharton duct is dilated, and an obstructive stone can be seen within the duct. (**C**) On sagittal reconstruction of the CT images, multiple obstructive stones in the Wharton duct are evident.

Imaging findings: Stones are more commonly associated with submandibular and sublingual glands. Thin-section CT imaging is the modality of choice for evaluation. A contrast-enhanced CT is sufficient for evaluation. Stones may occur anywhere along the course of the salivary duct or in the hilum of the gland. Secondary sialadenitis or sialodochitis may be present. Plain films may be of use in the assessment of a radiodense stone.

Differential diagnosis: None

Refer to Cummings chapter 85 for more details.

Further Reading

Kalia V, Kalra G, Kaur S, Kapoor R. CT scan as an essential tool in diagnosis of non-radiopaque sialoliths. *J Maxillofac Oral Surg.* 2015;14 (suppl 1):240–244.

Schwarz D, Kabbasch C, Scheer M, Mikolajczak S, Beutner D, Luers JC. Comparative analysis of sialendoscopy, sonography, and CBCT in the detection of sialolithiasis. *Laryngscope.* 2015;125(5):1098–1101.

CASE 39: SJÖGREN SYNDROME (Fig. 12.39)

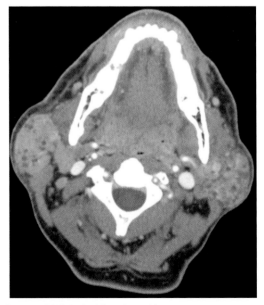

FIGURE 12.39 Sjögren Disease. Multiple tiny bilateral parotid cysts are seen on postcontrast axial CT imaging of the neck. No calcifications or volume loss of the glands were present for the stage of disease in this patient.

Imaging findings: Chronic multisystem autoimmune process, which may involve the salivary and lacrimal glands. Involvement of the parotid glands is a common finding. The early presentation is similar to parotitis. Typically, there is bilateral involvement of the salivary glands, which rules out simple sialadenitis. In the intermediate stage, intraductal strictures within the gland causing dilatation of the acinar sacs and microcysts are present, seen as honeycombing within the gland. Benign lymphoepithelial cysts or masses are present within the parotid gland, arising from the lymphoid tissue only found in the parotid glands. Calcifications may be present. In late-stage Sjögren syndrome, involution and fatty replacement of the glands may occur. Of note, there is a 44-times increased incidence of MALT-type of lymphoma in Sjögren syndrome. A dominant enlarged mass is worrisome for lymphoma and should be evaluated.

Differential diagnosis: Chronic obstruction of a salivary duct with chronic infection, human immunodeficiency virus disease, Warthin tumors, or lymphoma.

Refer to Cummings chapter 85 for more details.

Further Reading

Izumi M, Eguchi K, Ohki M. MR imaging of the parotid gland in Sjögren's syndrome: a proposal for new diagnostic criteria. *AJR.* 1996;166(6):1483–1487.

Ohbayashi N, Yamada I, Yoshino N, Sasaki T. Sjögren syndrome: comparison of assessments with MR sialography and conventional sialography. *Radiology.* 1998;209(3):683–688.

CASE 40: PLEOMORPHIC ADENOMA (Fig. 12.40)

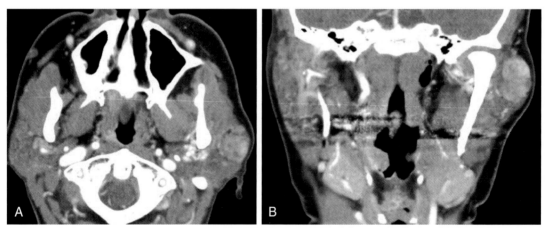

FIGURE 12.40 Pleomorphic Adenoma. (**A**) Postcontrast axial CT demonstrates a well-circumscribed lesion in the superficial lobe of the left parotid gland. This mass demonstrates moderate heterogeneous enhancement. (**B**) Coronal CT again demonstrates the well-circumscribed borders of the mass.

Imaging findings: Pleomorphic adenoma is the most common benign tumor of salivary gland origin. Well-circumscribed, heterogeneously moderate to avid enhancement is present. These lesions may demonstrate cystic change, calcification, and hemorrhage. The borders of the lesion are the best sign to determine benign from malignant salivary gland tumor. Benign tumors demonstrate well-marginated, sharp borders without stranding in the adjacent salivary parenchyma. Lack of facial paralysis for a parotid lesion is also useful. On MRI, the lesions are typically hyperintense on T2-weighted images and do not restrict on diffusion-weighted imaging.

Differential diagnosis: Warthin tumor, lymphadenopathy in the parotid gland, nerve sheath tumor, or malignant tumor (adenoid cystic carcinoma, mucoepidermoid carcinoma, lymphoma).

Refer to Cummings chapter 86 for more details.

Further Reading

Ikeda K, Katoh T, Ha-Kawa SK, Iwai H, Yamashita T, Tanaka Y. The usefulness of MR in establishing the diagnosis of parotid pleomorphic adenoma. *AJNR.* 1996;17(3):555–559.

O'Brien CJ. Current management of benign parotid tumors—the role of limited superficial parotidectomy. *Head Neck.* 2003;25(11): 946–952.

CASE 41: MUCOEPIDERMOID CARCINOMA (Fig. 12.41)

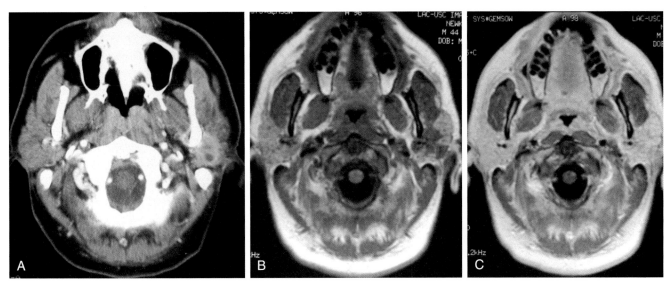

FIGURE 12.41 Mucoepidermoid Carcinoma. (**A**) Postcontrast CT demonstrates a complex mass with both solid and cystic components in the superficial lobe of the left parotid gland posterior to the ramus of the mandible. Note the ill-defined margins of the mass. (**B**) T1-weighted axial image demonstrates the mass is isointense to muscle signal intensity. Additionally, note the ill-defined borders of the lesion compared with the parotid signal intensity. The borders of the lesion are better appreciated on the CT study. (**C**) Postcontrast axial image demonstrates poor delineation of the enhancing mass to the hyperintense signal of the surrounding parotid parenchyma.

Imaging findings: The most common parotid malignancy and second most common in the remaining salivary glands. Ill-defined borders and associated pathological nodes are present though low-grade mucoepidermoid tumors may demonstrate a well-circumscribed border. On MRI, areas of lower signal intensity on T2-weighted images are characteristic but not pathognomonic. Perineural spread of tumor may be seen on MR imaging.

Differential diagnosis: Other malignant tumor (adenoid cystic carcinoma, acinic cell carcinoma, or lymphoma), pleomorphic adenoma, or Warthin tumor.

Refer to Cummings chapter 87 for more details.

Further Reading

Schlakman BN, Yousem DM. MR of Intraparotid masses. *AJNR.* 1993;14(5):1173–1180.

Shah GV. MR imaging of salivary glands. *Magn Reson Imaging Clin N Am.* 2002;10(4):631–662.

CASE 42: DERMOID OF FLOOR OF THE MOUTH (Fig. 12.42)

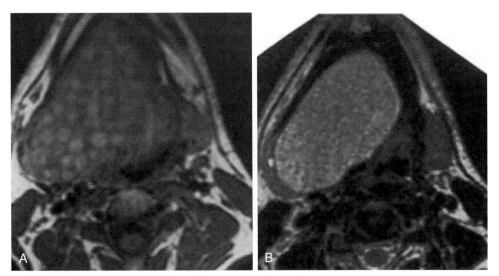

FIGURE 12.42 Dermoid of the Floor of the Mouth. (**A**) T1-weighted axial image demonstrates a mass in the floor of the mouth with a surrounding capsule. Note that within this lesion are numerous well-circumscribed hyperintense components representing fat globules. This is pathognomonic for a dermoid. (**B**) T2-weighted axial image demonstrates the mass to be hyperintense in signal intensity. The hyperintense components within the mass on the T1-weighted images are also hyperintense on the T2-weighted image consistent with fat.

Imaging findings: CT shows a well-circumscribed cystic lesion in the floor of the mouth. The wall is thin and may or may not enhance. Because of the presence of fat, the lesion may have as lower density compared with CSF. However, dermoids and epidermoid may not be distinguishable on CT.

MRI: Because of the presence of fat, the lesion may demonstrate hyperintense signal intensity on both T1- and T2-weighted images. On occasion, fat globules may be present and have the appearance of a sack of beads, which follow fat signal intensity. On postcontrast images, no enhancement is seen.

Differential diagnosis: Epidermoid, abscess, ranula, or Ludwig angina.

Further Reading

Meyer I. Dermoid cysts (dermoids) of the floor of the mouth. *J Oral Surg (Chic) O.* 1955;8(11):1149–1164.

Fujimoto N, Fujii N, Nagata Y, Uenishi T, Tanaka T. Dermoid cyst with magnetic resonance image of sack-of-marbles. *Br J Dermatol.* 2008;158(2):415–417.

NECK

CASE 43: THYROGLOSSAL DUCT CYST (Fig. 12.43)

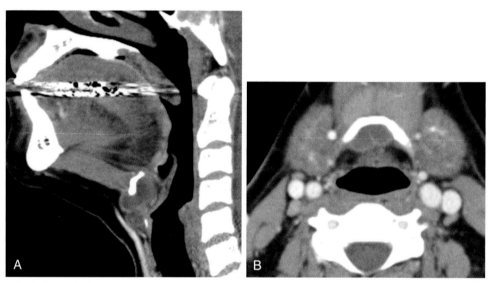

FIGURE 12.43 Thyroglossal Duct Cyst. (A) There is a lobulated cystic lesion posterior and inferior to the hyoid bone on sagittal postcontrast CT images of the neck. **(B)** In the axial plane, an internal septation is evident. The location is classic for a TGDC.

Imaging findings: As they arise from the primitive thyroglossal duct, these lesions tend to be midline, especially in the suprahyoid neck. A midline cystic lesion in the base of the tongue is pathognomonic for a TGDC. However, the majority of these lesions is in the infrahyoid neck and may lateralize to one side, and is deep, not superficial, to the strap muscles of the neck. Noninfected TGDC are well-circumscribed cystic lesions, unilocular, with a thin wall, which may or may not enhance. Infected TGDC may demonstrate increased density and have thick irregular walls that mimic an abscess. At the level of the hyoid bone, these lesions are associated with the anterior, inferior, and posterior aspect of the mid portion of the hyoid bone. Thyroid rests may be present within the TGDC, and malignancies (papillary carcinoma and squamous cell carcinoma) have been associated with these lesions, giving them a complex, aggressive appearance.

Refer to Cummings chapter 8 for more details.

Further Reading

Ewing CA, Kornblut A, Greeley C, Manz H. Presentations of thyroglossal duct cysts in adults. *Eur Arch Otorhinolaryngol.* 1999;256(3):136–138.

Lin ST, Tseng FY, Hsu CJ, Yeh TH, Chen YS. Thyroglossal duct cyst: a comparison between children and adults. *Am J Otolaryngol.* 2008;29(2):83–87.

CASE 44: SECOND BRANCHIAL CLEFT ANOMALY (Fig. 12.44)

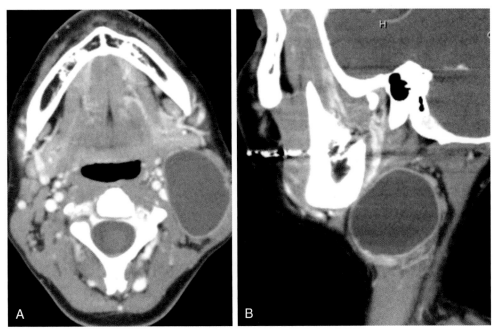

FIGURE 12.44 Second Branchial Cleft Anomaly. (**A**) There is a cystic mass in the left neck with a thin enhancing wall deep to the sternocleidomastoid muscle and lateral to the carotid artery. (**B**) On sagittal reconstruction, the simple nature of the cyst or anomaly is seen with no surrounding inflammatory change or nodularity. The cyst is located near the angle of the mandible.

Imaging findings: These are of embryologic origin from the second branchial cleft. The most common location is at the angle of the mandible posterior to the submandibular gland, lateral to the carotid space, and anterior to the sternocleido-mastoid muscle in the anterior cervical space. Noninfected cysts are well-circumscribed unilocular cystic lesions. The presence of septations or a solid component should raise the question of other etiologies. As all branchial cleft cysts have a sinus tract, the sinus tract for a second branchial cleft anomaly (BCA) is along the medial border and a teat sign may be present. The sinus tract is to the oropharynx. Infected cysts may demonstrate increased density on CT and variable signal on MRI, as well as a thickened irregular wall and stranding of the adjacent fat.

Differential diagnosis: Vasoformative malformation, thymic cyst, lymphadenopathy, abscess, or cystic metastatic disease.

Refer to Cummings chapter 181 for more details.

Further Reading

Harnsberger HR, Mancuso AA, Muraki AS, et al. Branchial cleft anomalies and their mimics: computed tomographic evaluation. *Radiology.* 1984;152(3):739–748.

Bailey H. The clinical aspect of branchial cysts. In: *Branchial Cysts and Other Essays on Surgical Subjects in the Facio-cervical Region.* London: H.K. Lewis; 1929:1–18.

CASE 45: THIRD BRANCHIAL CLEFT ANOMALY (Fig. 12.45)

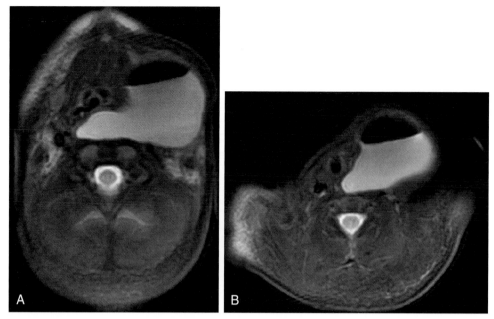

FIGURE 12.45 Third Branchial Cleft Anomaly in a Newborn with Stridor. (**A**) T2-weighted axial image demonstrating a cystic lesion in the left lateral neck extending medially into the retropharyngeal space. This lesion demonstrates an air-fluid level with the fluid component appearing hyperintense. (**B**) Axial image below A again demonstrates this large cystic lesion with air-fluid level. During surgery, a sinus tract was found to extend from this lesion to the apex of the piriform sinus, confirming the diagnosis.

Imaging findings: Arising from the third branchial cleft, these lesions are typically mistaken for an abscess in the upper posterior neck or lower anterior neck. The sinus tract for these cysts extends to the apex of the piriform sinus. CT and MRI findings are similar to the second BCA.

Differential diagnosis: second BCA, thymic cyst, abscess, lymphadenopathy, cystic metastatic disease, or external laryngocele.

Refer to Cummings chapter 181 for more details.

Further Reading

Mandell DL. Head and neck anomalies related to the branchial apparatus. *Otolaryngol Clin North Am.* 2000;33(6):1309–1332.

Mukherji SK, Fatterpekar G, Castillo M, Stone JA, Chung CJ. Imaging of congenital anomalies of the branchial apparatus. *Neuroimaging Clin N Am.* 2000;10(1):75–93.

CASE 46: LYMPHANGIOMA (Fig. 12.46)

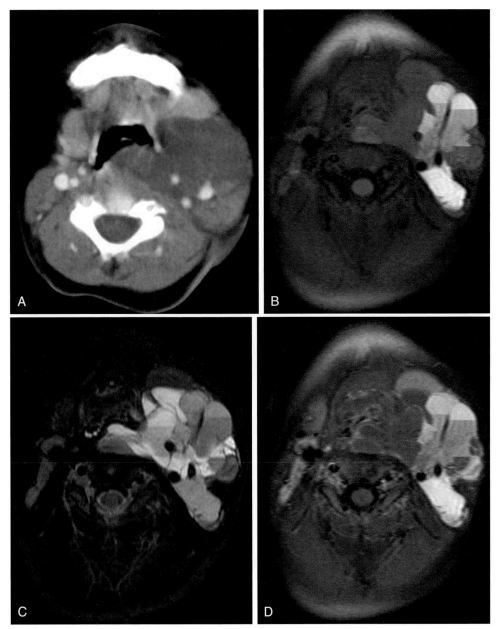

FIGURE 12.46 Neck Lymphangioma. (**A**) Postcontrast CT demonstrates a multicystic lesion in the left lateral neck with superior displacement of the submandibular gland. This lesion encircles the internal jugular vein, as well as the internal and external carotid arteries. (**B**) T1-weighted axial image demonstrates that this is a multicystic lesion with fluid-fluid levels. The fluid component appears to be predominantly hyperintense in signal intensity. (**C**) T2-weighted axial image demonstrates that the fluid component again exhibits intermediate to hyperintense signal intensity with fluid-fluid levels. (**D**) Postcontrast T1-weighted axial image demonstrates no enhancement.

Imaging findings: A form of vasoformative malformation—a multilocular thin-walled cystic lesion that may occur anywhere in the neck where lymph nodes occur. The cysts may contain fluid, proteinaceous material, or blood products, and the walls of the cystic components may enhance. On CT, these lesions are multicystic lesions with potential wall enhancement. On MRI, the cystic components may have variable signal intensities on T1- and T2-weighted images with fluid-fluid levels.

Differential diagnosis: Cystic metastasis, second branchial cleft anomaly (on CT), or abscess.

Refer to Cummings chapter 8 for more details.

Further Reading

Fageeh N, Manoukian J, Tewfik T, Schloss M, Williams HB, Gaskin D. Management of head and neck lymphatic malformations in children. *J Otolaryngol.* 1997;26(4):253–258.

Mulliken JB, Glowacki J. Hemangiomas and vascular malformations in infants and children: a classification based on endothelial characteristics. *Plast Reconst Surg.* 1982;69(3):412–422.

Zadvinskis DP, Benson MT, Kerr HH, et al. Congenital malformations of the cervicothoracic lymphatic system: embryology and pathogenesis. *Radiographics.* 1992;12(6):1175–1189.

CASE 47: LEMIERRE SYNDROME (Fig. 12.47)

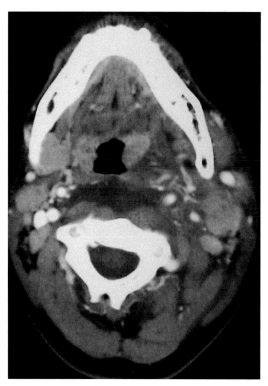

FIGURE 12.47 Lemierre Disease. Postcontrast CT of the neck at the level of the oropharynx demonstrates enlarged lymph nodes in the left level II region of the neck with stranding of the adjacent fat. There is partial thrombosis of the internal jugular vein with stranding of the fat around the carotid space structures. In addition, there is an effusion or abscess in the retropharyngeal space. Note the lack of enhancement of the collection in the retropharyngeal space. There is also edema associated with the left lateral OP wall.

Imaging findings: The imaging findings in Lemierre syndrome are thrombophlebitis of the internal jugular vein and presence of a retropharyngeal abscess. The most common organism is *Fusobacterium necrophorum*, although *Staphylococcus* and *Streptococcus* are also known causative agents. Because of the thrombophlebitis, the patient may go on to pulmonary thromboembolic disease. On CT, thrombosis of the internal jugular vein with thickening of the wall and stranding of the adjacent fat is present. A retropharyngeal abscess or fluid collection is also present.

Refer to Cummings chapter 10 for more details.

Further Reading

Righini CA, Karkas A, Tourniaire R, et al. Lemierre syndrome: study of 11 cases and literature review. *Head Neck.* 2014;36(7):1044–1051.

Kuwada C, Mannion K, Aulino JM, Kanekar SG. Imaging of the carotid space. *Otolaryngol Clin North Am.* 2012;45(6):1273–1292.

CASE 48: SUPPURATIVE LYMPHADENOPATHY (Fig. 12.48)

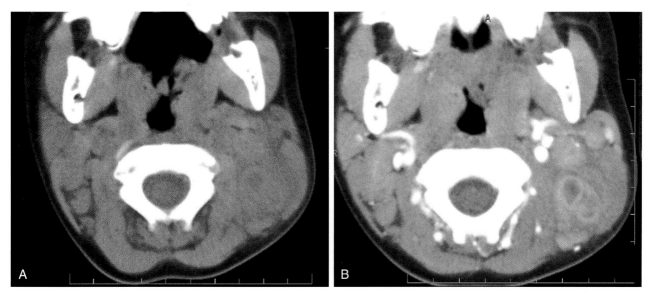

FIGURE 12.48 Suppurative Lymphadenitis. (A) Noncontrast axial CT at the level of the oropharynx demonstrates multiple bulky lymph nodes in the neck bilaterally. On the left side, there are hypoattenuating fluid collections noted and stranding of the adjacent fat. **(B)** Postcontrast CT demonstrates areas of necrosis within the lymph nodes on the left side. This pattern of lymphadenopathy is bacterial in origin in the setting of infection. Metastatic lymph nodes may also have this appearance.

Imaging findings: This is the sequela of a bacterial infection. Endo- and exotoxins cause necrosis within lymph nodes, which, once the lymph node ruptures, leads to formation of a neck abscess. On CT and MRI, cystic or fluid-filled areas are seen within the nodes with irregular borders on CT and MRI. The areas of necrosis may have variable signal intensity because of the presence of protein/exudate. Increased enhancement of the solid component of the lymph nodes, thickening of the capsule, and stranding of the adjacent fat are also present.

Differential diagnosis: Squamous cell carcinoma or other malignancies. Rarely, lymphoma may present with presence of cystic, necrotic lymph nodes.

Refer to Cummings chapter 8 for more details.

Further Reading

Coticchia JM, Getnick GS, Yun RD, Arnold JE. Age-, site-, and time-specific differences in pediatric deep neck abscesses. *Arch Otolaryngol Head Neck Surg.* 2004;130(2):201–207.

Luu TM, Chevalier I, Gauthier M, Carceller AM, Bensoussan A, Tapiero B. Acute adenitis in children: clinical course and factors predictive of surgical drainage. *J Paediatr Child Health.* 2005;41(5-6):273–277.

CASE 49: SQUAMOUS CELL CARCINOMA OF THE LARYNX (Fig. 12.49)

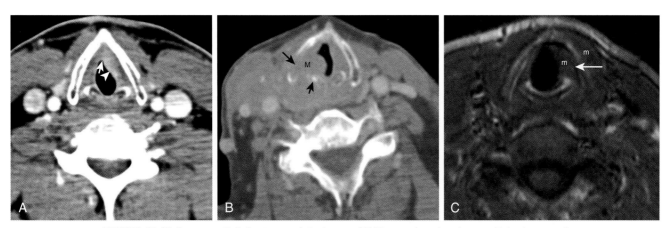

FIGURE 12.49 Squamous Cell Carcinoma of the Larynx. (A) True vocal cord carcinoma with involvement of anterior commissure on CT. Tumor of the left true vocal cord (*arrowheads*) extends anteriorly to involve the anterior commissure. **(B)** Thyroid cartilage destruction on CT. A large laryngeal soft-tissue mass (*M*) destroys both the right thyroid cartilage ala and the posterior right cricoid cartilage (*arrows*). **(C)** T1-weighted MRI shows thyroid cartilage invasion (arrow). A glottic carcinoma (*m*) extends into the left lamina of the thyroid cartilage. The invaded lateral cartilage has lost its hyperintensity because of tumor replacement. (From Flint PW, Haughey BH, Lund VJ, et al. *Cummings Otolaryngology—Head and Neck Surgery*. 6th ed. Philadelphia, PA: Saunders; 2015.)

Imaging findings: CT and MRI are excellent methods for evaluating the subsite involvement in squamous cell carcinoma of the larynx and determining the presence or extent of cartilage invasion for staging. True vocal fold paralysis and disease extension beyond the larynx may also be suggested on the basis of both CT and MRI.

Cartilage involvement of laryngeal squamous cell carcinoma may manifest as sclerotic change, erosion, destruction, or soft tissue extension through the cartilage on CT. MRI is more sensitive but less specific than CT for detection of cartilage involvement. Increased T2-weighted signal on fat suppressed images and contrast enhancement, particularly when the signal intensity is similar to the primary tumor, may indicate carcinoma invasion into the cartilage. More recent studies have also suggested diffusion-weighted imaging may be helpful in detecting cartilage invasion.

Differential diagnosis: Papilloma, laryngocele, hemangioma, or salivary gland neoplasm.

Refer to Cummings chapter 105 for more details.

Further reading

Becker M, Zbären P, Casselman JW, Kohler R, Dulguerov P, Becker CD. Neoplastic Invasion of Laryngeal Cartilage: Reassessment of Criteria for Diagnosis at MR Imaging. *Radiology.* 2008;249:551–559.

Taha MS, Hassan O, Amir M, Taha T, Riad MA. Diffusion-weighted MRI in diagnosing thyroid cartilage invasion in laryngeal carcinoma. *Eur Arch Otorhinolaryngol.* 2014;271:2511–2516.

CASE 50: CAROTID BODY TUMOR (Fig. 12.50)

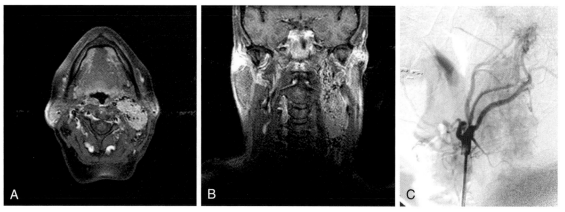

FIGURE 12.50 Glomus Jugulovagale/Carotid Body Tumor. (**A**) Enhanced axial MRI shows a vascular tumor with black flow voids that represent enlarged vessels, the so-called salt-and-pepper appearance that is characteristic of glomus tumors. (**B**) Coronal MRI shows the tumor extending from the left jugular foramen to the left common carotid bifurcation. Isolated carotid body tumor during embolization. (**C**) A common carotid artery injection showed the classic separation of the internal and external carotid trunks because of the hypervascular mass between them. (From Flint PW, Haughey BH, Lund VJ, et al. *Cummings Otolaryngology—Head and Neck Surgery.* 6th ed. Philadelphia, PA: Saunders; 2015.)

Imaging findings: A carotid body tumor is a vascular mass that occurs in the crotch between the origins of the internal and external carotid arteries, splaying them apart.

MRI: MRI demonstrates classic flow voids and the characteristic salt-and-pepper appearance. An isolated carotid body tumor can be differentiated from an isolated glomus vagale tumor by anterior displacement of both the internal and external carotid in the case of a glomus vagale tumor.

Angiography: Selective carotid angiography can be used both for diagnostic and for preoperative embolization.

Differential diagnosis: Glomus vagale, glomus jugulare, vagal schwannoma, or lymphadenopathy.

Refer to Cummings chapter 136 for more details.

Further reading

Griauzde J, Srinivasan A. Imaging of vascular lesions of the head and neck. *Radiol Clin North Am.* 2015 Jan;53(1):197–213.

Kuwada C, Mannion K, Aulino JM, Kanekar SG. Imaging of the carotid space. *Otolaryngol Clin North Am.* 2012 Dec;45(6):1273–1292.

Page numbers followed by *b*, *t*, or *f* refer to boxes, tables, or figures, respectively.